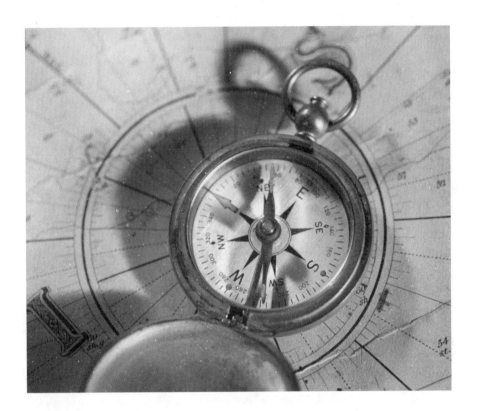

MEDICAL RECORD CHART ANALYZER

Documentation Rules and Rationales with Exercises

DEBORAH J. GRIDER

Medical Record Chart Analyzer
Documentation Rules and Rationales with Exercises

Internet address: www.ama-assn.org

This book is for informational purposes only. It is not intended to constitute legal or financial advice. If legal, financial, or other professional advice is required, the services of a competent professional should be sought.

For information regarding the reprinting or licensing of Medical Record Chart Analyzer,

Please contact:

CPT Intellectual Property Services
American Medical Association
515 N. State St.
Chicago, IL 60610
312 464-5022

Additional copies of this book may be ordered by calling 800 621-8335 or online orders can be taken at www.ama-assn.org/catalog. Mention product number OP084902.

ISBN 1-57947-269-9

BP40: 02-P-038: 07/02

Chapter 1

The Medical Record   1

Chapter 2

Documentation Basics

Chapter 3

Understanding the Evaluation and Management Codes and the Centers for Medicare and Medicaid Services (CMS) Documentation Guidelines

Chapter 4

Other Evaluation and Management Services

Chapter 5

Compliance in the Medical Practice

Chapter 6

Chart Audit Process—The Medical Record Review

Chapter 7

Analyzing the Office Medical Record   141

Chapter 8

Audit Recording Mechanisms   175

The American Medical Association (AMA) is pleased to present *Medical Record Chart Analyzer*. This book should serve as an important source of guidance to assist physicians and their office staff in responding to the increased non-clinical use of the medical record. It is important to provide physicians with information on proper medical record documentation.

A reality of modern medicine is that the medical record is no longer used solely to support patient care. Today, the medical record is used as an audit tool to demonstrate that services were provided and were reasonable and necessary, as well as a tool in the furtherance of documentation in malpractice cases. The AMA's policy: 1) opposes the use of the physician office medical record as a tool of the Centers for Medicare and Medicaid Services (CMS), as well as any other agency or third party, to regulate the financing and practice of medicine; 2) recognizes that the medical record is the property of the physician and the information contained therein, the property of the patient; and 3) believes that the physician's office medical record should be used solely to document the delivery of health care.

The AMA offers the *Medical Record Chart Analyzer* in recognition of the fact that physicians are audited and otherwise held accountable for information contained in the medical record. While the AMA policy does not support many of these practices and emphasizes privacy protections to maintain the confidentiality of this information, physicians need assistance in understanding what the medical record should contain so as to protect their patients and themselves.

Michael Beebe
Director CPT Editorial and Information Services
American Medical Association

Deborah J. Grider, CPC, CPC-H, CCS-P, CCP, is a Certified Professional Coder (CPC), a Certified Professional Coder–Hospital (CPC-H) with the American Academy of Professional Coders (AAPC), a Certified Coding Specialist–Physician (CCS-P) with the American Health Information Management Association (AHIMA), and a Certified Compliance Professional (CCP) with the Healthcare Fraud and Abuse Compliance Institute. Her background includes many years of practical experience in reimbursement issues, procedural and diagnostic coding, medical practice management, and compliance.

Ms Grider teaches and consults with private practices, physician networks, and hospital-based education programs. Under a federal retraining grant, she helped develop and implement a Medical Assisting Program for Methodist Hospital of Indiana (Clarian Health Partners, Inc). She conducts many seminars throughout the year on coding, reimbursement, and compliance issues and teaches several coding and insurance courses, including the Professional Medical Coder Curriculum licensed by the American Academy of Professional Coders. She is an approved instructor for the Professional Medical Coder Course. Ms Grider also co-developed and is the Program Director for a Reimbursement Specialist Certificate Program for Clarian Health Partners, Inc.

Ms Grider has been a speaker at several American Academy of Professional Coders national coding conferences, as well as for other nationally known organizations. Before becoming a consultant, Ms Grider worked as a marketing manager, a billing manager for 6 years, and a practice manager for 12 years.

As president of Medical Professionals, Inc, Ms Grider continues to provide consulting and educational services throughout the country. Her professional affiliations include the American Academy of Professional Coders (AAPC); the Central Indiana Chapter of the American Academy of Professional Coders (of which she was founder and president from 1996–1999 and current president for 2002–2004); the American Health Information Management Association (AHIMA); corporate sponsor for the Indiana Medical Group Management Association; member of the American Society of Training and Development; and member of the Indiana Chamber of Commerce. Ms Grider was awarded her bachelor's degree in business administration from Indiana University. She can be reached via e-mail at medprof@sprynet.com.

Documentation was traditionally generated and used only by the provider or physician as a source of information for patient care. The information was kept in the patient's medical record or chart, or on a card kept in a file. Until about 20 years ago, the only people who had access to the patient's medical record were the physician and his or her staff. Insurance carriers did not require the physician to submit documentation to support charges submitted. Chances of the medical record becoming a legal document in a malpractice case were minimal. Standards for recording the information in the patient's medical record did not exist. Physicians were not required to submit charges based on documentation.

The role of documentation today has changed dramatically. There are many reasons for the change in requirements. Medical malpractice claims have risen dramatically, the medical record serves as a legal document, the medical record serves as information about the patient's care, insurance carriers require documentation to support the level of service billed to them, and the medical record serves as evidence in defense of insurance fraud or malpractice.

PURPOSE OF ANALYZING THE MEDICAL RECORD

Given the increased scrutiny of the medical record in the physician's practice, developing standards for analyzing the medical record may help the provider maintain compliance with the government, insurance carriers, and other agencies that review medical records. Accrediting bodies responsible for rating a health care organization use contents of the medical record to evaluate services to the patient.

To effectively analyze the medical record, the health care professional should begin by learning the basics of the medical record, how to review the medical record for correct coding, and how to build auditing skills with continuous practice. This text will discuss the medical record structure, coding guidelines, documentation and its importance, review guidelines we use today, and give explanations and examples with tips to help along the way. In addition, chart-auditing fundamentals along with case studies are included in this publication.

Mastering the process of medical record analysis is a building-block process. It is building from the basics to the most complex medical record documentation. Basic rules, which remain constant and expand to include evaluation and management services through complex surgical procedures, will be reviewed. Tools that are essential to the analysis of the medical record will be described, along with detailed instructions on how to use them.

TEXT OBJECTIVES

Those completing this text will be able to understand how the medical record is structured, documentation and coding guidelines, the components of the medical record, a working knowledge of the Evaluation and Management Guidelines, and how to review medical record documentation to determine the level of service. Upon completion of this text, the health care professional not only will be able to review and analyze the medical record, but will gain valuable information regarding what to do after the analysis is completed, how to provide education to other health care professionals within an organization, and how to formulate a plan for improving coding and documentation.

HOW TO USE THIS BOOK

This book introduces the reader to principles of medical record documentation, and how to conduct a medical record chart review in the physician's or outpatient office. The information provided herein will prepare the reader to accomplish the following objectives:

- Understand the medical record
- Review documentation basics and formatting of chart notes
- Review documentation guidelines and elements required for each level of service
- Understand the medical record review process (auditing)
- Properly audit the medical record using tools provided
- Analyze and report results of the medical chart review (audit)
- Develop a mechanism for reporting and education
- Understand the importance of developing a performance improvement plan

Medical Record Chart Analyzer contains learning objectives at the beginning of each chapter that will offer an overview of chapter content and help measure progress. These objectives may also assist the instructor using this text in preparing lecture material. Medical chart review and coding tips are provided to help the reader understand the topic discussed. Key terms are found near the end of each chapter and in Appendix D, "Terminology." Application and checkpoint exercises are given in the chapters to allow the reader to learn each chapter, one at a time, building on the medical record analysis process. These exercises are presented in a variety of formats, including true/false, multiple choice, fill-in-the-blank, and short answer. "Test Your Knowledge," in Chapters 10 and 11, will ask the reader to analyze case histories and prepare a detailed analysis and summary report. These chapters may be used to analyze the reader's knowledge of the audit process or can be used as a final examination for instructors using this text in the classroom.

This book is designed to be used by community colleges, career colleges, and vocational school programs for training coders, medical insurance specialists, and other health care providers. It may also be used as an independent study training tool for physicians, coders, consultants, independent billing or reimbursement personnel, and any others in the health care field who want to learn additional skills.

ACKNOWLEDGMENTS

During my twenty-five years in the health care field, I have educated hundreds of students, physicians, colleagues, and instructors who have indirectly contributed to my career success. I wish to express my thanks to all of them. They all have truly enriched my life. I wish to particularly thank my students at Clarian Health for their comments and remarks that helped to make this book a better teaching tool.

In particular I wish to thank,

Elise Schumacher, Senior Acquisitions Editor, AMA Press, for her ideas, confidence in my abilities, and encouragement that enabled me to get this project started.

Patricia Lee, Technical Developmental Editor, AMA Press, who offered suggestions and encouragement to complete this project. She was instrumental in helping me meet my deadlines on the project and helped me through the rough spots.

I would like to also thank the many other people who participated in making this book a reality, also at the AMA Press:

Anthony J. Frankos, Vice President, Business Products

Mary Lou White, Executive Director, Editorial

Jean Roberts, Director, Production and Manufacturing

Boon Ai Tan, Senior Production Coordinator

Rosalyn Carlton, Senior Production Coordinator

Ronnie Summers, Senior Print Coordinator

Erin Kalitowski, Marketing Manager

Benita Ezerins, Administrative Assistant

But students, colleagues, production staff, and editors working alone do not make the project a book; there are others to whom I am deeply indebted. I wish to thank my husband, Jerry, who offered support, encouragement, and motivation throughout the preparation of this book along with his understanding of the priority this project took on my time and our personal life. Special thanks to my assistant Emily Stant, CPC, for without her day-to-day help I would not have been able to meet my deadlines.

Lastly, I wish to thank the consultants who reviewed each chapter and offered comments and suggestions. Without the knowledge of these reviewers and advisors, this text might not have been completed.

Deborah Grider

chapter 1

THE MEDICAL RECORD

LEARNING OBJECTIVES

- Understand the components of the medical record
- Understand how medical records are organized
- Review record retention recommendations
- Review examples of the components of the medical record
- Successfully complete end-of-chapter exercises

DEFINING THE MEDICAL RECORD AND THE ROLE OF THE MEDICAL RECORD ADMINISTRATOR

The medical record is a graphic record that is created for each patient at his or her first medical office visit. In the hospital, the medical record is created when the patient is admitted for services. The medical record serves a variety of purposes and is essential to the proper functioning of the medical practice—especially in today's complicated health care environment. The medical record is a key instrument used in planning, evaluating, and coordinating patient care in both the inpatient and the outpatient settings. The content of the medical record is essential for patient care, accreditation (if applicable to the practitioner), and reimbursement purposes. Your medical records (charts) should detail information pertinent to the care of the patient, document the performance of billable services, and serve as a legal document that describes a course of treatment. Periodic audits, whether internal or external, ensure that the record adequately serves these purposes and meets federal and state regulations.

Medical record employees are responsible for safeguarding the security of the patient record and maintaining confidentiality. Normally, one person is held responsible for overall supervision and maintenance of the medical record. It is the responsibility of each office employee, including the physician, to safeguard and protect the medical record. Safeguards should be implemented within the medical office to keep medical records secure and to prevent patients, vendors, or outside visitors from seeing a patient medical record.

The medical record administrator is responsible for filing patient information, eg, laboratory reports and test results, in the medical record. He or she is also responsible for knowing medical insurance contract requirements, legal requirements pertaining to privacy and confidentiality of the patient. The medical record administrator may be a clinician, billing manager, coder, or anyone assigned the responsibility in the medical office. The medical record administrator is also responsible for making sure the medical record is complete and that dates and signatures are evident in the medical record. Security and confidentiality of the medical record are another key responsibility. Medical records should be kept in the office and must be made available without delay. They should be kept in one location with easy access to all authorized personnel.

MEDICAL RECORD ACCOUNTABILITY AND PRIVACY AND RELEASE OF MEDICAL RECORD INFORMATION

Accountability for patient information and maintaining security of the information is an important aspect of a medical record position. The medical record administrator will be responsible for receiving and distributing faxes related to the patient record and distributing patient test results to the physician(s) to review before placing them in the medical record. The fax and/or test result should be attached to the front of the patient's medical record before the chart is given to the provider to review. The provider should date and sign and/or initial the test result, lab report, consultation report, etc, to attest that the information was reviewed. Once the physician has initialed the information, he or she becomes accountable for the information reviewed.

With the change in the Health Insurance Portability and Accountability Act (HIPAA), privacy and patient confidentiality are an important part of the medical record. The employee responsible for the medical record should:

- Appropriately respond to requests for medical records in a timely manner
- Safeguard against improper release
- Ensure that patient confidentiality is protected

Specific parameters concerning consent are as follows:

1. Consent must reference the individual to the covered entity's notice of privacy practices. A consent may not be combined in a single document with the notice.
2. The consent must indicate that the individual has the right to review the notice before signing the document. If the provider has reserved the right to change privacy policy, the consent must state that the notice may change and the method for obtaining the revised notice must be included.
3. If other legal permission is combined on the consent form, it must be separate from the consent for treatment and require separate signatures and dates.
4. The consent may combine other forms of legal permission or state law requirements.

5. Consent must state that the individual has the right to request restrictions on the use and disclosure of his or her personal medical information, but it must also state that the covered entity may refuse the request.

6. Consent may be combined with an authorization so that the patient's privacy may be breached when research involves treatment of the individual. This is the only circumstance when consent may be combined with an authorization.

7. Covered entities (providers of services) must document and retain any consent.

8. If the consent lacks the required elements, the consent is not valid.

COMPONENTS OF THE MEDICAL RECORD

The medical record has many components. Each component of the outpatient medical record will be reviewed with illustrations later in the chapter. At a minimum, the medical outpatient medical record should contain the following:

- Patient identification (patient registration form)
- Assignment of benefits and release of information
- Consent for treatment (evidence of appropriate informed consent)
- Medicare lifetime claim authorization (if applicable)
- Patient medical history (including drug allergies)
- Medication sheet
- Problem list
- Factors that affect learning
- Preventive medicine screenings
- Waiver of Medicare liability (if applicable)
- Invasive procedure consent (if applicable)
- Physical examination (encounter)
- Diagnostic and therapeutic orders
- Clinical observations, including progress notes, consultation reports, nursing notes, and entries by specified personnel
- Laboratory reports (reports of tests and their results)
- Reports of procedures and their results
- Conclusion if terminating treatment, including final disposition, condition at discharge, medications prescribed, and any instructions for follow-up care
- Preventive medicine services (primary care providers)
- Immunization records

The medical record in the physician's office should be consistently organized to allow information to be found promptly. Uniformity of the medical record is a key element in chart organization. Dividers may be used to separate sections of the medical record. For example, a medical record may have the patient registration form, consent for treatment, medication sheet, immunizations, screenings, and problem list on the left side of the chart, with the patient encounters (visit notes), nursing notes, operative reports, laboratory reports, old medical records, etc, on the right side of the chart.

MEDICAL RECORD ENTRIES

Medical record entries should be accurately dated and authenticated by the provider of service whether it is the physician, nurse practitioner, nurse, medical assistant, or any other health care provider who has access to the medical record. Legibility of recorded information is an important aspect for usefulness of the medical record. The auditor's motto is "not documented, not done," which also encompasses legibility. Pencil and blue ink should be avoided. The majority of documentation in the medical record is in black ink, which is the industry standard. Many states require the identity of the provider, signature, initials, and/or, in some states, a rubber stamp of an original will suffice. Rubber-stamped signatures are not permitted; however, as a substitute for written signatures or initials in many states, so when reviewing medical records, reference state regulations covering signature requirements.

Corrections to the medical record should be made by a single line drawn through the error, with the corrected text entered nearby. Each correction must be initialed and dated by the person who made the error. Review the example below:

Example:

10/20/2001 Sally Jones, RN

Tom, an established patient, is in the office today for follow-up of ~~otitis media~~ *bronchitis.*

All pages of the medical record must contain the date and patient's name. Medical records may be dictated, handwritten, or recorded on a form, typically referred to as a *patient encounter form.* All dictation, handwritten notes, and/or forms must show the date of service (examination and/or procedure) and the identity of the person recording the information. Dictation should also include the date of the dictation and the date of the transcription.

THE PATIENT REGISTRATION FORM

A new patient must complete a patient registration form at the first visit (Figure 1-1), which becomes part of the patient's permanent medical record. The registration form, sometimes referred to as the *patient information sheet,* is used to collect information regarding the patient's demographics. The patient and/or responsible party should complete the patient registration form. This is a legal record that can be used to hold the patient or guarantor (responsible party) accountable for the medical bill and allows the practice to collect payment from the guarantor.

The patient registration form should be updated periodically (at a minimum, once per year) to make sure accurate and updated information is available and to verify insurance information. The following information is normally included on the registration form:

FIGURE 1-1

Patient registration form

PATIENT INFORMATION

Patient name   First _____ Middle initial ___ Last _____

Address _____ City _____ State___ Zip code _____

Date of birth _____ Age_____ Sex ☐Male ☐Female Marital status ☐S ☐M ☐W ☐D

Social Security # _____ Phone # _____ Work # _____

Employer _____ Employer's address _____

Friend or relative not living with you _____ Phone # _____

RESPONSIBLE PARTY INFORMATION

Name First _____ Middle initial ___ Last _____

Address _____ City _____ State___ Zip code _____

Date of birth _____ Age _____ Sex ☐Male ☐Female Social Security # _____

Relationship to patient _____ Home telephone _____ Work # _____

Employer _____ Employer's address _____

Friend or relative not living with you _____ Phone # _____

INSURANCE INFORMATION

Primary insurance _____ Insurance company _____

Insurance company phone # _____ Insurance address _____

Insured name _____ Relationship ☐Self ☐Spouse ☐Dependent ☐Other

ID# _____ Group# _____ Is this an employer group plan? ☐Yes ☐No

If yes, name of employer _____ Insured's employer _____

Employer's address _____ Phone # _____

Insured Social Security # _____ Date of birth _____ Sex ☐Male ☐Female

Secondary Insurance Company _____Phone # _____

Insurance address _____ ID # _____ Group # _____

Insured name _____ Relationship ☐Self ☐Spouse ☐Dependent ☐Other

Is this an employer group plan? ☐Yes ☐No If yes, name of employer _____

Insured's employer _____ Address _____ Phone # _____

Insured Social Security # _____ Date of birth _____ Sex ☐Male ☐Female

- Patient name
- Address, including city, state, and zip code
- Date of birth
- Insurance information
- Previous practitioners who have treated the patient and/or referring physician
- Billing responsibility
- Other pertinent information

Registration forms can be customized on the basis of the medical practice's specific need. Review the example of a patient registration form in Figure 1-1. The registration form can be customized to the practice's needs, or a generic form can be purchased from a number of suppliers.

FINANCIAL RESPONSIBILITY AND ASSIGNMENT OF BENEFITS

As part of the medical record, the patient and/or guarantor will accept responsibility for any charges the insurance carrier does not pay (within insurance contract guidelines). This agreement must be in writing in order to collect any amount from the patient. The assignment of benefits authorizes the medical practice to file the insurance claim, accept payment from the insurance carrier, and collect patient charges directly from the patient and/or guarantor. Figure 1-2 gives one example of a financial responsibility/assignment of benefits form.

FIGURE 1-2

Financial responsibility/assignment of benefits form

FINANCIAL RESPONSIBILITY/ASSIGNMENT OF BENEFITS

For those health care providers who accept assignment, I hereby authorize any insurance carrier with whom I have a policy to pay directly to that provider any benefits of any policies of insurance to those health care providers who have rendered services to me and who accept such assignment. I agree to pay all charges that are not paid in full by assigned insurance. If such amounts due to the health care providers are not paid after reasonable notice, that account shall be deemed delinquent and a service charge shall be added to the amount due. In the event that I default on payment of my account, I agree to be responsible for collection fees and interest due on amounts in default, including court costs and reasonable attorney's fees. If the debt is assigned to a third party for collection, I agree to be responsible for collection fees and interest due on amounts in default.

James Doe
_____
Patient's Printed Name

James Doe
_____   06/01/2002
Patient's Signature   Date

Carrie Jones
_____   06/01/2002
Witness   Date

CONSENT FOR TREATMENT

Many medical practices will have the patient sign a "consent for treatment"
to allow the physicians in the group to provide medical treatment to the
patient. Obtaining a signed consent for treatment has become more
common in the medical office today as an added legal protection for the
practice in case of litigation. Figure 1-3 is one example of a general consent
for treatment. Release of information allows the provider to release

FIGURE 1-3

General consent to treat

CONSENT TO TREAT

The term "health care provider(s)" in this document means <u>Compliance Medical Group (CMG),</u> its agent and employees,
members of the medical staff, their agents and employees, and other health care practitioners who provide care to
patients.

I understand that as part of my health care, this organization originates and maintains health records describing my health
history, symptoms, examination and test results, diagnoses, treatment, and any plan for care including future treatment. I
understand that this information serves as:

1.   Basis for planning my treatment and care
2.   Information used to file my claim with the insurance company (procedure and diagnosis)
3.   Means by which a third-party payer can verify that billed services were actually provided
4.   A tool for routine health care operations including assessing quality and reviewing competency of your staff
     and/or other health care providers.

I understand that I have been provided with the Notice of Information Practices that provides more complete information
of uses and disclosures. I understand that I have the right to review the notice before signing this consent. I understand
that the organization reserves the right to change their notice and practices and before implementation will mail a copy of
any revised notice to the address I have provided. I understand that I have the right to restrict how my health information
may be used or disclosed to carry out payment, treatment, or health care operations and that the organization is not
required to agree to the restrictions requested. I understand that I have the right to revoke this consent in writing, except
to the extent that the organization has already taken action on my behalf.

Permission is hereby granted to all health care providers involved in my care to administer such examination, treatment,
testing, and procedures as are deemed necessary in the course of my care.

James Doe   06/01/2002
Patient Signature   Date

RELEASE OF INFORMATION

Information about me necessary to substantiate my insurance claims may be released by the health care provider involved
in my care.

☒ I am requesting the following restriction to the use or disclosure of my health information.

_____

James Doe   06/01/2002
Signature   Date

Carrie Jones   *Medical Assistant*   06/01/2002
Witness   Title   Date

F I G U R E   1-4

Medicare lifetime beneficiary claim authorization and information release

---

MEDICARE LIFETIME BENEFICIARY CLAIM AUTHORIZATION AND INFORMATION RELEASE

I request that payment of authorized medical benefits be made either to me or on my behalf to Compliance Medical Group for any services furnished me by the physician/supplier. I authorize any holder of medical information about me to release to the Centers for Medicare and Medicaid Services and its agents any information needed to determine benefits or the benefits payable for related services.

I understand my signature requests that payment be made and I authorize release of medical information necessary to pay the claim. If other health insurance is indicated on item 9 of the HCFA-1500 claim form or elsewhere on the approved claim form or electronically submitted claim, my signature authorizes release of information to the insurer or agency shown. In Medicare assigned cases, the physician or supplier agrees to accept the charge determination of the Medicare carrier as the full charge and the patient is responsible only for the deductible, co-insurance, and noncovered services. Co-insurance and deductible are based upon the charge determination of the Medicare carrier.

James Doe

SIGNATURE		06/01/2002
		DATE

Carrie Jones   *Medical Assistant*

WITNESS	Title	06/01/2002
		DATE

---

information to the insurance carrier if the insurance carrier requests all or a portion of the medical record.

MEDICARE LIFETIME BENEFICIARY CLAIM AUTHORIZATION

For Medicare patients, a Medicare claim authorization and information release can be signed yearly, or a lifetime claim authorization is available for the patient's signature (Figure 1-4). The lifetime claim authorization gives the provider permission to file claims on behalf of the patient to Medicare. The authorization further grants the provider authorization to provide to Medicare or any of its agents information, including requested medical records and/or chart documentation. Many times Medicare will request information regarding the claim, including the chart note, to determine if the claim was submitted appropriately. Further, the carrier will sometimes request a copy of the claim authorization and information release to ensure the provider obtained the patient's signature to release the information. The organization may use a form similar to Figure 1-5; use a standard claim authorization, which must be signed yearly; or have the patient sign the HCFA-1500 claim form each time the patient is seen by the provider.

Figure 1-5 is a combination consent for treatment and release of information form that can be used for a Medicare and/or non-Medicare patient and serves a dual purpose.

PATIENT MEDICAL AND INTERVAL HISTORY

Medical documentation regulations have become complex, and the physician's service must meet specific documentation requirements. The medical history form includes the patient's past medical history, family history, and social history. This information should be obtained during the patient's initial visit. If a full medical history is already on file, it is acceptable to obtain an interval history on subsequent visits. The patient

FIGURE 1-5

Combination consent for treatment and release of information

AUTHORIZATION AND CARE/RELEASE OF INFORMATION AND ASSIGNMENT OF BENEFITS

CONSENT TO TREAT

The term "health care provider(s)" in this document means Compliance Medical Group (CMG), its agent and employees, members of the medical staff, their agents and employees, and other health care practitioners who provide care to patients.

I understand that as part of my health care, this organization originates and maintains health records describing my health history, symptoms, examination and test results, diagnoses, treatment, and any plan for care including future treatment. I understand that this information serves as:

1. Basis for planning my treatment and care
2. Information used to file my claim with the insurance company (procedure and diagnosis)
3. Means by which a third-party payer can verify that billed services were actually provided
4. A tool for routine health care operations including assessing quality and reviewing competency of your staff and/or other health care providers

I understand that I have been provided with the Notice of Information Practices that provides more complete information of uses and disclosures. I understand that I have the right to review the notice before signing this consent. I understand that the organization reserves the right to change their notice and practices and prior to implementation will mail a copy of any revised notice to the address I have provided. I understand that I have the right to restrict how my health information may be used or disclosed to carry out payment, treatment, or health care operations and that the organization is not required to agree to the restrictions requested. I understand that I have the right to revoke this consent in writing, except to the extent that the organization has already taken action on my behalf. Permission is hereby granted to all health care providers involved in my care to administer such examination, treatment, testing, and procedures as are deemed necessary in the course of my care.

RELEASE OF INFORMATION

Information about me necessary to substantiate my insurance claims may be released by the health care provider involved in my care.

FINANCIAL RESPONSIBILITY/ASSIGNMENT OF BENEFITS

For those health care providers who accept assignment, I hereby authorize any insurance carrier with whom I have a policy to pay directly to that provider any benefits of any policies of insurance to those health care providers who have rendered services to me and who accept such assignment. I agree to pay all charges that are not paid in full by assigned insurance. If such amounts due to the health care providers are not paid after reasonable notice, that account shall be deemed delinquent and a service charge shall be added to the amount due. In the event that I default on payment of my account, I agree to be responsible for collection fees and interest due on amounts in default, including court costs and reasonable attorney's fees. If the debt is assigned to a third party for collection, I agree to be responsible for collection fees and interest due on amounts in default.

MEDICARE LIFETIME BENEFICIARY CLAIM AUTHORIZATION AND RELEASE OF INFORMATION

I request that payment of authorized medical benefits be made either to me or on my behalf to Compliance Medical Group for any services furnished me by the physician/supplier. I authorize any holder of medical information about me to release to the Centers for Medicare and Medicaid Services and its agents any information needed to determine benefits or the benefits payable for related services.

I understand my signature requests that payment be made and I authorize release of medical information necessary to pay the claim. If other health insurance is indicated on item 9 of the HCFA-1500 claim form or elsewhere on the approved claim form or electronically submitted claim, my signature authorizes release of information to the insurer or agency shown. In Medicare assigned cases, the physician or supplier agrees to accept the charge determination of the Medicare carrier as the full charge and the patient is responsible only for the deductible, co-insurance, and noncovered services. Co-insurance and deductible are based upon the charge determination of the Medicare carrier.

James Doe	06/01/2002
SIGNATURE	DATE
Carrie Jones *Medical Assistant*	06/01/2002
WITNESS Title	DATE

medical history form is a permanent part of the medical record. Figure 1-6 shows an example of a patient history form. It can be used to meet certain documentation requirements for past, family, and/or social history when

FIGURE 1-6
Patient history form

PATIENT MEDICAL HISTORY

Patient: Mary Thomas   DOB: 08/11/1951   Sex: Female

Check any past/current problems

☐ Confused	☐ Vision	☐ Abnormal Pap smears	☐ Difficulty walking
☐ Unresponsive	☐ Loose/chipped teeth	☐ Reproductive organs	☐ Frequent falls
☐ Eyes	☐ Capped/false teeth	☐ Dialysis	☐ Bones
☐ Ears	☐ Circulation problems	☐ Thyroid	☐ Weakness
☐ Nose	☐ Stomach problems	☒ Heart problems	☐ Immune system problems
☐ Mouth	☒ Weight loss	☐ Blood clots	☒ Too little sleep
☐ Sinus	☐ Weight gain	☐ Bleeding	☐ Too much sleep
☐ Throat	☐ Bowel problems	☒ High blood pressure	☐ Lung problems
☐ Skin problems	☐ Liver problems	☐ Stroke	☐ Breathing problems
☐ Rash	☐ Hepatitis	☐ Diabetes	☐ Chronic cough
☐ Hives	☐ Gallbladder	☐ Seizures	☐ TB
☐ Hearing	☐ Kidney	☐ Epilepsy	☐ Positive TB test
☐ Speech	☐ Pain:	☐ Cancer:	☐ Other:_____
	Location_____	Location_____	

☐ Implants/surgical or other metal inside the body: type_____ location_____
☐ Problems with anesthesia,

describe_____

Explain any checked items   Lost 20 lbs in 2 months; hypertension for 5 years and sleeps 4 hours per night for 10 years

List any previous hospitalizations/surgeries/invasive procedures: hysterectomy 1989

Date of last: pneumonia shot never had   tetanus shot 10/14/1976   flu shot 12/11/2000   TB test 12/11/2000

List any allergies   none

List any other problems you may have _____

FAMILY HISTORY

Father: ☒ living   ☐ dead   age at death (if   cause of death (if
                                 applicable) _____   applicable) _____
Mother: ☒ living   ☐ dead   age at death (if   cause of death (if
                                 applicable) _____   applicable) _____

Have you had a family member with any of the following? If so, check the appropriate box.

	Father	Mother	Children	Brother/Sister	Grandparent		Father	Mother	Children	Brother/Sister	Grandparent
Alcoholism	☐	☐	☐	☐	☐	Cancer	☐	☐	☐	☐	☐
Bleeding	☐	☐	☐	☐	☒	Asthma	☐	☐	☐	☐	☐
Thyroid	☐	☐	☐	☐	☐	Diabetes	☐	☒	☐	☐	☐
Heart disease	☐	☐	☐	☐	☐	Stroke	☐	☐	☐	☐	☐
Epilepsy	☐	☐	☐	☐	☐	Migraine	☐	☐	☐	☒	☐
Seizures	☐	☐	☐	☐	☐	TB	☐	☐	☐	☐	☐
Mental disorders	☐	☐	☐	☐	☐	Kidney disease	☐	☐	☐	☐	☐
High blood pressure	☒	☐	☐	☐	☐	Other	☐	☐	☐	☐	☐

SOCIAL HISTORY

Marital status: Married Children (list names): ☐ N/A John and Teresa   Do you live alone?   ☐ yes ☒ no
If you needed help to care for yourself, is there someone available to help you? ☐ yes ☐ no Tobacco: ☐ yes ☐ no
If yes, how much/day _____ x_____ years _____ Recreational drugs: ☐ yes ☐ no Alcohol: ☐ yes ☐ no
If yes, how much _____ / day _____ / week Caffeine: ☐ yes ☐ no If yes, how much /day _____ Exercise routine: _____ Occupation:_____
_____ Unusual dietary habits or herbal supplements: _____
Do you have an advanced directive?   ☐ yes ☐ no If yes, ☐ living will ☐ durable power of attorney ☐ health care directive
Would you like information about advanced directives?   ☐ Yes ☐ No (Staff use): ☐ Brochure given: date/initials: ____-____-____

Signature: *Mary Thomas*   Relationship to patient: self   Date: 06/01/2002

updated if applicable. The form may be designed to include a section for the physician to indicate that the patient's history has not been changed since last updated.

A complete past history should include both personal history and family history and should provide a complete review of body systems. Family history is important for identifying inherited and congenital conditions or diseases. The questions are pertinent for parents, siblings, grandparents, and natural children. Family conditions related to social problems the patient has been exposed to may also be pertinent.

The patient usually completes the form at the initial visit. The patient medical history form may be completed by the patient or by clinical or administrative personnel. The practitioner then has the opportunity to review the history during the patient visit. This information is valuable to the practitioner when determining the plan of care. Each medical practice may design its own form to meet its needs. Many styles and variations are also available through suppliers.

PROBLEM LIST AND MEDICATION SHEET

Many medical practices use a medication sheet and problem list to document current and past medications, medication failures, and chronic problems.

The problem list enables the practitioner to evaluate at a glance the chronic problems the patient encountered in the past to determine a course of treatment. Most practitioners do not document a patient problem unless the problem and/or condition has been evident for three patient encounters.

The practitioner may also choose to document current medications during each patient encounter. Figure 1-7 is an example of a problem list that includes allergies and medication failures. Figure 1-8 is an example of a medication sheet that lists medications in addition to the patient's pharmacy and telephone number, which is helpful to the practitioner when calling in medications for the patient.

The medication list gives the practitioner a complete list of current and past medications the patient is taking or has taken along with any medication failures and/or drug interactions. This tool is helpful when determining contraindications and effectiveness of medications prescribed. This tool also helps the provider avoid serious mistakes when prescribing medications.

FACTORS THAT AFFECT LEARNING (LEARNING NEEDS)

With so many legal and government regulations regarding patient rights, along with the practitioner's responsibility to his or her patient, it is important for the clinician to assess the patient's ability to understand his or

FIGURE 1-7
Problem list

PROBLEM LIST

Patient: Mary Thomas   DOB: 08/11/1951   Female

Date	Diagnoses and or Problems	Emp Initials	Date	Hospitalizations/Surgeries/Procedures	Emp. Initials
10/18/2001	Malignant hypertension	SLG	04/20/1985	Hysterectomy	SLG
12/20/2001	Malignant hypertension encephalopathy	SLG			

ALLERGIES   MEDICATION FAILURES

Date	Allergies (meds, food, iodine, latex, tape, etc)	Type of Allergic Reaction	Emp Initials	Date	Past Medications	Reason for Failure	Emp. Initials
10/01/1995	Codeine	Itching	DLS		none		

FIGURE 1-8
Medication sheet

Medication Sheet

Patient Name: <u>Mary Thomas</u>   Date of Birth: <u>08/11/1951</u>   Home Phone #: <u>(555) 555-5467</u>

Primary Care Physician: <u>Harrison Brinklemeyer</u>   Allergies: <u>Codeine</u>

Pharmacy Name: <u>XYZ Drug Stores</u>   Pharmacy Phone #: <u>(555) 545-5555</u>

Date	Medication (name, dose, and frequency)	Medication(s) Reviewed (dosage change/frequency) ☒=medication continued ☐=medication discontinued					Emp. Initials
10/18/01	Lasix 5 mg PO bid						CLK
10/18/01	Catapres 0.1 mg 1 PO qd						CLK
12/20/01	K-DUR 10 mEq PO qd						SLS

her condition and instructions for care in light of language barriers, physical or mental disabilities, and/or religious or cultural beliefs. Figure 1-9 is a valuable tool for assessing several elements that affect the patient's ability to understand the practitioner. The following key elements should be included when assessing factors that affect learning:

FIGURE 1-9

Form for assessing learning factors

Factors that may affect learning: Who is to be taught? ☒ patient ☐ other; If other, relationship to patient _____

Able to read: ☒ yes ☐no ☐ with difficulty   Comments: _____

Potential barriers to learning ☒ none ☐ blind ☐ poor vision ☐deaf ☐ decreased hearing ☐ unable to talk ☐ learning disability

☐ inability to understand ☐ memory loss   language, if other than English _____

Learns best by ☒reading ☐ talking ☐ verbal instructions ☐ practicing ☐ watching ☐ other _____

Are there any cultural or religious beliefs that need to be considered? ☐ yes ☒ no If yes, _____

Staff Review: date/initials <u>10/18/01-SLK</u>   date/initials <u>12/20/01 CLS</u> date/initials _____   date/initials _____
                 date/initials _____   date/initials _____   date/initials _____   date/initials _____

- Ability to read
- Potential barrier to learning
- Language barriers
- Cultural beliefs
- Religious beliefs

The practitioner or his or her clinical staff may assess this information and it should be periodically reviewed and updated. Review Figure 1-9 above.

PREVENTIVE SCREENINGS

To see that preventive services are effectively provided, it is recommended that an organization monitor these screenings on an ongoing basis. Preventive services may be delivered in a wide range of sites, including the medical office. They are intended to motivate and improve prevention service delivery within the organization and thus can be measured in any way useful to the individual organization. These preventive screenings were identified by the Centers for Disease Control and Prevention (CDC) on the basis of their review of the Guide to Clinical Preventive Services, Report of the US Preventive Services Task Force.

These measures were developed to improve prevention service delivery within an organization. The screenings identified were chosen on the basis of evidence supporting the benefit of the preventive service during the periodic health examination. Figure 1-10 contains the preventive screenings that were identified for adults, and Figure 1-11 identifies preventive screenings for children. Identified below are services for which there is good evidence to support the recommendation that these screenings be specifically considered in the periodic health examination.

ADVANCE BENEFICIARY NOTICE (MEDICARE WAIVER OF LIABILITY)

Certain patients will require additional forms. One form that is specific to Medicare patients is the Advance Beneficiary Notice, commonly referred to

FIGURE 1-10

Adult screening form

ADULT SCREENINGS

Screening	19–39 Years	40–64 Years	65+ Years	Comments/Findings	Emp. Initials
	✔=Recommended				
Diabetes Screen		✔			
Cholesterol	✔	✔	✔		
EKG		✔	✔		
Fecal Occult Blood		✔	✔		
Sigmoid		✔	✔		
TSH			✔		
PAP	✔	✔	✔		
Breast Exam Education	✔	✔	✔		
Mammogram		✔	✔		
PSA		✔	✔		
Testicular Exam Education	✔	✔	✔		

FIGURE 1-11

Pediatric screening form

PEDIATRIC SCREENINGS

	Growth	Denver	Anemia	UA	Lipids	Comments/Findings	Date	Emp. Initials
1–2 wks.	✔	✔						
1 mo.	✔	✔						
2 mo.	✔	✔						
4 mo.	✔	✔						
6 mo.	✔	✔						
9 mo.	✔	✔	✔					
12 mo.	✔	✔						
15 mo.	✔	✔						
18 mo.	✔	✔						
2 yr.	✔	✔						
3 yr.	✔	✔		✔				
4 yr.	✔	✔		✔				
5 yr.	✔			✔				
6 yr.	✔			✔				
7 yr.	✔			✔				
8 yr.	✔			✔				
9 yr.	✔			✔				
10 yr.	✔			✔	✔			
11 yr.				✔				
12 yr.				✔				
13 yr.				✔				
14 yr.				✔				
15 yr.				✔	✔			
16 yr.				✔				
17 yr.				✔				
18 yr.	✔			✔				

as the "Medicare Waiver of Liability form." See Figure 1-12. This form is used to meet Medicare's requirement for billing services that may not be covered. Medicare requires the use of advance notice that must be signed by the patient before the service is rendered. The form may be tailored specifically to the organization. However, Medicare requires the following:

■ Name of service or procedure

■ Statement that specifically states, "Medicare does not pay for the service"

■ Statement that the patient agrees to accept financial responsibility for the noncovered service.

Medicare has determined that a general financial responsibility statement is not specific enough to meet Medicare's regulation for billing services that do not meet its medical necessity requirements.

FIGURE 1-12

Medicare waiver of liability

Date: 01/21/2002   Patient's Name: Mamie Johnston   Medicare # (HICN): 555-55-5555A

ADVANCE BENEFICIARY NOTICE (ABN)

NOTE: You need to make a choice about receiving these health care items or services.

We expect that Medicare will not pay for the item(s) or service(s) that are described below. Medicare does not pay for all of your health care costs. Medicare only pays for covered items and services when Medicare rules are met. The fact that Medicare may not pay for a particular item or service does not mean that you should not receive it. There may be a good reason your doctor recommended it. Right now, in your case, Medicare probably will not pay for –

Items or Services:

G0001 Q0091

Because:

Screening Pap and pelvic exam performed 1 year ago; patient is not meet high-risk criteria

The purpose of this form is to help you make an informed choice about whether or not you want to receive these items or services, knowing that you might have to pay for them yourself. Before you make any decision about your options, you should:

• Read this entire notice carefully.

• Ask us to explain, if you don't understand why Medicare probably won't pay.

   • Ask us how much these items or services will cost you (Estimated Cost: $ 45.00   ), in case you have to pay for them yourself or through other insurance.

PLEASE CHOOSE ONE OPTION. CHECK ONE BOX. SIGN & DATE YOUR CHOICE.

☐ Option 1. YES.   I want to receive these items or services.

I understand that Medicare will not decide whether to pay unless I receive these items or services. Please submit my claim to Medicare. I understand that you may bill me for items or services and that I may have to pay the bill while Medicare is making its decision. If Medicare does pay, you will refund to me any payments I made to you that are due to me. If Medicare denies payment, I agree to be personally and fully responsible for payment. That is, I will pay personally, either out of pocket or through any other insurance that I have. I understand I can appeal Medicare's decision.

☒ Option 2. NO.   I have decided not to receive these items or services.
I will not receive these items or services. I understand that you will not be able to submit a claim to Medicare and that I will not be able to appeal your opinion that Medicare won't pay.

Date   01/21/2002   Signature of patient or person acting on patient's behalf

Mamie Johnston

NOTE: Your health information will be kept confidential. Any information that we collect about you on this form will be kept confidential in our offices. If a claim is submitted to Medicare, your health information on this form may be shared with Medicare. Your health information that Medicare sees will be kept confidential by Medicare.

OMB Approval No. 0938-0566   Form No. HCFA-R-131-G

CONSENT FORM FOR INVASIVE PROCEDURE

The medical record may contain consent for a procedure that is performed in the medical facility. By law, informed consent is required before any procedure with a significant risk of complication. The person granting consent must be of legal age or must meet legal requirement to sign the consent (parent and/or legal guardian). Figure 1-13 is an example of a consent form. Legal requirements may vary from state to state. Informed consent means the practitioner must inform the patient of possible risk, complication, benefits, and alternative forms of treatment (if applicable). Normally the practitioner will provide the patient with written information regarding the procedure before the patient signs the consent form. It is up to the practitioner to determine what type(s) of informed consent will be used.

PATIENT ENCOUNTERS

The medical record will contain patient encounters (visit notes) for each date of service. When the medical record is analyzed for correct coding, patient encounters are selected for review. The patient encounter may be dictated or handwritten, and/or a form may be used for recording the information. The level and type of procedure or service should be selected on the basis of the documentation. Documentation requirements will be reviewed in Chapter 2. Review the example of a handwritten patient encounter at top of next page.

Figure 1-14 illustrates a patient encounter that is dictated. Many practitioners still dictate chart notes. Since legibility is important when documentation is reviewed, dictation ensures that the note is easy to read.

FIGURE 1-13

Consent form

Patient Name Martin Smith   Date of Birth 10/14/1955   Medical Record # 405114
Date of Procedure 10/10/2001
I hereby authorize the performance upon me of a flexible sigmoidoscopy by Dr. John Stone.
I understand that this procedure involves the passage of a flexible tube through the rectum and into the lower part of the colon. The purpose is to examine that part of the colon for abnormalities. I have been provided with a pamphlet that explains the procedure, risks, and benefits.
I understand that the risks of this procedure include perforation (1 perforation in 1,000 procedures), bleeding (1 episode of bleeding per 1,000 procedures if a biopsy is taken), and the possibility of missing a small abnormality.

Signed : Martin Smith   Date   06/01/2002
Witness: Cynthia Thompson, RN   Date   06/01/2002

PHYSICIAN DECLARATION I have explained the contents of this document to the patient and have answered all the patient's questions, and to the best of my knowledge, I feel the patient has been adequately informed and has consented.
(Physician's signature): John Stone, MD   Date: 10/10/2001

For staff use only

JS   Chart has been reviewed and patient questioned regarding valvular heart disease before the procedure.

Kidermann, Nichole   Date of Service: 1/15/2001

Date of Birth: 04/10/72

This 28-year-old white established female is here with a complaint of severe diarrhea with abnormal bowel movements. Bowel movements occur every 10 minutes and there is fecal incontinence as well as nocturnal bowel movements. She complains of cramps and nausea, but no vomiting.   She denies chronic diarrhea. The patient has a past history of thyroid goiter. She is a nonsmoker; currently taking no medications. Patient denies excessive aspirin or antacid use. Denies dysphagia, gallbladder disease, liver disease, or pancreatitis, no history of peptic ulcer disease.

PHYSICAL EXAMINATION:
Her temperature is 98.6, pulse 88, respiratory rate 16, blood pressure 110/60, weight 130, height 5 feet, 7 inches. Heart regular rate with no murmurs. Lungs are clear to auscultation. No rales, rhonchi, or wheezing. Abdomen is soft with good bowel sounds, no pain or masses. No hepatosplenomegaly. Some lower abdominal tenderness. Extremities within normal limits; no edema.

PLAN:
Severe diarrhea and dehydration secondary to infectious colitis versus Clostridium difficile infection versus viral gastroenteritis versus inflammatory bowel disease, less likely. Obtain blood cultures, stool cultures. Await CBC with differential to determine whether the patient needs IV antibiotics.

Ima Caring, MD

Many practitioners are using forms to record the patient encounter (Figure 1-15). The primary reason is the escalating cost of transcription. All methods for recording the encounter are acceptable. Review Figure 1-14 and Figure 1-15.

LABORATORY REPORTS

Each medical record should include a separate identifiable section for laboratory reports if ordered by the physician. Figure 1-16 is an example of a laboratory report. When the laboratory report is received by the medical office, the medical records administrator or administrative or clinical personnel will locate the patient's medical record, attach the report to the chart, and give them to the practitioner for review. Normally the laboratory report is dated and initialed by the provider reviewing the record. All normal and abnormal findings should be reported to the patient. The person notifying the patient should document in the medical record that the patient was informed of laboratory or test results.

Example:

Patient notified via telephone of normal and abnormal test results

Jane Smith, CMA

FIGURE 1-14
FIGURE 1-14

Dictated patient encounter report

Mary Tyler   Date of Service: 5/01/02

This is the third office visit for this 65-year-old female who for the past 4-5 weeks has been having significant sharp stabbing pains of her anterior chest, primarily with movement, especially when lying down or sitting up. She does not have any palpitations or any significant shortness of breath, cough, wheezing, fever, or chills. She does have a history of COPD with chronic mild exertional dyspnea.

ALLERGIES: NKA.

MEDICATIONS: Lanoxin q day, inhaler as needed

ROS: Eyes: No diplopia or new visual disturbance. Ears, Nose, and Throat: No tinnitus, otalgia, or sore throat. Cardiac: No sustained chest pain or palpitations. Pulmonary: COPD with chronic mild exertional dyspnea. Gastrointestinal: No melena, hematochezia, vomiting, or diarrhea. Musculoskeletal: As per history of present illness. The remaining systems are negative.

Exam:

Well-developed, well-nourished female in mild distress. Skin has no gross abnormalities.
Pupils are equal, round, and reactive to light. Extraocular movements are intact. Sclerae are clear. Conjunctivae are pink. Ears are normal. Pharynx is clear. Anterior chest wall tenderness, primarily from the mid and lower left sternal border, extending laterally across the costal chondral cartilage. No associated deformity, swelling, erythema. No gross abnormalities.
Mildly diminished breath sounds bilaterally with no prominent rales, wheezing, or rhonchi. No rubs. Heart regular rate and rhythm. No murmurs, clicks or rubs.
Abdomen is soft and nontender. Bowel sounds are normal. No masses.
Extremities: Good color and warmth.

EKG: Dual chamber pacemaker, rate of 60. Rhythm—sinus. No significant ectopy noted.

Assessment & Plan:

Chest wall pain. We will be placing her on anti-inflammatory drugs and will start her on the first dose of Motrin here. It is recommended that she go on regular Motrin, limit activities that exacerbate her discomfort and will be back to see me in two weeks.

Ima Caring, MD

Dictated: 05/01/2002
Transcribed: 05/01/2002

REPORT OF PROCEDURES

The medical record may also contain reports of procedures or letters from consulting and/or referring physicians. Figure 1-17 is an example of an operative report that might be found in the medical record.

TERMINATION OR WITHDRAWAL OF TREATMENT

In some cases it may become necessary for the practitioner to discharge a patient from his or her care. Usually this occurs when the patient

ADULT PATIENT ENCOUNTER

Date of Service: 05/01/2001   Patient Name: Irma Doe   Date of Birth: 04/05/1935   Sex: ☐ M ☒ F

Vital Signs: *(record any three of the following)* Ht   5' 3"   Wt 120 lbs.   T 99.5   P 72   Resp   BP 125/85

	CURRENT MEDICATIONS
Chief Complaint: Patient is a 66-year-old Medicare patient here for annual exam HPI: Patient has a history of hypertension. She has had a 1-week history of raspy throat. OTC products have not helped. Patient has not had Pap and pelvic exam for past 3 years. Last mammogram was 4 years ago. Pain Assessed:☒ Yes ☐ No Location Duration:Pain Severity: 0/10 0	**See med sheet** ☐

REVIEW OF SYSTEMS: 1 system (213, 202) 2-9 systems (214, 203) 10 (215, 204, 205, preventive)

	+	−	**Abnormal Findings**	
Constitutional	X		Feverish	**Allergies reviewed** ☐
Eyes				
ENT	X		Sore throat; trouble swallowing	**None** ☐
CV		X		
Resp		X		
Endocrine		X		**PFSH** *see form front of chart*
Hemo/Lymph				☐ New Patient— form completed
GI		X		
GU		X		☒ Reviewed, No change
MS		X		
Skin		X		☐ Reviewed, Updated
Neuro		X		
Psych				
All/Immune				
All others neg				

EXAMINATION: 1-5 (212, 201) 6-11 (213, 202) 12-17 (214, 203) 18 (215, 204, 205, preventive)

Area/System	Normal=☆			Abnormal Findings
General	☐ WDWN	☒ Minimum 3 vitals		→ Temp; BP now controlled
Psych	☐ Insight	Orientation x 3 ☐	Memory Mood/ Affect	
Eyes	☐ Pupils	☐ Conjunctiva	☐ Ophthalmoscopic exam	
ENT	☒ TMs	☐ Nose	☒ Pharynx	Pharynx—red and swollen
Neck	☒ Supple	☐ Nodes	☐ Thyroid	
Respiratory	☒ Effort	☒ Auscultation	☒ Percussion	
Chest (Breasts)	☒ Inspection	☒ Palpation		
Cardiovascular	☒ Sounds	☒ Rate	☒ Rhythm	Regular rate and rhythm
Abdomen	☐ Soft ☒ Rectal Exam	☐ Nontender	☐ Masses ☐ Liver/Spleen	Rectal exam—normal
Extremities	☒ Edema	☒ Varicosities		
Skin	☐ Inspection	☐ Palpation		
Musculoskeletal	☐ Gait ☐ Muscle Strength	☐ Inspection	☐ ROM ☐ Stability	
GU Male	☐ Penis ☒ Genitalia	☐ Testicles ☒ Urethra	☐ Prostate ☐ Hemoccult ☒ Bladder ☒ Cervix	Pap smear obtained—Pelvic exam normal
Female	☒ Uterus	☒ Adnexa		
Neuro	☐ Cranial Nerves	☐ Deep Tendon Reflexes	☐ Sensation	

ASSESMENT/PLAN:
Dx: Hypertension—continue same meds; Pharyngitis; Orpharynx erythematous, few clear blisters noted in posterior pharynx. No purulent exudates noted. Amoxil 50 mg 1 PO TID x 10 days; increase fluids, gargle with warm salt water PRN. Tylenol or Advil PRN as indicated for pain/fever. Follow up 10 days. Pap obtained and sent to lab. Ordered TSH and Chem 7. Will call with lab and Pap results. Pt scheduled for

PATIENT EDUCATION
☒ Medication education/side effects reviewed with patient
☒ Educational materials given on: _____
☒ Other: _____

FIGURE 1-16

Laboratory report

9110 (555) 555-5555	Patient Name: John Doe
Harrison Brinklemeyer, MD	Sex: Male
10067 Anchor Mark Drive	Age: 61
Anytown, USA 46236	

ABC CLINICAL LABORATORIES

Test	Result	Units	Reference Range	Site Code
Lipid Panel				
Triglycerides	226H	MG/DL	10-190	JI
Cholesterol, Total	185	MG/DL	100-200	JI
HDL-Cholesterol	41	MG/DL	35-55	JI
LDL-Cholesterol	99	MG/DL		JI
===================				
LDL CHOLESTEROL				
< 130 DESIRABLE				
130-159 BORDERLINE/HIGH RISK				
> 130 HIGH RISK				
Chol/HDLC Ratio	4.51	(CALC)	< 4.98	JI
Urea Nitrogen (BUN)	18	MG/DL	6-19	JI
Ceatinine	1.1	MG/DL	0.5-1.2	JI
Potassium	4.3	MMOL/L	3.3-5.1	JI

>>END OF REPORT<<

moves or changes insurance companies, or the practitioner changes plan participation. Occasionally when a patient is noncompliant the practitioner may elect to discharge the patient from his or her care. The practitioner cannot abandon the patient and must provide written notice. When the practitioner discharges the patient for care, the following must apply:

■ Patient must be sent formal written notification
■ Patient must be given time to find another practitioner
■ The letter or notice should be sent by certified mail with a returned receipt request to ensure proof the patient received the notice

Figure 1-18 is an example of a patient discharge letter.

IMMUNIZATION RECORDS

The medical record may also contain a separate form for immunizations. Figure 1-19 is an example of an immunization form that may be found in a pediatric patient's medical record.

RECORD RETENTION

A medical practice should also include set policies regarding retention of compliance, business, and medical records. These records primarily include documents relating to patient care and the practice's business activities. A person designated by the practices should keep an updated binder or

FIGURE 1-17
Operative report

OPERATIVE REPORT

Patient Name: Mary Marsh   Date of Birth: 06/12/1954   Date of Surgery: 06/12/2002

PREOPERATIVE DIAGNOSIS: 4.1-cm infected sebaceous cyst, back. 2.5-cm infected sebaceous cyst, posterior neck

POSTOPERATIVE DIAGNOSIS: Same.

PHYSICIAN: James Mercer, MD

OPERATION PERFORMED: 1. Excision 4.1-cm benign cyst, back

                              2. Excision 2.5-cm benign cyst, neck

PROCEDURE: The patient was placed in the prone position, after which the back and posterior neck were prepped with Betadine scrub and solution. Sterile towels were applied in the usual fashion, and 0.25% Marcaine was injected subcutaneously in a linear fashion transversely over each of the cysts asynchronously. Additional local anesthetic was administered around the cysts. The lower cyst was excised. The cavity was irrigated with copious amounts of Marcaine solution and then the skin edges were loosely reapproximated throughout with #3-0 nylon suture. Following this, Marcaine was injected around the superior of the cyst and an incision was made transversely across this and the cyst was completely excised as well. Consequently, reexploration of the wound revealed scar tissue in the base of the wound, and this was excised as well as possible to ensure that the cyst was completely removed. The wound was irrigated with Marcaine and packed with Iodoform, and sterile dressings were applied. The patient was discharged with verbal and written instructions, as well as Tylenol #3 for pain and a prescription for 30 days. Return visit in 3 days for packing removal.

James Mercer, MD

Dictated: 06/12/2002
Transcribed: 06/13/2002

record of compliance-related activities. This involves, at a minimum, keeping track of compliance meetings, educational activities, and internal audit results.

The practice should establish policies and procedures regarding the creation, distribution, retention, and destruction of documents. In designing a record system, privacy concerns and federal and state regulatory requirements should be taken into consideration. In addition

FIGURE 1-18

Patient discharge letter

Harold Brinklemeyer, MD
10067 Anchor Mark Drive
Anytown, USA 46236

June 15, 2002

Jerry Greinhurst
4520 Pine Drive
Anytown, USA 47001

Dear Mr Greinhurst:

I regret to inform you that, together with the other physician of Compliance Medical Group, I must withdraw from providing services as your physician. Compliance Medical Group has withdrawn from participation in your health plan. Since your condition requires medical attention, I suggest you contact your medical insurance plan to arrange for a primary care physician. I will be available to provide you with medical care for a reasonable time after you receive this letter, but in no event for more than 30 days from the date of this letter.

This should give you sufficient time to select another physician from the physician roster of your medical plan. When you have selected a new physician, please request a release of records authorization from your new physician. Upon receipt of your written authorization, I will provide your new physician with your medical records.

Sincerely,

Harrison Brinklemeyer, MD

to maintaining appropriate and thorough medical records on each patient, it is recommended that the following types of documents be retained by the practice.

- All records and documentation (eg, billing and claims documentation) required for participation in federal, state, and private payer health care programs
- All records necessary to demonstrate the integrity of the physician practice's compliance process and to confirm the effectiveness of the program

While conducting its compliance activities, as well as its daily operations, a physician practice should document its efforts to comply with applicable federal health care program requirements. In short, all physician practices, regardless of size, should have procedures to create and retain appropriate documentation. The following record retention guidelines should be followed:

- The length of time that a physician's medical record documentation is to be retained should be specified in the physician practice's policies and procedures (federal and state statutes should be consulted for specific time frames).
- Medical records should be secured against loss, destruction, unauthorized access, unauthorized reproduction, corruption, and damage.
- Policies and procedures should stipulate the disposition of medical records in the event the practice is sold or closed.

FIGURE 1-19

Immunization form

IMMUNIZATIONS

Vaccine	Date	Age	Site***	Source of Vaccine*	Vaccine Manufacturer	Vaccine Lot Number	Vaccine Info Materials Publishing Date	Emp. Initials	Parent/ Guardian Initials
DT DTP DTaP 1									
DT DTP DTaP 2									
DT DTP DTaP 3									
DT DTP DTaP 4									
DT DTP DTaP 5									
DTP-Hib 1									
DTP-Hib 2									
DTP-Hib 3									
DTP-Hib 4									
Hib 1									
Hib 2									
Hib 3									
Hib 4									
Hib 1-Hep B 1									
Hib 2-Hep B 2									
Hib 3-Hep B 3									
Hep B 1									
Hep B 2									
Hep B 3									
OPV 1 IPV 1									
OPV 2 IPV 2									
OPV 3 IPV 3									
OPV 4 IPV 4									
MMR 1									
MMR 2									

*Vaccine Administrator Signature:

_____

_____

**Patient/Guardian Signature:

_____

_____

***Site Given Legend
RA= Right Arm
LA= Left Arm
RT= Right Thigh
LT= Left Thigh
O= Oral

****Source of Vaccine Legend
F=Federal
S=State
P=Private

Figure 1-20 shows a recommended schedule for record retention.

The medical record and all supporting documentation is important to support correct coding, billing, and compliance, which will be discussed further in Chapter 5.

KEY TERMS

Advance Beneficiary Notice (ABN)—A written notification that must be signed before services are rendered to a Medicare beneficiary that could potentially be denied or deemed "not medically necessary." A modifier must be used on the HCFA-1500 claim form to indicate to Medicare that the Advance Beneficiary Notice is on file. The notice is sometimes referred to as a "Medicare Waiver of Liability." Once an ABN is on file, the patient is lawfully liable for the charges if Medicare denies payment for the services.

FIGURE 1-20
Record retention schedule

RECORD RETENTION SCHEDULE

Records	Recommended Retention Period (years)
Accounts receivable ledger cards	4
Appointment schedules (sheets)	1
Balance sheets	5
Bank deposits and statements, reconciliations	6-8
Cash receipt records	10
Contracts and leases (expired)	7
Contracts with employees	6
Copies of estimated tax forms	6
Correspondence, general	1-5
Deceased patients' medical records	5
Depreciation schedules	3
Duplicate bank deposit slips	1
Employee time cards/sheets and schedules	5
Employee applications	3
Expense reports	7
Inventory records	7
Superbills, invoice, insurance, billing records	7
Medicare/Medicaid records	7
Payroll records	7
Petty cash vouchers	3
Postal and meter records	1

RECORD RETENTION SCHEDULE	
Records	**Recommended Retention Period (years)**
Accounts payable ledgers	Indefinite
Balance sheets	Indefinite
Bill of sale for important purchases	Indefinite
Canceled checks and check registers	Indefinite
Capital asset records	Indefinite
Cashbooks	Indefinite
Certified financial statements	Indefinite
Chart of accounts	Indefinite
Correspondence, legal	Indefinite
Credit history	Indefinite
Deeds, mortgages, contracts, leases, and property records	Indefinite
Equipment records	Indefinite
Inactive patient medical records purged from active files	Indefinite
Income tax returns and documents	Indefinite
Insurance policies and records	Indefinite
Journals	Indefinite
Magnetic tapes and disks	Indefinite
Patients medical records, including x-ray films	Indefinite
Property appraisals	Indefinite
Tax returns	Indefinite
Telephone records	Indefinite

Charge ticket—Routing slip, personalized for the medical group or practice, that encompasses patient demographics, charges, and Current Procedural Terminology (CPT®) codes, and may also include diagnosis codes (ICD-9-CM). A copy is normally given to the patient when he or she leaves the office.

Consent for treatment—An agreement that the patient signs allowing the provider to treat the patient.

CPT® Coding (Current Procedural Terminology)—The AMA publishes the CPT® (Current Procedural Terminology) book annually. The CPT® nomenclature is an alphanumeric coding system with two-digit add-on descriptors (modifiers) that designates medical services. It is a widely accepted method of communicating to payers descriptions of procedures and services that have been provided to patients.

Documentation—A method of recording facts chronologically including detailed observations about the patient's health status as seen in medical reports and chart notes.

HCFA-1500 Claim Form—The approved claim form, revised in December 1990, for providers to use to submit claims to Medicare Part B. Electronic submission is preferred; however, the HCFA-1500 claim form is the basis from which electronic transmissions are formatted. Thus, the claim filing instructions apply to all claims, whether paper or electronic. Most insurance carriers now accept the HCFA-1500 claim form. The Centers for Medicare and Medicaid Services (CMS), formerly the Health Care Financing Administration (HCFA), has determined that it is more cost-effective to process Medicare paper claims by means of the optical character recognition (OCR) system.

Medical history—History of the patient's past illnesses, surgical procedures, allergies, medications, and other pertinent facts related to the patient's illnesses and problems.

Medical record—Written or graphic information documenting facts and pertinent data during rendering of patient care.

Medication sheet—An up-to-date list of the patient's medications and/or failures. This information is located in the patient's medical record.

Patient encounter form—A form used to record the patient visit.

Patient registration form—A detailed form to record the patient demographic information and insurance information.

Problem list—A list of the patient's chronic medical problems and/or conditions. This information is located in the patient's medical record.

Record retention—Time limit that each individual state and/or insurance carrier requires records to be kept.

TEST YOUR KNOWLEDGE

True or False

1. _____ All states require that the physician either sign or rubber-stamp the chart entry.

2. _____ The nurse is responsible for filing patient information in the medical record.

3. _____ Patient confidentiality is important to ensure security and privacy of the medical record.

4. _____ Medical record entries should be accurately dated and signed by the provider of service.

5. _____ When correcting an error in the medical record, the provider only needs to draw a line through the error.

6. _____ It is not necessary to date the visit note.

7. _____ Medicare and Medicaid records should be retained for a minimum of 7 years.

Multiple Choice (circle the correct answer)

8. The patient registration form should include:
   a. Patient name, address, date of birth, insurance information, billing responsibility, and previous practitioner or referring physician.
   b. Patient name, address, date of birth, and insurance information.
   c. Patient name, address, date of birth, insurance information, billing responsibility, previous practitioner or referring physician, and consent for treatment.

9. Consent for treatment allows the practitioner to:
   a. Receive payment for services from an insurance company.
   b. Provide medical treatment to the patient.
   c. Collect charges from the patient.

10. The patient registration form is:
    a. A permanent part of the medical record.
    b. Used to collect patient demographic information.
    c. A legal record.
    d. All of the above.

11. The form that authorizes the medical practice to file the insurance claim is referred to as the:
    a. Patient registration form.
    b. Consent for treatment.
    c. Financial responsibility and assignment of benefits form.
    d. Past medical history form.

12. The form that includes the patient's social history, family history, and past medical history is the:
    a. Medicare lifetime beneficiary claim authorization.
    b. Content for treatment.
    c. Patient medical history form.
    d. Patient registration form.

13. The purpose of the problem list is to record:
    a. All minor problems.
    b. All chronic complaints.
    c. All diagnoses.
    d. The CPT® and ICD-9-CM codes in the patient record.

14. When a practitioner terminates or withdraws from a patient's care, he or she must:
    a. Notify the patient in person.
    b. Provide the patient with written notification, giving the patient time to find another practitioner.
    c. Send a letter by certified mail.
    d. Both b and c.

15. Factors that affect learning include:
    a. Ability to read, potential barriers to learning, and cultural beliefs.
    b. Ability to read, potential barriers to learning, religious beliefs, and cultural beliefs.
    c. Potential barriers to learning, language barriers, religious beliefs, cultural beliefs, and ability to read.
    d. Language barriers, cultural beliefs, religious beliefs, and ability to read.

chapter 2

DOCUMENTATION BASICS

LEARNING OBJECTIVES

■ Review the history of documentation
■ Review the SOAP format
■ Understand operative report documentation
■ Understand how documentation drives the coding process
■ Successfully complete end-of-chapter application exercises

A BRIEF HISTORY OF MEDICAL RECORD DOCUMENTATION

Documentation of medical recording began in ancient Egypt and contained details of surgery and prescriptions. There has always been a recognized need for those involved in healing or treatment to pass on details of successful procedures or potions either by written methods or through oral tradition. Individual practitioners most likely attempted to describe what they saw and what they did, but this was not widespread practice.

The earliest surviving records that described individual patients in the United Kingdom belonged to St Bartholomew's Hospital and dated from its foundation in 1123 AD. This occurred during the reign of Henry I, who established the first public records office in England. Physicians kept notes about their patients in books by the mid-19th century. As people became more interested in investigating illnesses and their causes, the importance of documenting past events became important to the health care community. The unit medical record was developed extensively at the Presbyterian Hospital in New York in 1916. Individual patient records were not fully realized yet.

Hospitals and institutions had attempted to influence the data collected within their walls, but there had always been resistance to standardization on the premise that freedom of the individual practitioner must be protected. In Britain, a system of primary and secondary care was instituted in 1948.

In 1957 a book called *The Doctor, His Patient and the Illness* was published that recognized the psychological basis of many problems. This book had a huge impact on medical practice. It indicated that the content of medical notes needed to contain information relevant to an individual's psychological well-being, including sources of stress, social interaction, and perceptions of illness.

As the United States and many European countries became more affluent in the second half of the 20th century, better education led to higher expectations of health care than previously were realized. To achieve a more comprehensive range of services, both primary and secondary care organizations became more complex, and the documentation became an important means of communication between physicians. The availability of continuous rather than episodic health care and recognition of the relationship between the physical, psychological, and social factors led to notes becoming a source of data from documentation with little structure to facilitate processing of the data.

A book published in 1969 entitled *Medical Records, Medical Education and Patient Care* introduced the method of structuring a record with the problem-oriented medical record (POMR). This included a format of recording information consisting of:

- Problem list
- History
- Examination
- Laboratory findings
- Plan of care (diagnostic, therapeutic, and educational)
- Daily SOAP (subjective, objective, assessment, and plan) progress note

The problem list was kept in the front of the medical record and served as an index for the practitioner so that each chronic problem could be followed up until resolved. This system influenced record keeping by recognizing four distinct elements of the clinical medical decision making process:

- Collecting data
- Formulating problems
- Devising a management plan
- Reviewing the medical problems and revising the plan when necessary

The POMR was not widely adopted because it proved to be too time consuming. The patient note entries were classified according to problems but were entered sequentially in chronological order, making it a time-consuming process to acquire a total picture of events within the problem.

With the expansion of education and greater awareness of civil liberties, the medical professional and the medical record have come under great scrutiny. Medical records are now used in claims form negligence and in supporting the level of service billed. Because medical records are used for auditing the medical practice, they must be understandable to the nonmedical reader and the rationale behind decision making must be clearly stated.

New developments in medical records include the popularity of hand-held devices that the practitioner can carry to record patient data, which are later transferred to the medical record. With the emerging popularity of the electronic medical record, documenting should become easier and more efficient in this century.

CODING AND REIMBURSEMENT

The process of assigning a CPT® code to a procedure or service is dependent on both the supporting documentation and the procedure recorded on an HCFA-1500 claim form. The rules or conventions for making this assignment come from the American Medical Association (AMA), which publishes the CPT® codes. An ICD-9-CM diagnosis code must be assigned to support medical necessity.

THE PURPOSE OF DOCUMENTATION

In the past, practitioners used documentation in the medical record to document the patient's problems and conditions. However, in recent years medical records have become a tool to document medical histories as well as to provide a method by which health statistics are tracked, act as a legal document, justify to insurance companies the charges billed on the basis of the medical care provided, and assess quality of care.

Medical records are currently kept in either paper or electronic format. Some examples of types of services found in the medical record are:

- Outpatient office visits
- Consultations
- Medications and prescriptions
- Immunization records
- Laboratory tests and results
- X-rays, imaging, and diagnostic studies
- Surgical services and operative reports
- Hospital records
- Pathology services

Organization and maintenance of the medical record is an important factor in providing quality of care. A well-organized and well-maintained medical record will provide a more user-friendly source of information for internal staff, physicians, auditors, and insurance carriers.

THE MEDICAL RECORD AS A LEGAL DOCUMENT

The medical record helps the practitioner to document care rendered to the patient. It is generally legally regulated by state regulatory or accrediting organizations and reflects the ethics of good clinical practice. The medical record must demonstrate competence through faithfulness to the mental process undertaken by the practitioner, and the synopsis of the care provided. The medical record can be released in certain situations such as professional liability cases, by third party payers, courts of law, or other entities as long as there is appropriate authorization.

The extent of the medical record depends largely on the health care facility and the service(s) offered. There is, however, agreement that the primary purpose of the record is to benefit the patient by creating a record of medical care that supports the provision of care by the same or other practitioner in the future. The medical record assists with audits. Medical audits by the insurance carriers are a major growth area in health care today. The retrospective data collection used in the past is fast changing to a protocol-based recording using standardized forms and other data.

The insurance carriers review medical records to support the level(s) of service billed by the practitioner. The carrier can determine based on the medical record documentation whether the documentation supports the intensity of the services billed or not. The auditor is also looking for medical necessity. Was it medically necessary to bill a comprehensive level of service with the presenting problems(s) and the diagnoses billed? With so many regulations and with increased government scrutiny, the medical record has become one of the most important tools in a health care organization.

PROGRESS AND SOAP NOTES

The medical record is the repository of all information generated in the patient's clinical encounter with the practitioner and other health care providers within the practice. It has three main purposes: an aid to memory; support for continuity of care; and provision of a record of witness to an event or care for legal, financial, and regulatory purposes.

The record should be organized chronologically and should contain a detailed account of the patient's encounter (visit) with the practitioner. Visit notes can be handwritten, typed, or dictated, or a form may be used to record the encounter. In the medical practice, records are usually paper-based. Computerized or electronic medical records are now emerging with the latest technology and may be used more widely in the future. Although there are substantial differences between practitioners and practices in format, content, and layout of the medical record, it typically contains similar information.

The most popular note style is the SOAP note. SOAP stands for **S**ubjective, **O**bjective, **A**ssessment, and **P**lan. It prompts the practitioner to include the following key components:

- History
- Examination
- Medical decision making

Following is an overview of the components of a SOAP note. Review the following clinical note.

Example:

Patient here for follow-up for chest pain and jaw pain. Patient began having chest and right jaw pain upon walking to get the newspaper 2 days ago. The pain was relieved with rest, but it lasted 10–15 minutes. Patient has no complaints of stomach, bowel, or urinary symptoms. Patient has history of

COPD. Medications: Humibid LA 2 bid, Tagamet 400 mg bid, Senokot 25 at hs. Nebulizer with Atrovent and Albuterol qid, Ativan, Diazide 1 day, Aerorbid two puffs bid, Biaxin 500 mg bid. Father—history of COPD and diabetes mellitus; mother—died of myocardial infarction. Patient has history of previous smoking, quitting 5 years ago. Blood pressure 136/60. Pulse 92, Weight 185. Heart rate 100 to 120. There was II/VI systolic murmur in the precordium. Abdomen was soft, nontender. No edema of the feet. EKG, performed in office, showed atrial fibrillation with rapid ventricular response and was positive for new anterior wall infarction. Acute myocardial infarction with the elevation of troponin. Admit patient to hospital (critical care unit). Will maintain on Imdur 30 mg daily. Metroprolol 50 mg in am and 25 mg in pm. Also, add Nitro-Dur. Order chest x-ray to rule out pneumonia. Patient is critical but stable in critical care unit; will reevaluate tomorrow.

When the elements are broken apart, you will see the note follows the progression of the SOAP format. Review the same example below:

- Subjective
  - Patient's chief complaint (reason for visit)
    Example: Patient here for follow-up for chest pain and jaw pain.
  - History of present illness (HPI)
    - Patient began having chest and right jaw pain upon walking to get the newspaper 2 days ago. The pain was relieved with rest but lasted 10–15 minutes.
  - Review of systems
    Example: Patient has no complaints of stomach, bowel, or urinary symptoms.
  - Past medical history
    Example: Patient with history of COPD. Medications: Humibid LA 2 bid, Tagamet 400 mg bid, Senokot 25 at hs. Nebulizer with Atrovent and Albuterol qid, Ativan, Diazide 1 day, Aerorbid two puffs bid, Biaxin 500 mg bid.
  - Family history
    Example: Father—history of COPD and diabetes mellitus; mother—died of myocardial infarction.
  - Social history
    Example: Patient has history of previous smoking, quitting 5 years ago.
- Objective
  - Vital signs
    Example: Blood pressure 136/60. Pulse 92, Weight 185.
  - Physical examination
    Example: Heart rate 100 to 120. There was II/VI systolic murmur in the precordium. Abdomen was soft, nontender. No edema of the feet.
- Assessment
  - Review of pertinent data
    Example: EKG, performed in office, showed atrial fibrillation with rapid ventricular response and was positive for new anterior wall infarction.

○ Diagnosis

Example: Acute myocardial infarction with the elevation of troponin.

- Plan
  ○ Treatment

  Example: Admit patient to hospital (critical care unit).

    ■ Medications

    Example: Will maintain on Imdur 30 mg daily. Metroprolol 50 mg in am and 25 mg in pm. Also, add Nitro-Dur.

    ■ Tests ordered

    Example: Order chest x-ray to rule out pneumonia.

    ■ Referrals to other providers
  ○ Discharge plan

    ■ Return visit

    ■ Hospitalization

    Example: Patient is critical but stable in critical care unit; will re-evaluate tomorrow.

Subjective

The subjective element includes the reason for the visit and all pertinent history elements including the patient's history of present illness, the review of systems, and past, family, and social history.

Examples:

1. Patient complains of abdominal pain for 4 days.
2. Patient states he has congestion, has been running a temperature for 2 days and has trouble sleeping.
3. Patient complains of sore throat, runny nose, and fever that has lasted a week.
4. Patient states she feels lousy in general, does not have any energy, and has not slept well for the past 6 months.

Objective

The objective element includes the examiner's (practitioner's) findings, including abnormal and pertinent normal findings from the examination.

Examples:

1. Temp 99.6, BP 140/80, respirations 18.
2. Heart: regular rate and rhythm, lungs clear to auscultation and percussion.
3. Abdomen nontender, rash on right forearm.
4. Urinalysis indicates a trace of blood, EKG normal.

Assessment

The assessment component includes the thought process and the practitioner's conclusions based on the history and examination. Included in the assessment is the definitive diagnosis, significant findings, signs, and/or symptoms. The practitioner's thought process during the assessment, which is an important component of medical decision making that will be discussed further in Chapter 3, may be documented in the medical record. When the practitioner indicates that a condition is suspected and/or the need to rule out a problem or diagnosis, the practitioner must code only signs and symptoms when submitting a claim to an insurance carrier.

Examples:

Ordered renal x-ray UA and labs. Acute pyelonephritis and nausea with vomiting.

1. Type II diabetes mellitus, uncontrolled.
2. Unstable angina. Recommend heart catheterization.
3. This patient has chronic otitis media, which has recurred within a 3-month period.
4. It is determined that the patient has lobar pneumonia and will be placed on oral antibiotics.

Plan

The plan component is the practitioner's plan for care, including tests, treatments, procedures, medications, and directions given to the patient during a course of treatment. Recommendations and orders for consultations and/or follow-up visits are also recorded in the plan.

Examples:

1. Suture removal today, return in 3 months for follow-up.
2. I have given the patient a refill for Ultram 1 tablet qid and will see her back in the office prn.
3. The patient will be scheduled for a heart catheterization tomorrow.
4. We will get an A1C today. Increase insulin to 3 shots per day. I think we can improve his condition and make him feel a little better. I will see him back in the office in 3 months.

Review the SOAP note example below:

Example:

S—Patient presents with cough; 13-year-old male with 7 days of worsening cough and earache. OTC medications have not improved the cough. The cough is described as dry and hacky. He has had a low-grade fever along with the cough. Patient denies sputum production and wheezing but does admit to feeling of lower respiratory congestion and fullness and mild shortness of breath. Past medical history is negative for significant illnesses or surgeries. Child has no known allergies and is not currently taking any medications other than OTC meds for cough.

O—WT: 145 lbs; BP: 130/80; P: 82 and regular. Lungs are clear with upper respiratory sound, with no wheezing. Cerumen is noted in right ear canal. Left ear canal is bulging and translucent. Heart: Regular rate and rhythm; no murmurs, thrills, gallops, or rubs. Extremities are negative for cyanosis, edema, or clubbing.

A—Otitis media left ear and upper respiratory infection.

P—Treat with Zithromax 200 per 5. Auralgan suspension, three drops to left ear for 7 days. The patient will return in 1 week to recheck ears.

CHECKPOINT EXERCISES

Indicate if the statement is subjective (S), objective (O), an assessment (A), or a plan (P) by using the letter of the SOAP format.

1. _____ Well-developed, well-nourished female in no acute distress.

2. _____ We will start patient on Pen VeeK 250 mg to be taken qid for 10 days.

3. _____ Chest is clear, no wheezing or rales noted.

4. _____ Impression right upper quadrant pain.

5. _____ HEENT: Tympanic membranes were clear bilaterally.

6. _____ She is to take the strain off her elbows and lower back. Patient given instruction sheet on low cholesterol diet and I will see her for recheck in 2 weeks.

7. _____ This 50-year-old male presented to the office with complaint of weakness, malaise, and dyspnea on exertion for approximately 3 weeks.

8. _____ Esophageal reflux; will refer patient to gastroenterologist for treatment.

9. _____ The patient is a nonsmoker with a family history of cardiovascular disease and stroke.

10. _____ Neck: no jugular venous distention, no goiter.

THE OPERATIVE REPORT

Operative reports vary according to the circumstance. An operative report can be a short narrative description of a minor procedure that is performed in a physician's office to a more formal report dictated by a surgeon in a format required by hospitals and ambulatory or free-standing surgery centers.

The office operative note may be formal or informal, depending on the organization needs and type of procedures performed. Review a simple office operative note below:

Patient presents with a lesion on the left arm. Patient states the lesion appeared approximately 6 weeks ago and has been getting larger. Exam reveals a 1.0-cm lesion on the left arm. The left arm was prepped with Betadine and draped in a sterile fashion. Local anesthesia: 1% Xylocaine with epinephrine was used. The dermis was undermined for distance of approximately 2.0 cm around the wound. Skin was closed with a running horizontal mattress suture of 5-0 Ethilon. Antibiotic ointment and sterile dressing were placed over the incision. The patient tolerated the procedure well. He will return in 1 week for suture removal.

Institutional formats may vary slightly, but all contain the following information in the same general format in outline form. There are two parts to a surgical note: the heading and the body. Review the two parts of the surgical note and its contents. (See next page.)

- Date of surgery
- Patient identification (name and/or medical record number)
- Preoperative diagnosis(es)
- Postoperative diagnosis(es)
- Name of the procedure(s) performed
- Name of the primary surgeon
- Co-surgeons or assistant surgeons (if applicable)

The body of the report outlines the detailed narrative of the surgery.

- Positioning and draping of the patient
- Anesthesia administration
- Detailed description of the actual procedure performed, including:
  - surgical approach
  - identification of incision
  - instruments, drains, dressings, and/or special packs
  - identification of abnormalities during surgery
  - description of how hemostasis was obtained
  - closure of surgical site(s)
- Condition of patient when he or she left operating room
- Signature of surgeon

Review Figure 2-1, an example of a formal operative report.

DOCUMENTATION GUIDELINES

The following suggestions are provided for the documentation of each patient encounter:

- The beneficiary's name and date should appear on each page of the patient's record.
- All handwritten notations, names, and signature of the professional must be legible. Also, the therapist's credentials should be present and legible.
- If the therapist is billing as "incident to a physician's services," the name of the physician who is on the premises and is responsible for that patient should appear on each page of documentation for that date of service.
- The therapist and/or physician should make a notation as to the beginning and ending times of any therapy session. Never leave blank lines in any form of documentation.
- Address each blank space with an appropriate notation. It is permissible to draw a line through the blank space or indicate N/A for not applicable.
- Draw a line through any space between the last notation and the therapist's or physician's signature. This ensures that no one else can use that space to make an entry with your name as being the responsible professional.
- Mark any "out of sequence" entries with the notation "Late Entry." Also, the appropriate date, time, and signature and credentials of the therapist or physician must be noted.

FIGURE 2-1

Formal operative report

Patient: Margo Peterson   Date of Procedure: 06/10/2002

Preoperative Diagnosis: Mass, right breast

Postoperative Diagnosis: Same

Procedure: Excision of mass, right breast, with prior localization in
                               the radiographic suite

Surgeon: Emily Stant, MD

Anesthesia: Local 1% Xylocaine with epinephrine

The patient was prepped and draped in the usual fashion. The patient had previously
had an abnormality in the right breast localized in the radiographic suite by Dr Ray
Gunn. The skin overlying the insertion site of the needle was infiltrated with 1%
Xylocaine. The incision was made through the skin and subcutaneous tissue down to
the wire. The breast tissue contained in the hook of the wire was dissected
circumferentially free from the surrounding breast tissue and excised. This was sent
for specimen mammogram, which revealed the abnormality to be present within the
resected specimen. Hemostasis was obtained with cautery. The incision was closed
with 3-0 Vicryl to approximate the subcutaneous tissue and 4-0 Vicryl to close the
skin. A sterile bulky pressure was applied, and the patient was taken to the recovery
room in stable condition.

Addendum: Pathology report
             Diagnosis based on gross and microscopic examination is
             fibroadenoma

Surgeon: *Emily Stant, MD*   06/10/2002

Dictated: 06/11/2002

- Do not black out any entry on a patient record. (The blacking out of
  entries is not acceptable on legal documents.)
- To correct any error, draw a line through the error and note "error" and
  initial it. You may then enter the correct information.
- Patient records must not contain "cut and paste" entries. Cut and paste
  entries cannot be supported as valid for that patient's record.

■ Documentation entered by nonlicensed personnel must be co-signed by
the appropriate licensed practitioner and dated. This ensures that the
licensed professional responsible for that patient has seen and evaluated
the entry. Also, it denotes active participation by the key members of
the treatment team.

HOW DOCUMENTATION AFFECTS THE CODING PROCESS

One of the most important documents in the medical record is the progress
note, which updates the patient's clinical course of treatment and
summarizes the assessment and plan of care. Good progress notes can
be written in a variety of styles or methods. The SOAP note is just one
example.

It is important to understand what the insurance carrier wants in relation to
documentation. Because the insurance carrier has a contractual obligation
to its enrollees, each carrier may require reasonable documentation that
services are consistent with the insurance coverage provided.

CODING AND COMPLIANCE TIPS

1. Use current CPT®, ICD-9-CM, and HCPCS codebooks as well
   as the current rules, regulations, and provider manuals for Medicare
   and for private payers with whom you have a contractual
   arrangement.
2. Educate yourself on CPT® guidelines as well as the rules and
   regulations of your payers. The Health Insurance Portability and
   Accountability Act (HIPAA) indicates that nothing is an excuse for
   lack of knowledge for incorrect coding.
3. When using an encounter form/superbill/charge ticket, specify the
   exact CPT® code and description. Always have an area on the
   encounter form to add procedure and diagnosis codes.
4. Code directly from the chart note or operative note.
5. Update codes annually. Remember that guidelines and codes are
   added, deleted, and revised each year.
6. Avoid fragmented billing. Use your encounter form as the key to
   correct coding. You might add a star next to the starred procedures
   and "SP" next to the separate procedures on your encounter form.
7. Make sure physicians provide the person coding the encounter with
   complete documentation and concise information. Consult the
   physician if documentation is not adequate or if documentation will
   not support the code selected.
8. Use correct modifiers to clarify or append circumstances that can arise
   within the global package.
9. Coders must exercise caution when reporting integral procedures.
   Medicare and Medicaid closely monitor physicians' billing practice for
   possible abuse or fraudulent billing. Private payers also have the
   mechanisms in place to scrutinize claims.
10. Have an independent medical record review (audit) a minimum of
    twice a year to identify coding and documentation errors.

KEY TERMS

Ambulatory surgery center—An independent surgical facility licensed by the state health department for the purpose of performing outpatient surgeries on patients expected to be discharged the same day.

Diagnosis/impression—The impression or condition of the patient after the history and examination are performed.

Encounter form—A form used to record all services and diagnoses applicable to an individual patient encounter.

Key components—History, examination, and medical decision making are considered key components in selecting a level of E/M (evaluation and management) services. These are the first components considered when the level of E/M service to report is determined.

Medical coding—The act of assigning a code to a medical service to submit to an insurance carrier.

Medical necessity—When a service is rendered to a patient by a practitioner, the service(s) should be necessary to effect a cure or a change in the condition for which the patient is being seen.

Operative note—A formal or informal (depending on setting) form of documentation indicating the procedure performed, including all pertinent details of the surgery.

Outpatient services—Services provided in the physician's or other outpatient setting or ambulatory facility.

SOAP—Acronym for a method of documentation: subjective, objective, assessment, and plan.

Treatment plan—Plan of care involving the complexity of the physician's medical decision making.

TEST YOUR KNOWLEDGE

Fill in the Blanks

1. Where were the earliest surviving records describing individual patient care from? _____ How old were they? _____

2. What book indicated that medical notes need to contain information relevant to an individual's psychological well-being?

    _____

3. What does POMR stand for?

    _____

4. What information is included in the POMR?

    _____

5. What are the elements of the clinical medical decision making
    process?_____

    _____

6. What are the two parts of a surgical note called? _____
    and _____

7. What is the correct way to correct an error in the medical record?

    _____

    _____

8. What does the term *SOAP* stand for?_____

    _____

9. What three elements are the level of service based on?

    _____

10. What is the main purpose of the progress note?

    _____

    _____

11. Give three examples of the types of services found in a medical
    record.

    _____

    _____

    _____

12. Name three ways medical records are used in the modern world.

    _____

    _____

    _____

chapter 3

UNDERSTANDING THE EVALUATION AND MANAGEMENT CODES AND THE CENTERS FOR MEDICARE AND MEDICAID SERVICES (CMS) DOCUMENTATION GUIDELINES

LEARNING OBJECTIVES

■ Review the Centers for Medicare and Medicaid Services (CMS) 1995 and 1997 Evaluation and Management guidelines

■ Understand the differences between the CMS 1995 and 1997 Evaluation and Management guidelines

■ Understand key terms in the chapter

■ Successfully complete the end-of-chapter application exercises

EVALUATION AND MANAGEMENT DOCUMENTATION GUIDELINES FROM CMS

The Centers for Medicare and Medicaid Services (CMS), formerly the Health Care Financing Administration (HCFA), revised the guidelines for documentation of evaluation and management (E/M) services in 1992. The guidelines were further expanded with the 1995 documentation guidelines. The 1995 guidelines are less cumbersome than the 1997 documentation guidelines, which went into effect in November 1997. One of the main reasons the 1997 guidelines were created was because medical records lacked enough detail to support the level of services billed. Eliminating or alleviating ambiguity was the goal.

Because many medical societies and practitioners voiced concerns over the 1997 guidelines, indicating the guidelines were missing valid detail and were too burdensome, *CMS has instructed practitioners and auditors to use either the 1995 or 1997 guidelines, whichever is the most advantageous to the provider.*

An auditor or reviewer of medical records for E/M services has a challenge when reviewing medical records to review both sets of guidelines. Both the 1995 and 1997 CMS guidelines will be examined in this chapter. The definite differences between the 1995 and 1997 guidelines are indicated in the key components, including the examination, with minimal differences in the history and medical decision making components. Specific differences will be reviewed in this chapter, along with examples to help you understand both sets of guidelines.

MEDICAL RECORD DOCUMENTATION AND ITS IMPORTANCE

Medical record documentation is required to record pertinent facts, findings, and observations about an individual's health history, including past and present illnesses, examinations, tests, treatments, and outcomes. The medical record chronologically documents the care of the patient and is an important element contributing to high-quality care. An appropriately documented medical record can reduce many of the "hassles" associated with claims processing and may serve as a legal document to verify the care provided if necessary. Because payers have a contractual obligation to enrollees, they may require reasonable documentation that services are consistent with the insurance coverage provided.

They may request information to validate:

- The site of service
- The medical necessity and appropriateness of the diagnostic and/or therapeutic services provided
- That services provided have been accurately reported on the claim form using the correct CPT® and ICD-9-CM and/or HCPCS codes.

The principles of documentation listed below are applicable to all types of medical and surgical services in all settings. For E/M services, the nature and amount of physician work and documentation vary by type of service, place of service, and the patient's status. These general principles may be modified to account for the variable circumstances in providing E/M services.

1. The medical record should be complete and legible.
   a. When notes are not legible and cannot be read clearly, the service may be considered not properly documented and therefore not billable. The carrier may disallow the service and ask for a refund. The encounter should be legible; use of a form and/or dictation is acceptable. It is also acceptable to hand-write chart notes as long as they can be read.
2. The documentation for each patient encounter should include:
   a. Reason for the encounter and relevant history, physical examination findings, and prior diagnostic test results
      (1) The reason for the encounter should support medical necessity and should be clearly stated in the chief complaint. Avoid using phrases such as "follow up" without a definite reason, or "patient has no complaints." The statement should be concise and complete.
      Example: follow-up for otitis media or follow-up for hypertension

    b. Assessment, clinical impression, or diagnosis
        (1) The practitioner's clinical impression or diagnosis(es) should be clearly documented in the chart note for each visit.

    c. Plan for care
        Example: Will obtain A1C today, order mammography and PA and lateral chest x-ray. Will see patient back in 1 week.

    d. Date and legible identity of the observer
        (1) The date of service should be clearly indicated on each patient encounter. Many states require initials and/or signatures, while some will accept a signature stamp for the identity of the observer. It is good practice to check with your individual state for signature requirements.

3. If not documented, the rationale for ordering diagnostic and other ancillary services should be easily inferred.
    a. It is important that the reason for ordering tests and/or services be clearly stated in the chart note, even though the guidelines indicated it may be inferred. Inferring the rationale for ordering test, labs, etc, leaves it up to the reviewer to determine if the rationale is present, which makes the decision too subjective.

4. Past and present diagnoses should be accessible to the treating and/or consulting physician.

5. Appropriate health risk factors should be identified.
    a. Example: Identify patients with family history of a condition or past medical history in the chart note during the visit. If a patient has a family history of heart disease, any risk factors, tests ordered, and/or screening should be noted as to the risk factor.

6. The patient's progress, response to and changes in treatment, and revision of diagnosis should be documented.

7. The CPT® and ICD-9-CM codes reported on the health insurance claim form or billing statement should be supported by the documentation in the medical record.
    a. All CPT®, ICD-9-CM, and/or HCPCS codes must be supported in the medical record. This is why documentation is key to each encounter.

MEDICAL NECESSITY AND DIAGNOSIS CODING (ICD-9-CM) FOR PHYSICIAN SERVICES

ICD-9-CM codes form a crucial partnership with CPT® procedural codes by supporting the medical necessity of the CPT® procedure or service performed. Diagnosis codes identify the medical necessity of services provided by describing the circumstances of the patient's condition. Most third-party payers use claims "edits" or automatic denial/review commands within the computer software to review claims. These edits ensure that payment is made for specific procedure codes when provided for a patient with a specific diagnosis code or predetermined range of ICD-9-CM codes. An important point to realize when filing claims is that neither the CPT® codes nor the ICD-9-CM codes can stand alone.

Apply the following principles to diagnosis coding to properly demonstrate medical necessity:

1. List the principal diagnosis, condition, problem, or other reason for the medical service or procedure.

2. Assign the code to the highest level of specificity.

3. For office and/or outpatient services, never use a "rule-out" statement (a suspected but not confirmed diagnosis); a clerical error could permanently tag a patient with a condition that does not exist. Code symptoms, if no definitive diagnosis is yet determined, instead of using rule-out statements.

4. Be specific in describing the patient's condition, illness, or disease.

5. Distinguish between acute and chronic conditions, when appropriate.

6. Identify the acute condition of an emergency situation, eg, coma, loss of consciousness, or hemorrhage.

7. Identify chronic complaints, or secondary diagnoses, only when treatment is provided or when they impact the overall management of the patient's care.

8. Identify how injuries occur.

These facts must be substantiated by the patient's medical record, and that record must be available to payers upon request.

EVALUATION AND MANAGEMENT SERVICES

Every practitioner in health care today will use E/M services. These services are categorized in CPT® and include:

- Office visits
- Hospital visits
- Observation care
- Emergency department services
- Preventive medicine services
- Consultations (inpatient, outpatient, and confirmatory)
- Home care services
- Nursing home care
- Rest home, domiciliary care
- Hospital discharge services
- Critical care services
- Neonatal intensive care
- Prolonged physician services
- Physician standby services
- Care plan oversight
- Telephone calls
- Team conferences
- Newborn care
- Basic life and/or disability evaluation services
- Work-related or medical disability evaluation services

Most of the E/M services are further categorized into new and established patient services. Review the following CPT® definitions for new and established patients:

New patient—A new patient is one who has not received any professional services from the physician or another physician of the same specialty who belongs to the same group practice within the past 3 years.

Established patient—An established patient is one who has received professional services from the physician or another physician of the same specialty who belongs to the same group practice within the past 3 years. In the instance where a physician is on call for and/or covering for another physician, the patient encounter is classified as if it would have been by the physician who is not available.

A practitioner in the same specialty with the same tax identification number, even though each practitioner has his or her own provider number, would be considered part of the same group. Many practitioners are physically located in different parts of a city, state, or country, but are of the same group.

If a practitioner has the same tax identification number, but is of a different specialty, the patient would not be considered an established patient unless the practitioner has seen the patient within the past 3 years. The *CPT® Assistant* is the American Medical Association's (AMA's) authoritative coding newsletter on CPT® changes and an excellent source for a correct coding reference. Review the following diagram (Figure 3-1), published in the *CPT® Assistant* in 1999, which clarifies new and established patient status.

KEY COMPONENTS AND CONTRIBUTORY FACTORS

In the past, the reporting of the physician's professional encounters was subjective, undefined, and easily manipulated for better description. With the implementation of new methods of payment, the entire structure of an encounter had to meet measurable standards. In 1992, all narratives and components changed, forcing the measurement of service intensity into the selection process. Intensity of service is measured as graduated levels of service but is not given names equivalent to the terminology used in the past (eg, brief, intermediate). Within each level, CPT® lists specific components to measure service intensity. The descriptors for the levels of E/M services recognize seven components that are used in defining the levels of E/M services. Three of these components are considered key to the selection of a service level. Four more components are considered contributory to the choice of the service level. Exceptions include critical care and neonatal care services, among others; these will be discussed in a later chapter. The focus of this chapter will be the key components and documentation requirements.

The three key components are as follows:

- History, relative to the patient's clinical picture
- Examination, relative to present and concurrent problems
- Physician's medical decision making process in managing the patient

FIGURE 3-1

Decision tree for new vs established patient

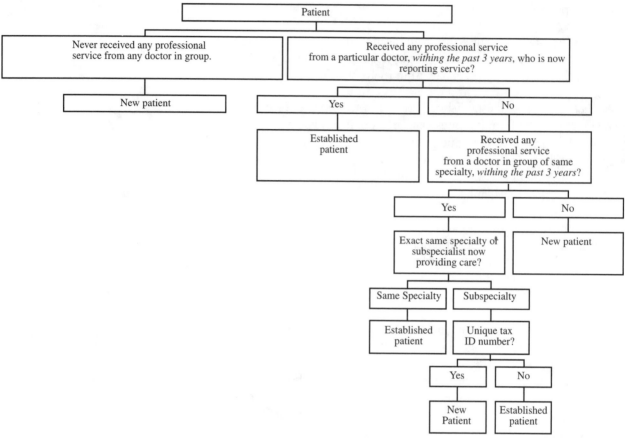

Source: *CPT Assistant,* June 1999

The following are the four contributory elements:

- ■ Counseling with the patient and/or family
- ■ Coordination of care with other health care professionals or facilities
- ■ Nature of the patient's presenting problem
- ■ Time

The three key components are the primary components in selection of the level of E/M services. An exception to this rule is the case of visits that consist predominantly of counseling or coordination of care. Because the level of E/M service is dependent on two or three key components, performance and documentation of one component (eg, examination) at the highest level does not necessarily mean that the encounter in its entirety qualifies for the highest level of E/M service. In the case of visits that consist predominantly of counseling or coordination of care, time is the key or controlling factor to qualify for a particular level of E/M service.

The three key components—history, examination, and medical decision making—are used most often to determine the level of service rendered. Some levels of E/M services in CPT® require only two of the three key components to be met or exceeded, while other services require all three key components to qualify for a given level of service. Key component requirements are given in the instructions in the next section.

INSTRUCTIONS FOR SELECTING A LEVEL OF E/M SERVICE

Definitions for the levels of E/M service for history, examination, and medical decision making in the CPT® guidelines are found in the current edition of the CPT® book and reproduced below.

1. Determine the extent of history obtained, which is dependent on clinical judgment and on the nature of the presenting problem(s). The levels of E/M service recognize four types of history:

   - Problem focused (chief complaint; brief history of present illness or problem)

   - Expanded problem focused (chief complaint; brief history of present illness; problem pertinent system review)

   - Detailed (chief complaint; extended history of present illness; problem pertinent system review extended to include a review of a limited number of additional systems; **pertinent** past, family, and/or social history **directly related to the patient's problems**)

   - Comprehensive (chief complaint; extended history of present illness; review of systems which is directly related to the problem(s) identified in the history of the present illness plus a review of all additional body systems; **complete** past, family, and social history)

   Note: The comprehensive history obtained as part of the preventive medicine E/M service is not problem oriented and does not involve a chief complaint or present illness. It does, however, include a comprehensive system review and comprehensive or interval past, family, and social history, as well as a comprehensive assessment/history of pertinent risk factors.

2. Determine the extent of examination performed, which is dependent on clinical judgment and on the nature of the presenting problem(s). The levels of E/M services recognize four types of examination that are defined as follows:

   - Problem focused (a limited examination of the affected body area or organ system)

   - Expanded problem focused (a limited examination of the affected body area or organ system and other symptomatic or related organ system[s])

   - Detailed (an extended examination of the affected body area[s] and other symptomatic or related organ system[s])

   - Comprehensive (a general multi-system examination or a complete examination of a single organ system)

   Note: The comprehensive examination performed as part of the preventive medicine E/M service is multi-system, but its extent is based on age and risk factors identified.

3. Determine the complexity of medical decision making. This refers to the complexity of establishing a diagnosis and/or selecting a management option as measured by the number of possible diagnoses and/or the number of management options that must be considered; the amount and/or complexity of medical records, diagnostic tests, and/or other information that must be obtained, reviewed, and analyzed; and the risk of significant complications, morbidity, and/or

mortality, as well as comorbidities, associated with the patient's presenting problem(s), the diagnostic procedure(s), and/or the possible management options. Four types of medical decision making are recognized:

- Straightforward
- Low complexity
- Moderate complexity
- High complexity

Note: Comorbidities/underlying conditions, in and of themselves, are not considered in selecting a level of E/M services unless their presence significantly increases the complexity of the medical decision making.

4. Select the appropriate level of E/M services based on the following:

   a. For the following categories/subcategories, **all of the key components** (ie, history, examination, and medical decision making) must meet or exceed the stated requirements to qualify for a particular level of E/M service: office, new patient; hospital observation services; initial hospital care; office consultations; initial inpatient consultations; confirmatory consultations; emergency department services; comprehensive nursing facility assessments; domiciliary care, new patient; and home, new patient.

   b. For the following categories/subcategories, **two of the three key components** (ie, history, examination, and medical decision making) must meet or exceed the stated requirements to qualify for a particular level of E/M services: office, established patient; subsequent hospital care; follow-up inpatient consultations; subsequent nursing facility care; domiciliary care, established patient; and home, established patient.

   c. When counseling and/or coordination of care dominates (more than 50%) of the physician/patient and/or family encounter (face-to-face time in the office or other outpatient setting or floor/unit time in the hospital or nursing facility), then time may be considered the key or controlling factor to qualify for a particular level of E/M services. This includes time spent with parties who have assumed responsibility for the care of the patient or decision making whether or not they are family members (eg, foster parents, person acting in locum parentis, legal guardian). The extent of counseling and/or coordination of care must be documented in the medical record.

See Table 3-1 for selection of E/M codes for office visits. (Documentation requirements for the level of service selected for hospital visits, emergency department visits, and consultations are given in Appendix A.) The last column of the table shows the average time it takes to perform a level of E/M service, but time is not the controlling factor unless counseling and/or coordination of care dominates at least 50% of the visit.

DEFINITIONS OF KEY COMPONENTS

In addition to restating the difference between new and established patients, terms have been structured to fit in with the numerical measurement of visits. These terms progress in description, allowing graduated relative value units that proportionately reflect greater intensity in the service required.

TABLE 3-1

Evaluation and management office visit selection grid

E/M Code	History	Physical Exam	Medical Decision Making	Average Time
Office Visit—New: 3 of 3 components must be met or exceeded				
99201	PF	PF	S	10
99202	EPF	EPF	S	20
99203	D	D	L	30
99204	C	C	M	45
99205	C	C	H	60
Office Visit—Established: 2 of 3 components must be met or exceeded				
99212	PF	PF	S	10
99213	EPF	EPF	L	15
99214	D	D	M	25
99215	C	C	H	40

Key: PF=Problem Focused   EPF=Expanded Problem Focused
D=Detailed   C=Comprehensive   S=Straightforward
L=Low Complexity   M=Moderate Complexity   H=High Complexity

As mentioned, the Centers for Medicare and Medicaid Services (CMS) implemented Evaluation and Management Documentation Guidelines in 1995 and expanded the guidelines in 1997. Since both guidelines are currently in effect, it is up to the practitioner to decide which set of guidelines to follow. It is important to maintain consistency so as not to get confused when documenting the patient encounter.

History

Following is a detailed review of the components of history for the CMS Evaluation and Management Documentation Guidelines.

Chief Complaint

Chief complaint is included in all history levels and must be clearly documented in the medical record. It is defined by CPT® as "a concise statement describing the symptom, problem, condition, diagnosis, or other factor that is the reason for the encounter, usually stated in the patient's words."

Review the following two examples of a definitive chief complaint:

Example 1: This is the first visit for this 2-year-old female patient with a complaint of 11/2 days of cough and fever.

Example 2: Tom, a 15-year-old established patient, returns for follow-up of diabetes mellitus.

History of Present Illness

The next important step in determining the history is the history of present illness (HPI). The HPI is defined by the CPT® book as "a chronological description of the

CODING TIP

Do not state "Patient here for follow-up." The specific reason the patient is visiting the practitioner must be clearly stated.

development of the patient's present illness from the first sign and/or symptom to the present." Normally this information is derived from the patient's own words.

Elements included in the HPI are:

- Location—where problem, pain, or symptom occurs (leg, chest, back, etc)
- Quality—description of problem, symptom, or pain (dull, itching, constant, etc)
- Severity—description of severity of symptom or pain (1–10 rating, mild, moderate, etc)
- Duration—how long problem, symptom, or pain has persisted (one week, since last night, etc)
- Timing—when a problem, symptom, or pain occurs (morning, after eating, while lying down, etc)
- Context—instances that can be associated with the problem, symptom, or pain (while standing for long periods of time, when sitting, etc)
- Modifying factors—actions taken to make the problem, symptom, or pain better or worse (pain relievers help dull pain, nausea after eating, etc)
- Associated signs and symptoms—other problems, symptoms, or facts that occur when primary problem, symptom, or pain occurs (stress causes headache, burning during urination, etc)

There are two levels of HPI for both the 1995 and 1997 CMS documentation guidelines. The HPI for both sets of guidelines is similar; however, the 1997 guidelines allow documentation of the status of three or more chronic conditions, whether they are stable or have worsened, as acceptable documentation for the HPI.

Brief and extended HPI are differentiated by the amount of detail documented on the basis of the patient's clinical and/or presenting problem(s). One to three elements are documented in a brief HPI. Extended HPI requires the documentation of four or more elements, or the status of three or more chronic or inactive conditions (1997 guidelines).

Review the following two examples of an HPI.

Example 1:   Patient's cough is nonproductive and "nonbarky" and has worsened today. Patient also has rhinorrhea, which began yesterday.

Four elements have been identified in this example of the HPI:

- Location—cough
- Quality—nonproductive
- Context or modifying factors—nonbarky and has worsened today
- Associated signs and symptoms—rhinorrhea

Notice that the statement "nonbarky and has worsened today" could be viewed as either context or modifying factors in example 1.

Example 2:   This 15-year-old male is doing very well on his insulin regimen. His insulin dose remains low, 29N +1R in the morning and 6N at night. I note that he is having a few lows in the middle of the night even though he cut back his insulin at night to +4N on game days. This has been an issue. Even though he eats well, he goes low at night because of the activity level.

- Duration—cut back on insulin at night to +4N on game days
- Context—insulin dose remains low
- Quality—few lows in the middle of night
- Modifying factors—even though he eats well, he goes low at night because of the activity level

Review of Systems

The next important element contained in the history is the review of systems (ROS). The ROS is defined by CPT® as "an inventory of body systems obtained through a series of questions seeking to identify signs and/or symptoms which the patient may be experiencing or has experienced." The review of systems is normally a series of questions and answers related to the patient's complaints and/or problems. The review of systems may also be recorded on a form or completed by the patient, as long as it is referenced in the chart note. The review of systems requirements are the same for both the 1995 and 1997 CMS guidelines.

For the purposes of ROS, the following systems are recognized:

- Constitutional symptoms (eg, fever, weight loss)
- Eyes (eg, double vision, pain, eye strain)
- Ears, Nose, Mouth, Throat (eg, ear pain, sinus drainage, pain when swallowing)
- Cardiovascular (eg, chest pain, edema, palpitations)
- Respiratory (eg, shortness of breath, wheezing)
- Gastrointestinal (eg, bowel movement, appetite, bloating, stomach pain)
- Genitourinary (eg, burning when urinating, discharge, hematuria)
- Musculoskeletal (eg, pain, stiffness, swelling, pain)
- Integumentary (skin and/or breast) (eg, pain, itching, rash)
- Neurological (eg, seizures, headaches, tremors)
- Psychiatric (eg, sleeping habits, awareness, feelings)
- Endocrine (eg, thryoid problems, excessive thirst or sweating)
- Hematologic/Lymphatic (eg, bleeding, bruising, anemia)
- Allergic/Immunologic (eg, allergies, reactions, immune symptoms or problems)

The ROS is defined in graduated levels:

- Problem Pertinent (1 system)—directly related to the patient's problem
- Extended (2–9 systems)—directly related to the patient's problem identified in the HPI and limited number of additional systems
- Comprehensive (10 or more systems)—directly related to the patient's problem in the HPI plus all additional body systems

A problem-pertinent ROS is composed of documentation of only one system, whereas an extended ROS is composed of two to nine systems. A complete review of systems, which is required for a comprehensive history, is composed of 10 or more systems or body areas based on the systems listed previously.

A practitioner is expected to document all positive and pertinent and negative responses to some systems and may include a phrase "all other systems negative" when documenting a comprehensive or complete ROS. The practitioner must actually review all systems for the statement to apply.

+DOCUMENTATION TIP

Caution: do not count elements previously counted and used in the HPI. If an element was used in the HPI, it cannot be used again in the ROS.

The following two examples will give you an understanding of what elements are present with an ROS.

Example 1:   Mother denies any diarrhea or other GU complaints. Patient's sleep pattern was poor last night and appetite was down today. Patient is positive for fever and cough with trouble breathing at night.

Systems reviewed:

- Diarrhea—Genitourinary (GU)
- Sleep patterns poor—Neurological system
- Appetite down today—Gastrointestinal system
- Patient positive for fever—Constitutional
- Cough—Respiratory system

In example 1, five systems were reviewed, which indicates an extended ROS.

Example 2:   Review of systems from 4 months previously reveals that he is doing well. He has experienced no GI or GU symptoms and no neurological complaints. He has minor joint aches following extensive practices or games. His mood and affect are good.

Systems reviewed:

- Gastrointestinal system (GI)
- Genitourinary (GU)
- Neurological system
- Joint aches—Musculoskeletal system
- Mood and Affect—Psychiatric

In example 2, five systems are reviewed, which indicates an extended ROS.

Past, Family, and/or Social History

The last element that makes up history is the past, family, and/or social history (PFSH). Both the 1995 and 1997 CMS guidelines for this element of history are the same. The PFSH consists of three elements that are defined in the CPT® guidelines:

- Past history: a review of the patient's past experiences with illnesses, operations, injuries, and treatments
- Family history: a review of medical events in the patient's family, including diseases which may be hereditary or place the patient at risk
- Social history: an age-appropriate review of past and current activities

At least one specific item from any of the three history areas must be documented for a pertinent PFSH. A complete PFSH is a review of two or all three PFSH areas, depending on the category of the E/M service, with at least one specific item being documented from the history area reviewed. For certain categories of E/M services that include only an interval history, it is not necessary to record information about the PFSH. Those categories are subsequent hospital care, follow-up inpatient consultations, and subsequent nursing facility care.

NOTE: The medical records of infants, children, and adolescents may have additional or modified information recorded in each history area. As an example, newborn records may include under medical history details of the mother's pregnancy and the infant's status at birth; social history will focus on family structure; family history will focus on congenital anomalies and hereditary disorders in the family. In addition, information on growth and development and/or nutrition will be recorded. Although not specifically defined in these documentation guidelines, these patient group variations on history are appropriate.

Review both examples of PFSH.

Example 1: Patient finished Keflex for cellulitis 1 week ago and was doing well. Mother has given patient Tylenol and Robitussin for cough. Patient has a history of RAD and mother ran out of albuterol 1–2 weeks ago, but states she didn't believe it helped. Patient has a history of URI symptoms on and off for past 3 months.

Past medical history—past illness: cellulitis, Tylenol and Robitussin for cough. Patient has a history of RAD. Patient has a history of URI symptoms on and off for the past 3 months.

The example above is confined to the past medical history related to the patient's illness

Example 2: PFSH remains unchanged from history form date 7/1/99 (see form).

This example indicates that the patient's PFSH was recorded on a form dated 12/06/2000 and has not changed since that date. Review the PFSH from 12/06/2000 in Figure 3-2. Notice that at the bottom of the historical summary form, a date and initials of a staff member are apparent, and there is no question that the medical history form was reviewed. Also notice that all history areas are identified, including past medical history, family history, and social history. This form, completed and updated, does meet the requirement for a comprehensive history, which includes all three history areas and would meet comprehensive documentation requirements for new as well as established patients.

Table 3-2 is an excellent tool for a practitioner or auditor to use to review at a glance what elements are required for a level of history.

Using a Form to Record Historical Summary
Using a form is acceptable practice, but the practitioner must indicate in the note that the past history form and/or review of systems was reviewed with

FIGURE 3-2

Adult screening form

PATIENT MEDICAL HISTORICAL SUMMARY

Patient Name: Mary Jones   **Date of Birth: 08/11/1951**   Sex: ☐M ☒F

Check any past/current problems

☐Confused	☐Vision	☐Abnormal Pap smears	☐Difficulty walking
☐Unresponsive	☐Loose/chipped teeth	☐Reproductive organs	☐Frequent falls
☐Eyes	☐Capped/false teeth	☐Dialysis	☐Bones
☒Ears	☐Circulation problems	☐Thyroid	☐Weakness
☐Nose	☒Stomach problems	☒Heart problems	☐Immune system problems
☐Mouth	☐Weight loss	☐Blood clots	☐Too little sleep
☐Sinus	☐Weight gain	☐Bleeding	☐Too much sleep
☐Throat	☐Bowel problems	☒High blood pressure	☐Lung problems
☐Skin problems	☐Liver problems	☐Stroke	☐Breathing problems
☐Rash	☐Hepatitis	☐Diabetes	☐Chronic cough
☐Hives	☐Gallbladder	☐Seizures	☐TB
☐Hearing	☐Kidney	☐Epilepsy	☐Positive TB test
☐Speech	☐Pain:	☐Cancer:	☐Other:_____
	Location_____	Location_____	

☐ Implants/surgical or other metal inside the body: type_____ location_____

☐ Problems with anesthesia, describe_____

Explain any checked items _____

List any previous hospitalizations/surgeries/invasive procedures: hysterectomy 1985

Date of last: pneumonia shot <u>12/06/2000</u> tetanus shot: <u>not sure</u> flu shot <u>12/06/2000</u> TB test <u>Unknown</u>

List any allergies <u>None</u>_____

List any other problems you may have _____

FAMILY HISTORY

Father: ☒living ☐dead age at death (if   cause of death (if

                              applicable)   applicable)

Mother: ☒living ☐dead age at death (if   cause of death (if

                              applicable)   applicable)

Have you had a family member with any of the following? If so, check the appropriate box.

	Father	Mother	Children	Brother/Sister	Grandparent		Father	Mother	Children	Brother/Sister	Grandparent
Alcoholism	☐	☐	☐	☐	☒	Cancer	☐	☐	☐	☐	☐
Bleeding	☐	☐	☐	☐	☐	Asthma	☐	☐	☐	☐	☐
Thyroid	☐	☒	☐	☐	☐	Diabetes	☒	☐	☐	☒	☐
Heart disease	☐	☐	☐	☐	☒	Stroke	☐	☐	☐	☐	☐
Epilepsy	☐	☐	☐	☐	☐	Migraine	☐	☐	☐	☐	☐
Seizures	☐	☐	☐	☐	☐	TB	☐	☐	☐	☐	☐
Mental disorders	☐	☐	☐	☐	☐	Kidney disease	☐	☐	☐	☐	☐
High blood pressure	☒	☐	☐	☐	☐	other	☐	☐	☐	☐	☐

SOCIAL HISTORY

Marital Status Married Children (list names): <u>Nancy, Susan, and John</u>   ☐N/A

_____

Do you live alone? ☐yes ☒no If you needed help to care for yourself, is there someone available to help you? ☒yes ☐no

Tobacco: ☐yes ☒no If yes, how much/day _____ x _____ years _____ Recreational drugs: ☐yes ☐no

Alcohol: ☐yes ☒no If yes, how much _____ / day _____ / week Caffeine: ☒yes ☐no

If yes, how much day <u>2 cups of coffee day</u> Exercise routine: <u>None</u> Occupation: <u>Bank Examiner</u>

Unusual dietary habits or herbal supplements: _____

Do you have an advanced directive? ☐Yes ☒No If yes, ☐ living will ☐ durable power of attorney ☐ health care directive

Would you like information about advanced directives? ☒Yes ☐No (Staff use): ☒ Brochure given: date/initials: <u>12/2/2001</u>

Staff Review: date/initials <u>12/2/2001 SLM</u> date/initials _____ date/initials _____

TABLE 3-2

1997 E/M guidelines (CMS)

Type of History	History of Present Illness (HPI)	Review of Systems (ROS)	Past, Family, and/or Social History (PFSH)
Problem focused (PF)	Brief (1–3 elements)	N/A	N/A
Expanded problem focused (EPF)	Brief (1–3 elements)	Problem pertinent	N/A
Detailed (D)	Extended (≥ 4 elements [1995 and 1997] or status of ≥ 3 multiple chronic or inactive conditions [1997 only])	Extended (2–9 systems)	Pertinent (1 history area)
Comprehensive (C)	Extended (≥ 4 elements [1995 and 1997] or status of ≥ 3 multiple chronic or inactive conditions [1997 only])	Complete (10 systems or some systems with statement "all others negative")	Complete (2 history areas for established; 3 history areas for new patient)

the patient. The location of the form must be referred to in the chart. Any changes, updates, or additions to the information on the form should be noted, and the form should be dated and initialed by the person updating the information, whether it is ancillary staff or the practitioner. It is acceptable for a nurse and/or ancillary staff member to complete the history for the practitioner.

CMS Documentation Guidelines for History

1. The chief complaint, ROS, and PFSH may be listed as separate elements of history, or they may be included in the description of the HPI.

2. An ROS and/or a PFSH obtained during an earlier encounter does not need to be rerecorded if there is evidence that the physician reviewed and updated the previous information. This may occur when a physician updates his or her own record or in an institutional setting or group practice where many physicians use a common record. The review and update may be documented by:

   ■ Describing any new ROS and/or PFSH information or noting there has been change in the information
   ■ Noting the date and location of the earlier ROS and/or PFSH

3. The ROS and/or PFSH may be recorded by ancillary staff or on a form completed by the patient. To document that the physician reviewed the information, there must a notation supplementing or confirming the information recorded by others.

4. If the physician is unable to obtain a history from the patient or other source, the record should describe the patient's condition or other circumstance which precludes obtaining a history.

5. To qualify for a given type of history, all three elements in the table must be met; a chief complaint is indicated at all levels. Notice that a PFSH is not required for a problem focused and expanded problem focused history.

TABLE 3-3

CMS 1995 vs 1997 examination documentation guidelines

Documentation Requirement	Problem Focused	Expanded Problem Focused	Detailed	Comprehensive
1995 body areas or organ systems	1 body area or organ system	2-4 body areas or organ systems	5-7 body areas or organ systems	8 or more body areas or organ systems OR comprehensive single organ system
1997 performance and documentation of elements identified by a bullet	1–5 elements identified by a bullet from one or more body areas or organ systems	6 elements identified by a bullet from one or more body areas or organ systems	2 elements identified by a bullet from six body areas or organ systems OR 12 elements from two more body areas or organ systems	2 elements identified by a bullet from nine body areas or organ systems

Examination

The second key component that is part of the E/M documentation guidelines is the examination. Identical graduated terms or phrases are used to measure the extent of an examination. The documentation in this key area is often assumed in the dictation or writing of the progress note. Without thorough documentation, however, there is no actual evidence of examination during the patient encounter.

The 1995 CMS documentation guidelines are based on systems and/or body areas, whereas the 1997 documentation guidelines for examination are based on either a multisystem or single organ system exam table. All the 1997 exam tables are located in Appendix A, and the 1995 systems and/or body areas are located in Appendix B.

See Table 3-3 to identify documentation requirements for both 1995 and 1997 guidelines. The examination is the largest difference between the two sets of guidelines. Also see Appendix B.

CMS Documentation Guidelines

1. Specific abnormal and relevant negative findings of the examination of the affected or symptomatic body area(s) or organ system(s) should be documented. A notation of "abnormal" without elaboration is insufficient.
2. Abnormal or unexpected findings of the examination of any asymptomatic body area(s) or organ system(s) should be described.
3. A brief statement or notation indicating "negative" or "normal" is sufficient to document normal findings related to unaffected area(s) or asymptomatic organ system(s).

CMS Guidelines for 1995

The following body areas and organ systems are recognized in the CMS guidelines for 1995 (Table 3-4).

TABLE 3-4

Body areas and organ systems according to 1995 CMS guidelines

Body Areas	Organ Systems
Head, including the face	Constitutional (vital signs, general appearance)
Neck	Eyes
Chest, including breast and axillae	Ears, nose, mouth, and throat
Abdomen	Cardiovascular
Genitalia, groin, buttocks	Respiratory
Back, including spine	Gastrointestinal
Each extremity	Musculoskeletal
	Skin
	Neurologic
	Psychiatric
	Hematologic/Lymphatic/Immunologic

CMS Guidelines for 1997

The type(s) of examinations for 1997 have been defined for general multisystem examinations and the following single organ systems:

- Cardiovascular
- Ears, Nose, Mouth, and Throat
- Eyes
- Genitourinary (Female)
- Genitourinary (Male)
- Hematologic/Lymphatic/Immunologic
- Musculoskeletal
- Neurological
- Psychiatric
- Respiratory
- Skin

A general multi-system examination or a single organ system examination may be performed by any physician regardless of specialty. The type (general multi-system or single organ system) and content of examination are selected by the examining physician and are based on clinical judgment, the patient's history, and the nature of the presenting problem(s).

The content and documentation requirements for each type and level of examination are summarized below; the exam tables are located in Appendix A.

In the tables, organ systems and body areas recognized by the CPT® nomenclature for purposes of describing examinations are shown in the left column. The content, or individual elements, of the examination pertaining to that body area or organ system are identified by bullets (•) in the right column.

Documentation for each element must satisfy any numeric requirements (such as "Measurement of any three of the following seven vital signs in

Constitutional") included in the description of the element. Elements with multiple components but with no specific numeric requirement (such as "Examination of liver and spleen") require documentation of at least one component. It is possible for a given examination to be expanded beyond what is defined here. When that occurs, findings related to the additional systems and/or areas should be documented.

General Multi-system Examination

The general multi-system exam table is located in Appendix A. Study the table carefully. To qualify for a given level of multi-system examination, the following content and documentation requirements should be met:

- Problem-Focused Examination—should include performance and documentation of one to five elements identified by a bullet (•) in one or more organ system(s) or body area(s).
- Expanded Problem-Focused Examination—should include performance and documentation of at least six elements identified by a bullet (•) in one or more organ system(s) or body area(s).
- Detailed Examination—should include at least six organ systems or body areas. For each system/area selected, performance and documentation of at least two elements identified by a bullet (•) are expected. Alternatively, a detailed examination may include performance and documentation of at least 12 elements identified by a bullet (•) in two or more organ systems or body areas.
- Comprehensive Examination—should include two elements identified by a bullet in at least nine organ systems or body areas with a total of 18 exam elements. For each system/area selected, all elements of the examination identified by a bullet (•) should be performed, unless specific directions limit the content of the examination. For each area/system, documentation of at least two elements identified by a bullet is expected.

Single Organ System Examinations

The single organ system exam tables recognized by the CPT® nomenclature are found in Appendix A. Variations among these examinations in the organ systems and body areas identified in the left columns and in the elements of the examinations described in the right columns reflect differing emphases among specialties. To qualify for a given level of single organ system examination, the following content and documentation requirements should be met:

- Problem-Focused Examination—should include performance and documentation of one to five elements identified by a bullet (•), whether in a box with a shaded or unshaded border.
- Expanded Problem-Focused Examination—should include performance and documentation of at least six elements identified by a bullet (•), whether in a box with a shaded or unshaded border.
- Detailed Examination—examinations other than the eye and psychiatric examinations should include performance and documentation of at least 12 elements identified by a bullet (•), whether in box with a shaded or unshaded border.
- Eye and psychiatric examinations—should include the performance and documentation of at least nine elements identified by a bullet (•), whether in a box with a shaded or unshaded border.

■ Comprehensive Examination—should include performance of all elements identified by a bullet (•), whether in a shaded or unshaded box. Documentation of every element in each box with a shaded border and at least one element in each box with an unshaded border is expected.

Review the example below and compare the 1995 exam guidelines (organs and/or body systems) and the 1997 guidelines using the multisystem exam table in Appendix A.

Example 1: General, alert, NAD; throat, nonerythematous; neck, supple, no adenopathy; heart, RRR without murmurs; lungs, CTA, no wheezes, no crackles; Abd, soft/nontender.

1995 Systems/Body Areas	**1997 Multi-system Exam Table**
Constitutional—General, Alert, NAD	Constitutional—General appearance
ENT—throat	ENT—Throat, examination of oropharynx
Neck—supple, no adenopathy	Neck—examination of thyroid
Heart—RRR without murmurs	Heart—auscultation of heart with notation of abnormal sounds and murmurs
Respiratory—Lungs CTA	Respiratory—auscultation of lungs

On the basis of the 1995 CMS guidelines, the exam elements are composed of five systems and/or body areas: constitutional, ENT, neck, heart, and respiratory. On the basis of the 1997 CMS guidelines, there are six elements identified by a bullet from the multisystem exam table that would be problem focused for the examination. For 1995, the level of services based on the documentation guidelines is detailed (five to seven systems or body areas) (Table 3-5). For 1997, the level of services would be problem focused (one to five elements identified by a bullet) (Table 3-6).

Example 2: Weight, 137 lbs; Ht, 165 cm; BP, 96/60; HEENT, normal; neck, supple; chest, clear to auscultation. Cardiac exam is benign. Shot sites look to be all buttocks, but look good.

Review Tables 3-5 and 3-6 and determine, according to both 1995 and 1997 guidelines, what level of examination is documented in example 2.

1995 Systems/Body Areas	**1997 Multi-system Exam Table**
Constitutional—three vitals	Constitutional—three vitals
Neck—supple	Neck—supple
Respiratory—chest clear	Respiratory—chest clear to auscultation
Cardiac—exam benign	Cardiovascular—exam benign
Skin—buttocks	Skin—inspection of skin

Note that under cardiovascular or cardiac the documentation indicates benign. Since this element is not listed on the multi-system exam table, the practitioner may receive credit for only one element.

For the encounter in example 2, according to the 1995 guidelines the examination is detailed and according to the 1997 guidelines the examination is problem focused (one to five elements identified by a bullet using the multi-system exam table).

DOCUMENTATION TIP

It is recommended that when using the 1997 documentation guidelines for E/M services, the practitioner document specific exam elements by using the multi-system or single organ system exam table(s) as a guide.

TABLE 3-5

CMS examination documentation guidelines for 1995

Documentation Requirement	Problem Focused	Expanded Problem Focused	Detailed	Comprehensive
1995 body areas or organ systems	1 body area or organ system	2–4 body areas or organ systems	5–7 body areas or organ systems	8 or more body areas or organ systems OR comprehensive single organ system

TABLE 3-6

CMS examination documentation guidelines for 1997

Documentation Requirement	Problem Focused	Expanded Problem Focused	Detailed	Comprehensive
1997 performance and documentation of elements identified by a bullet	1–5 elements identified by a bullet from one or more body areas or organ systems	6 elements identified by a bullet from one or more body areas or organ systems	2 elements identified by a bullet from 6 body areas or organ systems OR 12 elements from 2 more body areas or organ systems	2 elements identified by a bullet from 9 body areas or organ systems

Medical Decision Making

The last key component is medical decision making, which is composed of the following:

- The presenting problem
- Amount and/or complexity of data to be reviewed
- Risk

Treatment of a patient is not entirely counseling, care coordination, examination, and history taking. On the basis of all subjective, objective, and assessment data available, as well as concurrent injuries or illnesses, the physician must evaluate and recommend options to the patient before pursuing a treatment protocol or therapy.

The levels of E/M service in the CPT® book recognize four types of medical decision making:

- Straightforward
- Low complexity
- Moderate complexity
- High complexity

Medical decision making refers to the complexity of establishing a diagnosis and/or selecting a management option, as measured by:

- The number of possible diagnoses and/or the number of management options that must be considered

- The amount and/or complexity of medical records, diagnostic tests, and/or other information that must be obtained, reviewed, and analyzed
- The risk of significant complications, morbidity, and/or mortality, as well as comorbidities, associated with the patient's presenting problem(s), the diagnostic procedure(s), and/or the possible management options (see Table 3-7).

The level of medical decision making for a given visit actually depends on the highest two out of three of the elements stated above. Review each category in the risk table. Notice that for each category, the more complex problems addressed, the more complex tests and/or diagnostic procedures ordered or reviewed, and the more complex management options, the higher the level of decision making.

Table 3-8 shows the progression of the elements required for each level of medical decision making. To qualify for a given type of decision making, two of the three elements in the table must be met or exceeded.

The number of possible diagnoses and/or the number of management options that must be considered is based on the number and types of problems addressed during the encounter, the complexity of establishing a diagnosis, and the management decisions that are made by the physician.

1. For each encounter, an assessment, clinical impression, or diagnosis should be documented. It may be explicitly stated or implied in documented decisions regarding management plans and/or further evaluation.
   - For a presenting problem with an established diagnosis the record should reflect whether the problem is (a) improved, well controlled, resolving or resolved; or (b) inadequately controlled, worsening, or failing to change as expected.
   - For a presenting problem without an established diagnosis, the assessment or clinical impression may be stated in the form of differential diagnoses or as a "possible," "probable," or "rule out" (R/O) diagnosis.
2. The initiation of, or changes in, treatment should be documented. Treatment includes a wide range of management options including patient instructions, nursing instructions, therapies, and medications.
3. If referrals are made, consultations requested, or advice sought, the record should indicate to whom or where the referral or consultation is made or from whom the advice is requested.

Since it is impossible for the auditor to know what the practitioner was thinking regarding the medical decision making, Tables 3-9 to 3-11 were designed to help with the process. The methods shown in Tables 3-9 to 3-11 are tools to calculate medical decision making. The number of diagnoses or management options is set up as a point system. Review Table 3-9 on page 67. You will check the risk table (Table 3-7) to determine what a self-limited minor problem is vs a new problem with additional workup required for the examining practitioner. In Table 3-9, notice that the greater the intensity of the diagnoses or management options, the more point value is given to this category. Also note that there are maximum point values for

TABLE 3-7

Table of risk

Level of Risk	Presenting Problem(s)	Diagnostic Procedure(s) Ordered	Management Options Selected
Minimal	▪ One self-limited or minor problem, eg, cold, insect bite, tinea corporis	▪ Laboratory tests requiring venipuncture ▪ Chest x-rays ▪ ECG/EEG ▪ Urinalysis ▪ Ultrasound, eg, echocardiography ▪ KOH prep	▪ Rest ▪ Gargles ▪ Elastic bandages ▪ Superficial dressings
Low	▪ Two or more self-limited or minor problems ▪ One stable chronic illness, eg, well-controlled hypertension, noninsulin-dependent diabetes, cataract, BPH ▪ Acute uncomplicated illness or injury, eg, cystitis, allergic rhinitis, simple sprain	▪ Physiologic tests not under stress, eg, pulmonary function tests ▪ Noncardiovascular imaging studies with contrast, eg, barium enema ▪ Superficial needle biopsies ▪ Clinical laboratory tests requiring arterial puncture ▪ Skin biopsies	▪ Over-the-counter drugs ▪ Minor surgery with no identified risk factors ▪ Physical therapy ▪ Occupational therapy ▪ IV fluids without additives
Moderate	▪ One or more chronic illnesses with mild exacerbation, progression, or side effects of treatment ▪ Two or more stable chronic illnesses ▪ Undiagnosed new problem with uncertain prognosis, eg, lump in breast ▪ Acute illness with systemic symptoms, eg, pyelonephritis, pneumonitis, colitis ▪ Acute complicated injury, eg, head injury with brief loss of consciousness	▪ Physiologic tests under stress, eg, cardiac stress test, fetal contraction stress test ▪ Diagnostic endoscopies with no identified risk factors ▪ Deep needle or incisional biopsy ▪ Cardiovascular imaging studies with contrast and no identified risk factors, eg, arteriogram, cardiac catheterization ▪ Obtain fluid from body cavity, eg lumbar puncture, thoracentesis, culdocentesis	▪ Minor surgery with identified risk factors ▪ Elective major surgery (open, percutaneous, or endoscopic) with no identified risk factors ▪ Prescription drug management ▪ Therapeutic nuclear medicine ▪ IV fluids with additives ▪ Closed treatment of fracture or dislocation without manipulation
High	▪ One or more chronic illnesses with severe exacerbation, progression, or side effects of treatment ▪ Acute or chronic illnesses or injuries that pose a threat to life or bodily function, eg, multiple trauma, acute MI, pulmonary embolus, severe respiratory distress, progressive severe rheumatoid arthritis, psychiatric illness with potential threat to self or others, peritonitis, acute renal failure ▪ An abrupt change in neurologic status, eg, seizure, TIA, weakness, sensory loss	▪ Cardiovascular imaging studies with contrast with identified risk factors ▪ Cardiac electrophysiological tests ▪ Diagnostic endoscopies with identified risk factors ▪ Discography	▪ Elective major surgery (open, percutaneous, or endoscopic) with identified risk factors ▪ Emergency major surgery (open, percutaneous, or endoscopic) ▪ Parenteral controlled substances ▪ Drug therapy requiring intensive monitoring for toxicity ▪ Decision not to resuscitate or to de-escalate care because of poor prognosis

TABLE 3-8

Medical decision making

Type of Decision Making	Number of Diagnoses or Treatment Options	Amount and/or Complexity of Data to Be Reviewed	Risk of Complications and/or Morbidity or Mortality
Straightforward	Minimal	Minimal	Minimal
Low complexity	Limited	Limited	Low
Moderate complexity	Multiple	Moderate	Moderate
High complexity	Extensive	Extensive	High

TABLE 3-9

Number of diagnoses or management options

Number of Diagnoses/Management Options	Points
Self-limited or minor (stable, improved, or worsened) → Maximum 2 points in this category	1 point
Established problem (to examining MD); stable or improved	1 point
Established problem (to examining MD); worsening	2 points
New problem (to examining MD); no additional workup planned → Maximum 3 points in this category	3 points
New problem (to examining MD); additional workup (eg, admit/transfer)	4 points
Total	

the self-limited or minor problem (maximum, 2 points) even if minor problems are documented. Also, a new problem to the examining practitioner with no additional workup planned only allows a maximum of 3 points even if more than three new problems are identified by the practitioner.

The next element in medical decision making is the amount and/or complexity of data reviewed. The amount and complexity of data to be reviewed are based on the types of diagnostic testing ordered or reviewed. A decision to obtain and review old medical records and/or obtain history from sources other than the patient increases the amount and complexity of data to be reviewed.

Documentation Guidelines

1. If a diagnostic service (test or procedure) is ordered, planned, scheduled, or performed at the time of the E/M encounter, the type of service, eg, lab or x-ray, should be documented.

2. The review of lab, radiology, and/or other diagnostic tests should be documented. A simple notation such as "WBC elevated" or "chest x-ray unremarkable" is acceptable. Alternatively, the review may be documented by initialing and dating the report containing the test results.

3. A decision to obtain old records or decision to obtain additional history from the family, caretaker, or other source to supplement that obtained from the patient should be documented.

TABLE 3-10

Amount and/or complexity of data reviewed

Amount and/or Complexity of Data Reviewed	Points
Lab ordered and/or reviewed (regardless of number ordered)	1 point
X-ray ordered and/or reviewed (regardless of number ordered)	1 point
Medicine section (90701–99199) ordered and/or reviewed	1 point
Discussion of test results with performing physician	1 point
Decision to obtain old record and/or obtain history from someone other than patient	1 point
Review and summary of old records and/or obtaining history from someone other than patient and/or discussion with other health provider	2 points
Independent visualization of image, tracing, or specimen (not simply review of report)	2 points
Total	

4. Relevant findings from the review of old records, and/or the receipt of additional history from the family, caretaker, or other source to supplement that obtained from the patient, should be documented. If there is no relevant information beyond that already obtained, that fact should be documented. A notation of "old records reviewed" or "additional history obtained from family" without elaboration is insufficient.

5. The results of discussion of laboratory, radiology, or other diagnostic tests with the physician who performed or interpreted the study should be documented.

6. The direct visualization and independent interpretation of an image, tracing, or specimen previously or subsequently interpreted by another physician should be documented.

Review Table 3-10 above. The table is set up with a point value for each element. Under labs ordered or reviewed and x-rays ordered or reviewed, the number of labs or x-rays is not considered when allowing credit for these elements. Only the point value in column 2 of the grid is allowed for the element. The practitioner is given credit for each section if performed, ordered, and/or documented.

The risk of significant complications, morbidity, and/or mortality is based on the risks associated with the presenting problem(s), the diagnostic procedure(s), and the possible management options. A table of risk may be used to determine whether risk of significant complications, morbidity, and/or mortality is minimal, low, moderate, or high. Because the determination of risk is complex and not readily quantifiable, the table includes common clinical examples rather than absolute measures of risk. The assessment of risk of the presenting problem(s) is based on the risk related to the disease process anticipated between the present encounter and the next one. The assessment of risk of selecting diagnostic procedures and management options is based on the risk during and immediately after any procedures or treatment. The highest risk in any one category (presenting problem[s], diagnostic procedure[s], or management option[s]) determines the overall risk. See Table 3-11.

TABLE 3-11

Results of final medical decision making

	Straight-forward	**Low**	**Moderate**	**High**
Number of diagnosis or treatment options	1	2	3	4
Amount and/or complexity of data to be reviewed	1	2	3	4
Risk of complications, morbidity, mortality	Minimal	Low	Moderate	High
E/M level=2 out of 3				

Documentation Guidelines

1. Comorbidities/underlying diseases or other factors that increase the complexity of medical decision making by increasing the risk of complications, morbidity, and/or mortality should be documented.

2. If a surgical or invasive diagnostic procedure is ordered, planned, or scheduled at the time of the E/M encounter, the type of procedure, eg, laparoscopy, should be documented.

3. If a surgical or invasive diagnostic procedure is performed at the time of the E/M encounter, the specific procedure should be documented.

4. The referral for or decision to perform a surgical or invasive diagnostic procedure on an urgent basis should be documented or implied.

Final Medical Decision Making Results

When selecting the level of service for medical decision making, remember it is two out of three elements that compose overall medical decision making. Table 3-11 identifies a point value for each level selected. For example, if the number of diagnoses or treatment options is moderate, the complexity of data ordered or reviewed is low, and the risk of complications, comorbidity, and/or mortality is moderate, the medical decision making would be moderate. The highest level attained in two out of three categories will determine the level of E/M code as it relates to medical decision making.

Examine the medical decision making examples below.

> Example 1: Possible sinusitis due to Keflex that seemed to help last URI. Pediazole 4 cc po qid × 14 days. Continue Tylenol. Return in 2 weeks if symptoms persist.

Sinusitis-one self-limited or minor problem; minimal complexity

Number of Diagnoses/Management Options	**Points**
Self-limited or minor (stable, improved, or worsened) → Maximum 2 points in this category	1 point
Established problem (to examining MD); stable or improved	1 point
Established problem (to examining MD); worsening	2 points
New problem (to examining MD); no additional work-up planned → Maximum 3 points in this category	3 points
New problem (to examining MD); additional workup (eg, admit/transfer)	4 points
Total	**1**

Amount and/or complexity of data to be reviewed: none

Amount and/or Complexity of Data Reviewed	Points
Lab ordered and/or reviewed (regardless of number ordered)	1 point
X-ray ordered and/or reviewed (regardless of number ordered)	1 point
Medicine section (90701–99199) ordered and/or reviewed	1 point
Discussion of test results with performing physician	1 point
Decision to obtain old record and/or obtain history from someone other than patient	1 point
Review and summary of old records and/or obtaining history from someone other than patient and/or discussion with other health provider	2 points
Independent visualization of image, tracing, or specimen (not simply review of report)	2 points
Total	**0**

Risk of complications/morbidity/mortality (risk table): moderate; prescription drug management

Final Results of Medical Decision Making

The highest level attained in two out of three categories will determine your level of E/M code as it relates to medical decision making.

	Straight-forward	Low	Moderate	High
Number of diagnosis or treatment options	**1**	2	3	4
Amount and/or complexity of data to be reviewed	**1**	2	3	4
Risk of complications, morbidity, mortality	**Minimal**	Low	**Moderate**	High
E/M Level=2 out of 3	x			

Medical decision making: straightforward complexity (2 of 3)

Example 2:   Diagnosis: diabetes mellitus, uncontrolled. We will get an A1c today. Will change him to three shots, leaving insulin at 9N +1R alone at night, but drop him back to 4–5N at bedtime. I think we can improve him, make the peak of his insulin that will probably make him feel a little better. I will see him back in 3 months.

Number of diagnoses or management options: diabetes mellitus, established problem, worsening, low complexity

Number of Diagnoses/Management Options	Points
Self-limited or minor (stable, improved, or worsened) → Maximum 2 points in this category	1 point
Established problem (to examining MD); stable or improved	1 point
Established problem (to examining MD); worsening	2 points
New problem (to examining MD); no additional workup planned → Maximum 3 points in this category	3 points
New problem (to examining MD); additional workup (eg, admit/transfer)	4 points
Total	**2**

Amount and/or complexity of data to be reviewed: ordered A1C; minimal

Amount and/or Complexity of Data Reviewed	Points
Lab ordered and/or reviewed (regardless of number ordered)	1 point
X-ray ordered and/or reviewed (regardless of number ordered)	**1 point**
Medicine section (90701–99199) ordered and/or reviewed	1 point
Discussion of test results with performing physician	1 point
Decision to obtain old record and/or obtain history from someone other than patient	1 point
Review and summary of old records and/or obtaining history from someone other than patient and/or discussion with other health provider	2 points
Independent visualization of image, tracing, or specimen (not simply review of report)	2 points
Total	**1**

Risk of complications/morbidity/mortality (risk table): moderate; prescription drug management

Final Results of Medical Decision Making
The highest level attained in two out of three categories will determine your level of E/M code as it relates to medical decision making.

	Straight-forward	Low	Moderate	High
Number of diagnosis or treatment options	1	**2**	3	4
Amount and/or complexity of data to be reviewed	**1**	2	3	4
Risk of complications, morbidity, mortality	Minimal	Low	**Moderate**	High
E/M Level=2 out of 3		**x**		

Medical decision making: low complexity (2 of 3)

Review the following two examples. These two examples will be broken down into the key components to select the level of service. As the key components are reviewed, the elements and documentation requirements should become clear.

Example 1:   This is the first visit for this 2-year-old female patient with complaint of 1½ days of cough and fever. Patient's cough is nonproductive and nonbarky and has worsened today. Patient also has rhinorrhea, which began yesterday. Mother denies any diarrhea or other GU complaints. Patient's sleep pattern was poor last night and appetite was down today. Patient is positive for fever and cough with trouble breathing at night. Patient finished Keflex for cellulitis 1 week ago and was doing well. Mother has given patient Tylenol and Robitussin for cough.

Patient has a history of RAD and mother ran out of albuterol 1–2 weeks ago, but states she didn't believe it helped. Patient has a history of URI symptoms on and off for past 3 months.

Exam: General, alert, NAD; throat, nonerythematous; neck, supple, no adenopathy; heart, RRR without murmurs; lungs, CTA, no wheezes, no crackles; Abd, soft/nontender. Possible sinusitis due to Keflex that seemed to help last URI. Pediazole 4 cc po qid × 14 days. Continue Tylenol. Return in 2 weeks if symptoms persist.

Review examples 1 and 2 using both the 1995 and 1997 CMS E/M guidelines to select the appropriate level of service.

Example 1:   **Chief complaint:** This is the first visit for this 2-year-old female patient with complaint of 1½ days of cough and fever.

History of present illness: Patient's cough is nonproductive and nonbarky and has worsened today. Patient also has rhinorrhea, which began yesterday.

Review of systems: Mother denies any diarrhea or other GU complaints. Patient's sleep pattern was poor last night and appetite was down today. Patient is positive for fever and cough with trouble breathing at night.

PFSH: Patient finished Keflex for cellulitis 1 week ago and was doing well. Mother has given patient Tylenol and Robitussin for cough. Patient has a history of RAD and mother ran out of albuterol 1–2 weeks ago, but states she didn't believe it helped. Patient has a history of URI symptoms on and off for past 3 months.

Examination: General, alert, NAD; throat, nonerythematous; neck, supple, no adenopathy; heart, RRR without murmurs; lungs, CTA, no wheezes, no crackles; Abd, soft/nontender.

Medical decision making: Possible sinusitis due to Keflex that seemed to help last URI. Pediazole 4 cc po qid × 14 days. Continue Tylenol. Return in 2 weeks if symptoms persist.

History:	Detailed—HPI, extended; review of systems, 5 systems; PFSH, past medical history reviewed
Examination:	Detailed—1995 guidelines Expanded problem focused—1997 guidelines
Medical decision making:	Straightforward
Level of service:	99201—1995 guidelines 99201—1997 guidelines

Notice that it did not make a difference which guidelines were used with this patient encounter. This was a new patient visit, which requires all three key components to be met or exceeded. Since the medical decision making was straightforward, the highest level of service reached is a problem focused visit (99201) or a level 1 visit.

Example 2:   Tom, a 15-year-old established patient, returns for follow-up of otitis media. This 15-year-old male is doing very well on his insulin regimen. His insulin dose remains low, 29N +1R in the morning and 6N at night. I note that he is having a few lows in the middle of the night even though he cut back his insulin at night to +4N on game days. This has been an issue. Even though he eats well, he goes low at night because of the activity level. Review of systems from 4 months prior reveals that he is doing well. He has experienced no GI or GU symptoms and no neuro complaints. He has minor joint aches following extensive practices or games. His mood and affect are good. Remains unchanged from history form dated 7/1/99 (see form). Weight, 137 lbs; Ht, 165 cm; BP, 96/60. HEENT, normal. Neck, supple. Chest, clear to auscultation. Cardiac exam is benign. Shot sites look to be all buttocks, but look good. We will get an A1c today. Will change him to three shots, leaving insulin at 9N +1R alone at night, but drop him back to 4-5N at bedtime. I think we can improve him, make the peak of his insulin that will probably make him feel a little better. I will see him back in 3 months.

Example 2: **Chief complaint:** Tom, a 15-year-old established patient, returns for follow-up of otitis media.

History of present illness: This 15-year-old male is doing very well on his insulin regimen. His insulin dose remains low, 29N +1R in the morning and 6N at night. I note that he is having a few lows in the middle of the night even though he cut back his insulin at night to +4N on game days. This has been an issue. Even though he eats well, he goes low at night because of the activity level.

Review of systems: Review of systems from 4 months prior reveals that he is doing well. He has experienced no GI or GU symptoms and no neuro complaints. He has minor joint aches following extensive practices or games. His mood and affect are good.

PFSH: Remains unchanged from history form dated 7/1/99 (see form).

Examination: Weight, 137 lbs; Ht, 165 cm; BP, 96/60. HEENT, normal. Neck, supple. Chest, clear to auscultation. Cardiac exam is benign. Shot sites look to be all buttocks, but look good.

Medical decision making: We will get an A1c today. Will change him to three shots, leaving insulin at 9N + 1R alone at night, but drop him back to 4–5N at bedtime. I think we can improve him, make the peak of his insulin that will probably make him feel a little better. I will see him back in 3 months.

History:	Detailed—HPI, extended; detailed review of systems, 5 systems reviewed; PFSH, comprehensive; three history areas reviewed (reviewed and updated history form)
Examination:	Detailed—1995 guidelines Problem focused—1997 guidelines

Medical decision making: Moderate complexity
1 chronic condition: diabetes mellitus with mild exacerbations; ordered labs; minimal data to review and management options: managing insulin (prescription drug management)

Level of service: 99214—1995 guidelines
99214—1997 guidelines

Notice that it did not make a difference which guidelines were used with this patient encounter. This was an established patient visit, which requires two out of three key components to be met or exceeded. With this encounter the history was detailed with moderate-complexity decision making, so the examination was not the driving force behind the level of service selected.

VISITS DOMINATED BY COUNSELING AND/OR COORDINATION OF CARE

The inclusion of time as an explicit factor beginning in the CPT® nomenclature in 1992 is to assist physicians in selecting the most appropriate level of E/M services. It should be recognized that the specific times expressed in the visit code descriptors are averages and therefore represent a range of times, which may be higher or lower depending on actual clinical circumstances.

In the case where counseling and/or coordination of care dominates (more than 50%) of the physician-patient and/or family encounter (face-to-face time in the office or other outpatient setting or floor/unit time in the hospital or nursing facility), then time is considered the key or controlling factor to qualify for a particular level of E/M services. The extent of counseling and/or coordination of care must be documented in the medical record.

Example: A 10-year-old has had recurrent ear infections and comes in to the office for a recheck of the latest infection. A problem focused history and exam are performed and documented, which reveal that the acute otitis media is improving but not resolved (99212 based on key components). The physician spends an additional 20 minutes, beyond the time required to perform the key components, counseling the patient's parents regarding strategies to decrease the incidence of ear infections, treatment options, and allaying parent anxiety concerning the child's condition (10 minutes visit +20 minutes counseling = 35 minutes total).

99213   E/M selected on the basis of time criteria (more than 50% of face-to-face encounter dominated by counseling)

THE FUTURE OF THE CMS E/M DOCUMENTATION GUIDELINES

In June 2000, the Centers for Medicare and Medicaid Services (CMS), then the Health Care Financing Administration, issued draft Evaluation and Management Documentation Guidelines. These guidelines were revised in December 2000. They focused on correct documentation of E/M encounters with Medicare beneficiaries and offered an alternative approach through clinical examples. CMS contracted with Aspen Systems Corporation to develop clinical examples that were intended to illustrate acceptable E/M documentation practices, provide guidance for clinical practitioners, and promote consistent medical review of E/M claims by Medicare carriers. The clinical examples were to illustrate the guidelines for various levels of physical examination and medical decision making. Aspen developed clinical examples for 16 medical specialties from de-identified medical records obtained from Medicare carriers throughout the country. In May 2001, Aspen introduced the examples and their methods to organized medicine to begin an in-depth review by physicians and carrier medical directors.

At the time of the introduction, specialty societies had many questions regarding how the clinical examples would be used in practice, the availability of carrier feedback to the specialties, coordination between carriers and specialty societies, and next steps. Also, the possibility that the clinical examples were based on medical records that were "downcoded" was raised as a serious concern. Since medical records were not available for some specialties, including pediatrics, the issue was raised of the ability to develop sufficient clinical examples for all E/M services for all specialties. The participating specialty societies and carriers were given a short time frame (60 days) to review a large volume of clinical examples.

On June 26, 2001, the AMA hosted a specialty society meeting designed to collect broad specialty society reaction to the CMS/Aspen clinical examples. This meeting resulted in a specialty sign-on letter to Thomas Scully, administrator of CMS. The letter attempted to capitalize on the Bush Administration's efforts to reduce the regulatory burden on physicians and called on CMS to reexamine the need for documentation guidelines and their commitment to the development of clinical examples. The letter made the point that it would be more appropriate for organized medicine to develop their own examples that accurately reflect appropriate levels of patient care, rather than use those suggested by the CMS contractor.

On July 19, 2001, the Department of Health and Human Services responded to medicine's concerns, indicating that they were willing to address the E/M documentation burden. CMS stopped all work on the Aspen project and the 2000 Documentation Guidelines (carriers will continue to use either the 1995 or the 1997 documentation guidelines). The announcement was a direct response to advocacy efforts by the AMA and the specialty societies and represents a significant concession to the physician community. In follow-up statements, CMS indicated that they believed that E/M coding should also be reviewed, and it was their belief that physicians may be having problems with the E/M descriptors and CPT® coding guidelines.

The AMA, through the CPT® Editorial Panel, is responsible for maintaining CPT® codes, and thus the preferred approach would be to address ambiguities with the code descriptors and coding guidelines through the established CPT® Panel process. The Panel opted to form an E/M

Workgroup to address CMS's concerns. Initial discussions were held with CMS on the proposed scope and composition of the Workgroup. The Federal Advisory Committee Act (FACA) has prevented CMS from organizing its own task force, and the Workgroup provides a viable approach to resolve CMS's coding concerns. CMS is supportive of the Workgroup and will participate in its deliberations. In November 2001, at the CPT® Annual Advisory Committee and Editorial Panel Meeting, the issue of a Panel E/M Workgroup was discussed. Advisors from the specialty societies were given the Workgroup's prospective charge and scope of work that was developed through detailed discussions with CMS. After the advisors' discussion, the Panel voted unanimously to form a workgroup that would report back to the Panel in November 2002 through the normal Advisory Committee process.

The Panel E/M Workgroup will include representatives from several specialties, the Practicing Physician Advisory Commission (PPAC), a carrier medical director, the Blue Cross Blue Shield Association, and the AMA Board Ad Hoc Task Force on E/M Documentation Guidelines. The charge of the Workgroup is to enhance the functionality and utility of CPT® E/M codes by recommending changes in code descriptors, code selection criteria, and/or code levels in order to improve understanding among physicians. E/M codes must reflect current clinical practice and continue to describe physician work, while reducing the need for documentation guidelines and ensuring that any remaining documentation guidelines are oriented toward facilitating patient care. To assist in their examination of E/M coding, the Workgroup will collect data through physician surveys and oral and written testimony, and will analyze existing and alternative coding structures.

KEY TERMS

Common Evaluation and Management Terminology

The E/M section of the CPT® book is divided into broad categories such as office visits, hospital visits, and consultations. Most of the categories are further divided into two or more subcategories. The basic format of the levels of E/M services is the same for most categories. Certain key words and phrases are used throughout the E/M section.

Chief complaint—A concise statement describing the symptoms, problems, diagnosis, or other factor that is the reason for the encounter, usually stated in the patient's words.

Comprehensive exam—A general multi-system examination or a complete examination of a single organ system. The comprehensive examination performed as part of the preventive medicine E/M service is multi-system, but its extent is based on age and risk factors identified.

Counseling—A discussion with the patient and/or family members regarding diagnostic results, impressions, and/or recommended diagnostic studies; prognosis; risks and benefits of management (treatment) options; and instructions for management (treatment) and/or follow-up.

Critical care services—Defined by the CPT® nomenclature as "the direct delivery by a physician(s) of medical care for a critically ill or critically injured patient. A critical illness or injury acutely impairs one or more vital organ systems such that there is a high probability of imminent or life threatening deterioration of the patient's condition."

Detailed exam—An extended examination of the affected body area(s) and other symptomatic or related organ system(s).

Detailed history—Chief complaint; extended history of present illness; problem-pertinent system review extended to include a review of a limited number of additional systems; pertinent past, family, and/or social history directly related to the patient's problems.

Domiciliary care—CPT® codes are used to report care given to patients residing in a long-term care facility that provides room, board, and other personal assistance services, generally on a long-term basis. The facility's services do not include a medical component.

Emergency Department Services—CPT® codes used to report E/M services provided in the emergency department. No distinction is made between new and established patients in the emergency department.

Established patient—An eatablished patient is one who has received professional services from the physician or another physician of the same specialty who belongs to the same group practice within the past 3 years. In the instance where a physician is on call for and/or covering for another physician, the patient encounter is classified as it would have been by the physician who is not available.

Expanded problem focused examination—A limited examination of the affected body area or organ system and other symptomatic or related organ system(s).

Family history—A review of medical events in the patient's family that includes significant information about the health status or cause of death of parents, siblings, and children; specific diseases related to problems identified in the chief complaint or history of present illness, and/or system review; diseases of family members which may be hereditary or place the patient at risk.

High severity—A type of presenting problem in which the risk of morbidity without treatment is high to extreme; there is moderate to high risk of mortality without treatment; or high probability of severe, prolonged functional impairment.

History of present illness—A description of the chronological development of the patient's present illness from first onset of symptoms. This includes a description of location, quality, severity, timing, duration, modifying factors, and associated signs and symptoms related to the present problem(s).

Home services—CPT® codes used to report the E/M services in a private residence.

Hospital observation—CPT® codes used to report the E/M services provided to patients designated/admitted as "observation status" in the hospital. It is not necessary that the patient be located in an observation area designated by the hospital.

Initial hospital care—CPT® codes used to report the first hospital inpatient encounter with the patient by the admitting physician.

Low severity—A problem where the risk of morbidity without treatment is low; there is little to no risk of mortality without treatment; full recovery without functional impairment is expected.

Medical decision making—Refers to the complexity of establishing a diagnosis and/or selecting a management option measured by the number of possible diagnosis and/or the number of management options that must be considered; the amount and/or complexity of medical records, diagnostic tests, and/or other information that must be obtained, reviewed, and analyzed; and the risk of significant complications, morbidity, and/or mortality, as well as comorbidities, associated with the patient's presenting problem(s), the diagnostic procedure(s), and/or the possible management options.

Minimal severity—A type of presenting problem that may not require the presence of a physician, but in which services are rendered under a physician's supervision.

Moderate severity—A type of presenting problem in which the risk of morbidity without treatment is moderate; there is a moderate risk of mortality without treatment, or there is uncertain prognosis or increased probability of prolonged functional impairment.

New patient—A new patient is one who has not received any professional services from the physician or another physician of the same specialty who belongs to the same group practice within the past 3 years.

Past history—A review of the patient's previous experiences with illness, injuries, and treatments that includes significant information about prior major illnesses and injuries; prior operations; prior hospitalizations; current medications; allergies (eg, drug, food); age-appropriate immunization status; and age-appropriate feeding/dietary status.

Problem focused exam—A limited examination of the affected body area or organ system.

Social history—An age-appropriate review of past and current activities that include significant information about marital status and/or living arrangements; current employment; occupational history; use of drugs, alcohol, and tobacco; level of education; sexual history; and other relevant social factors.

Special E/M services—CPT® codes used to report evaluations performed to establish baseline information prior to issuance of life or disability insurance certificates.

Systems review—An inventory of body systems obtained through a series of questions seeking to identify signs and/or symptoms, which a patient may be experiencing or has experienced.

TEST YOUR KNOWLEDGE

True or False

1. _____ Documentation of examination at the highest level means that the encounter in its entirety qualifies for the level of E/M service.

2. _____ A "chief complaint" is defined as an inventory of body systems obtained through a series of questions seeking to identify signs and/or symptoms that the patient may be experiencing or has experienced.

3. _____ Services performed by the physician must be consistent with the symptoms or diagnoses of the illness or injury under treatment. This is considered medical necessity.

4. _____ Social history is an age-appropriate review of past and current activities.

5. _____ An HPI is required to be recorded only at the detailed and comprehensive level of history.

6. _____ Context is the situation associated with the symptom of pain (eg, dairy products, large meals, etc). This is recorded in the HPI.

7. _____ The 1997 documentation guidelines for examination utilize systems or body areas vs an exam table.

8. _____ Medical decision making is determined on the basis of exam findings alone.

9. _____ To qualify for the first element identified by a bullet under "constitutional" on the General Multisystem Exam table, you must perform and document a minimum of three vital signs.

10. _____ One to five elements identified by a bullet on the General Multisystem Exam table indicate a problem focused examination (1997 guidelines).

Select the appropriate E/M CPT® code(s) for the following by using the 1997 E/M guidelines.

11. _____ Established patient with wheezing. Parent questions allergic reaction to Pediazole. No fever. Woke up with itchy rash over face and trunk. She is currently taking Pediazole. Skin: rash partially gone. Wheezing continued with RR of 36. HEENT, clear; weight, 21 lbs 2 oz; 1 year old. Asthma secondary to viral URI. Albuterol syrup

2.5 mL q 4–6 hours. Recheck prn. D/C Pediazole. Allergic to sulfa.

12. _____   Tom is a 16-year-old with a ganglion cyst on the dorsum of the right hand that apparently was much bigger last week. This is Tom's first visit. Exam: Cyst at this time is hard to palpate at all. Apparently it has been causing him some discomfort on lifting weights, but it is so hard to identify at this point that I told him he needs to return when it gets bigger. We will certainly consider scheduling for surgery if it gets bigger.

13. _____   Mandy is here for follow-up for back pain. She continues to complain of pain especially after carrying heavy books and running around during school. Examination shows that she continues to have round back posture. Otherwise no significant findings. Neurological examination is unremarkable. X-rays were taken in the office. Standing lateral of the spine shows she has continued curvature of 57 degrees, unchanged from previous exam. Impression: Scheuermann's kyphosis, moderately symptomatic. I have discussed with the mother the options for treatment. If she continues to have pain after not carrying heavy books and modifying her activities during the summer, she will be a candidate for thoracolumbar orthosis.

14. _____   A follow-up examination in the office for a 40-year-old insulin-dependent male diabetic revealed rectal bleeding after use of the bathroom and pain from prolonged sitting. The patient is to have a fasting blood sugar and stool cultures for analyses. Patient history is expanded problem focused. A detailed examination was performed on the patient. Currently the patient has multiple diagnoses that must be considered with a moderate risk of complication since he is a diabetic.

15. _____   A 33-year-old new patient comes into the office for his annual physical examination. After a comprehensive history and examination, the doctor recommended that the patient decrease his weight, watch his cholesterol level, and start a modified exercise program.

16. _____   An ENT specialist saw a new patient in the office for recurrent otitis media unresponsive to medical management. The patient had a detailed history.

The physical exam is as follows: Patient is a 10-year-old well-nourished well-developed white male in no acute distress. Minimal cerumen noted in the ear canals. Otoscopic examination revealed bulging and redness of the left ear. Nose and throat appeared normal. There were no masses or tenderness of the neck. The chest is clear to auscultation. The patient is being placed on antibiotics. The medical decision making is of low complexity.

17. _____   A new patient, a 10-year-old girl, presents to the office with acute contact dermatitis, which she has never had before. The physician documents a brief HPI and records the following examination: VS: T, 98.0; Wt, 67 lbs; Ht, 55″; skin, erythematous streaks on right forearm; ears, clear. The patient was given a prescription for the dermatitis with instructions to return to the office if the condition does not improve in a few days. Medical decision making for this case is of moderate complexity.

chapter 4

OTHER EVALUATION AND MANAGEMENT SERVICES

LEARNING OBJECTIVES

- Review documentation criteria for consultations
- Understand exam requirements for preventive medicine services
- Review prolonged services guidelines
- Understand key terms in the chapter
- Successfully complete the end-of-chapter application exercises

CONSULTATION GUIDELINES

The following CMS definition of consultation distinguishes a consult as a request for advice—not transfer of care or treatment: "A consult is a request of another physician to obtain advice or opinion on patient care. A consulting physician may initiate diagnostic and/or therapeutic services. When the referring physician orally or in writing transfers complete responsibility of treatment at the time of the request for a specific problem and/or suspected problem, at the time of the request for consult and/or referral, the receiving physician may not bill a consult."

Example:

Consult: Family practitioner asked the opinion of a pulmonologist regarding treatment options for a patient newly diagnosed with left-lower-lobe pneumonia and cough.

Referral: Family practitioner requests that a pulmonologist take over the treatment of a patient newly diagnosed with left-lower-lobe pneumonia. The chart notes indicate that the family physician will continue to manage the patient's leukemia (initial reason for admission).

It is up to the requesting physician to decide who will treat the patient in the case of a consultation, based on the advice offered by the consultant.

Documentation for Consultation

The request for the consult from the attending physician and the need for a consult must be documented in the patient's medical record by the attending physician.

The consulting physician must provide a written report to the requesting physician for his/her opinion or treatment advice. With inpatient consultations, the request may be documented as part of a plan written in the attending physician's progress notes, an order in the hospital record, or a specific written request for a consultation. In an office setting, the requirement can be met by a reference in the medical record to the request.

Consultation (Codes 99241–99275)

A consultation may be paid for when all the criteria for the use of a consultation code are met. Specifically, a consultation is distinguished from a visit or referral because it is provided by a physician whose advice or opinion regarding evaluation and/or management of a specific problem is requested by another physician or other appropriate source (unless it is a patient-generated confirmatory consultation).

A request for a consultation from an appropriate source and the need for the consultation must be documented in the patient's medical record. After the consultation is provided, the consultant prepares a written report of his/her findings, which is provided to the physician requesting the consultation. In the instance that the encounter is provided in the hospital setting, documentation in the hospital medical record is sufficient.

When consultation is followed by treatment, the initial consultation may be paid for if all the criteria for a consultation are satisfied, unless a transfer of care occurs. A transfer of care occurs when the referring physician transfers the responsibility of the patient's care to the receiving physician at the time of the referral, and the receiving physician documents approval of care in advance. This could be for a portion of medical management or a complete transfer of care.

The receiving physician would report a new or established patient visit depending on the E/M documentation criteria (new vs established patient). A physician consultant may initiate diagnostic and/or therapeutic services at an initial or subsequent visit.

Subsequent visits (not performed to complete the initial consultation) to manage a portion or all of the patient's condition should be reported as an established patient office or hospital visit, depending on the setting.

A consultation may be paid for if one physician in a group practice requests a consultation from another physician in the same group practice, as long as all the requirements for use of the consultation codes are met.

A request for a consultation from an appropriate source and the need for consultation must be documented in the patient's medical record. A written report must be furnished to the requesting physician (office setting).

In the emergency department or an inpatient or outpatient setting, in which the medical record is shared between the referring physician and the consultant, the request may be documented as part of the plan that is written in the requesting physician's progress note, an order in the medical record, or a specific written request for consultation. In this setting, the consultation report may consist of an appropriate entry in the medical record.

The following examples *do not* satisfy the criteria for consultation:

- Standing orders in the medical record for consultation
- No order documented for a consultation by the requesting physician
- No written report sent back to the requesting physician from the consultation
- Statements in the medical record such as, "Patient referred by Dr Jones for consultation"

Consultation vs Referral

Determining the difference between a consultation and referral is sometimes difficult because coders are not provided with enough information in the patient's chart to make the determination. A referral is the transfer of the total or specific care of a patient from one physician to another. This is not a consultation. The physician accepting a patient on a referral basis knows he/she will be managing either a portion of or all of the patient's care. Table 4-1 presents CMS' distinctions between these two services.

TABLE 4-1

CMS' distinctions between consultation vs referral

Consultation	Referral
Suspected problem or known problem	Known problem
Undetermined course of treatment	Prescribed and known course of treatment
Only opinion or advice sought	Transfer of partial or total patient care for the specific problem
Written request for opinion or advice received from attending physician, including the specific reason the consultation is required	Patient appointment made for the purpose of providing treatment, diagnostic, and/or therapeutic services
Written opinion returned to attending physician (if telephone call made, there must be documentation of the call by both physicians in the patient record)	No further communication required (or limited contact) with referring physician
Primary (attending) physician will decide who will manage patient care	Physician is managing the known problem from the beginning
Patient advised to follow up with attending physician	Patient advised to return for appointment; testing, treatment, or continuation of treatment
Final diagnosis is probably unknown	Final diagnosis is typically known at time of referral
Consulting physician must submit a written report to the original physician	No written letter or report required
Recommended documentation: Please examine patient and provide me with your **opinion** on his/her condition	Recommended documentation: Patient is referred to your office for evaluation and **treatment** of his/her condition

PREVENTIVE MEDICINE SERVICES

Preventive services are services performed in the absence of complaints or symptoms for the purpose of detecting any new diseases, as well as to protect by way of risk factor reduction against future disease.

Preventive services have been receiving increasing coverage in the past few years because insurance companies are recognizing the benefits in cost control. Approximately 50% of commercial insurance companies have some coverage for preventive services, and Medicare is expanding coverage yearly.

Preventive medicine services codes 99381 through 99429 are used to report the preventive medicine E/M of infants, children, adolescents, and adults. Codes are based on patient status (new or established) and age. Immunizations and ancillary studies involving laboratory, radiology, or other procedures are reported separately. The extent and focus of the services will largely depend on the age of the patient.

The following are the descriptions of basic preventive medicine services codes from the CPT® book.

> Codes 99381–99387—Initial comprehensive preventive medicine evaluation and management of an individual including an age and gender appropriate history, examination, counseling/anticipatory guidance/risk factor reduction interventions, and the ordering of appropriate immunization(s), laboratory/diagnostic procedures, new patient [ages under 1 year through 65 years and over]

> Codes 99391–99397—Periodic comprehensive preventive medicine reevaluation and management of an individual including an age and gender appropriate history, examination, counseling/anticipatory guidance/risk factor reduction interventions, and the ordering of appropriate immunization(s), laboratory/diagnostic procedures, established patient [ages under 1 year through 65 years and over]

The preventive medicine guidelines were changed in the CPT® 2002 book to further clarify that the comprehensive nature of the preventive medicine services codes 99281 through 99387 reflects an age- and gender-appropriate history/exam and is not synonymous with the "comprehensive" examination required in the E/M codes 99201 through 99350.

Immunizations and ancillary studies involving laboratory, radiology, other procedures, or screening tests identified with a specific CPT® code are reported separately.

Use preventive services codes to report the routine evaluation and management of a patient when the patient is healthy and has no complaint or when the patient has a chronic condition/disease that is controlled but has planned yearly routine physical examinations.

Preventive medicine services are used to identify comprehensive services, not a single system examination, such as a yearly gynecologic examination. Just because a patient schedules an appointment for a "yearly physical" does not necessarily mean the encounter would not qualify for an E/M "problem" visit.

Distinguishing between preventive and problem-specific E/M services is a dilemma that continues to plague users of CPT® coding. First, does a "yearly physical" or "annual examination" need to be coded with a preventive medicine code? The answer is simply no! There are situations when an annual exam/physical should be coded with a preventive medicine code. However, there are many situations when an annual exam/physical would be coded with a "problematic" E/M code. Problematic is defined as an E/M visit in which the patient has chronic medical problems that warrant a yearly complete physical, eg, hypertension, insulin-dependent diabetes mellitus, chronic obstructive pulmonary disease, rheumatoid arthritis, and congestive heart failure. Following is an overview of the components required to make this determination.

Components Used to Distinguish Between Preventive and Problem-Related Services

History

When the higher-level E/M codes (eg, 99204 and 99205 and 99214 and 99215) are used, the history criteria are as follows:

- Chief complaint
- Extended history of present illness
- Extended/complete review of systems
- Pertinent/complete past family and social history
  - 1 history area for established patients, 2 history areas for new patients (99204 or 99214)
  - 2 history areas for established patients, 3 history areas for new patients (99205 or 99215)

For preventive services, the history is not problem oriented and does not involve a chief complaint or history of present illness. This fact cannot be overlooked when determining the service being rendered.

Examination

A preventive medicine exam is multi-system, but the extent of the exam is based on the age and gender of the patient and the risk factors identified.

A problematic visit is based on the same E/M criteria as stated above, but the expectation is that problems identified in the history will be examined in the encounter. For example, if the patient is complaining of chest pain, the expectation is that one of the systems examined will be the cardiovascular and/or respiratory system.

Medical Decision Making

The element that should not be overlooked is medical decision making. When a preventive medicine service is provided, medical decision making is not determined because it is not in the criteria for codes. When coding problematic visits, medical decision making is a factor that must be considered. For problematic visits, the criteria to quantify medical decision making are as follows:

- Number of diagnoses and management options
- Amount and complexity of data to be reviewed
- Risk

A preventive medicine visit involves counseling, risk factor reduction, and interventions. An insignificant or minor problem/abnormality that is encountered in the process of performing the preventive medicine E/M service and that does not require additional work should not be reported separately.

The CPT® book states that if an abnormality is encountered or a preexisting problem is addressed in the process of performing the preventive medicine E/M service and the problem/abnormality is significant enough to require additional work to perform the key components of a problem oriented E/M service, then the appropriate office/outpatient code 99201 through 99215 should also be reported. Modifier -25 should be added to the office/outpatient code to indicate that a significant, separately identifiable E/M service was provided by the same physician on the same day as the preventive medicine service. The appropriate preventive medicine service is additionally reported.

Keep in mind, however, that many insurance carriers and managed care plans will not pay for a preventive medicine visit and a problematic visit on the same day. Each carrier may have a policy to determine what service they pay for on the basis of the patient's coverage.

Ask yourself if the documentation includes the following information:

- Is the patient presenting for an annual examination because of medical problems that warrant a complete physical once per year?
- Is there a chief complaint and a history of present illness(es)?
- Is there an extended/complete review of systems?
- Is there a pertinent/complete past, family, and social history?
- Was a detailed/complete physical done?
- Is the medical diagnosis(es) clearly indicated in the assessment?
- Are medical problems being managed?

If the documentation includes all of the above, the code selected would most likely be a problematic E/M service. If the documentation states that the patient came for a physical and no medical problems, history of present illness(es), or management of medical problems is indicated, select a preventive medicine service code.

Diagnosis

The diagnosis must coincide with the code selected.

- If a preventive medicine code is used, the diagnosis selected will be from the "V" category: "Persons without reported diagnosis encountered during the examination."
- If the patient has chronic medical problems, list the diagnoses that coincide with the condition treated.

Example: Preventive Visit: A 33-year-old new patient comes into the office for his annual physical examination. After a comprehensive history and examination, the doctor recommended that the patient decrease his weight, watch his cholesterol level, and start a modified exercise program.

Example: Problematic Visit: A 35-year-old patient arrives for her annual physical examination. The patient complains of headache and rhinitis of 4 days' duration. The patient has a history of problems with allergies during this season for years. An expanded problem focused history and examination are performed and documented by the physician. The patient is prescribed Claritin for her allergy symptoms and advised to return to the office in 4 weeks for reevaluation.

PROLONGED PHYSICIAN SERVICE WITH DIRECT (FACE-TO-FACE) PATIENT CONTACT

Codes 99354 through 99357 are used when a physician provides prolonged service involving direct (face-to-face) patient contact that is beyond the usual service in either the inpatient or outpatient setting. This service is reported in addition to other physician service, including E/M services at any level. Appropriate codes should be selected for supplies provided or procedures performed in the care of the patient during this period.

Codes 99354 through 99357 are used to report the total duration of face-to-face time spent by a physician on a given date providing prolonged service, even if the time spent by the physician on that date is not continuous. Code 99354 or 99356 is used to report the first hour of prolonged service on a given date, depending on the place of service. Either code also may be used to report a total duration of prolonged service of 30 to 60 minutes on a given date. Either code should be used only once per date, even if the time spent by the physician is not continuous on that date. Prolonged service of less than 30 minutes in total duration on a given date is not separately reported because the work involved is included in the total work of the E/M codes.

Threshold for Billing Prolonged Services (Face-to-Face)

You can use prolonged service codes (99354 and 99355) with visits if they exceed the typical time for the service by 30 minutes or more. Table 4-2 gives CPT® code threshold times for outpatient and/or office visits.

TABLE 4-2

CPT® code threshold times

CPT® Code	Typical Time Spent for E/M Service	Threshold Time for 99354	Threshold Time to Bill 99354 and 99355
99201	10	40	85
99202	20	50	95
99203	30	60	105
99204	45	75	120
99205	60	90	135
99212	10	40	85
99213	15	45	90
99214	25	55	100
99215	40	70	115

Example: An 11-year-old established patient with a history of asthma presents in respiratory distress with acute asthmatic bronchitis. A detailed history and examination are performed and documented; treatment that includes aerosol treatment is initiated. This visit requires intermittent physician face-to-face time with the patient over a period of 2 hours (which includes 30 minutes to provide the E/M service), during which the child's condition improves significantly.

99214	E/M service (30 minutes + 90 minutes prolonged service)	493.90
99354	First hour of prolonged service (face-to-face contact)	493.90
99355	Each additional 30 minutes of prolonged service (face-to-face contact)	493.90
94640	Nonpressurized inhalation treatment for acute airway obstruction	493.90

(also bill for medications with CPT® supply code 99070 or HCPCS "J" code)

KEY TERMS

Consultation—A service provided by a physician whose opinion or advice concerning the evaluation and/or management of a specific problem is requested by another physician or other appropriate source.

Critical care services—Defined by the CPT® book as "the direct delivery by a physician(s) of medical care for a critically ill or critically injured patient." A critical illness or injury acutely impairs one or more vital organ systems such that there is a high probability of imminent or life threatening deterioration of the patient's condition."

Domiciliary care—Care given to patients residing in a long-term care facility that provides room, board, and other personal assistance services, generally on a long-term basis. The facility's services do not include a medical component.

Preventive medicine—CPT® codes used to report the preventive medicine evaluation and management of infants, adolescents, and adults. The extent and focus of the services largely depend on the age of the patient.

Prolonged services—CPT® codes used to report when a physician provides prolonged services involving (face-to-face) patient contact that is beyond the usual service in either the inpatient or outpatient setting. This service is reported in addition to other physician services, including evaluation and management services at any level.

TEST YOUR KNOWLEDGE

Determine whether the visit is a preventive medicine service (P), consultation (C), prolonged service (PS), problematic E/M visit (E/M), or a combination of preventive and problematic E/M service (PP). Use the abbreviations in parentheses to indicate the appropriate type of service.

1. _____ A 2-year-old patient presents to a physician for administration of pneumococcal vaccine because of chronic otitis media. The physician performs an expanded problem focused history and examination with medical decision making of low complexity. This is an established patient. Provide the appropriate CPT® code(s) for the services rendered.

2. _____ A 16-year-old receives routine tetanus prophylaxis with TD. Provide the appropriate CPT® code(s) for the service rendered.

3. _____ A 24-month-old female established patient presents to her physician for examination. A detailed history and expanded problem focused examination are performed. Medical decision making is straightforward. During the visit, the patient is given a DT and influenza vaccine. Provide the appropriate CPT® code(s) for the services rendered.

4. _____ Michael, a 7-year-old boy, presents today after falling from a tree in the yard and breaking his cast. This is the first time that this physician has seen the patient. He originally went to an urgent care center for fracture care 10 days ago, when the left leg was casted. During the current visit, the mother indicates that the child has been complaining of a sore throat that has gotten progressively worse for the past 3 days. After performing an expanded problem focused history and problem focused exam, the physician determines that the patient has acute tonsillitis and prescribes appropriate antibiotic therapy. The medical decision making is moderate. A new cast is applied to the leg and the patient is to return in 10 days for follow-up. Provide the appropriate CPT® code(s) for the services rendered.

5. _____ This is the first time I have seen 4-year-old Stephen, and he is accompanied by his mother. They have recently moved here from Cleveland. Mom reports that Stephen has had an epigastric hernia since shortly after birth. Recently the patient has been experiencing some discomfort. A detailed history and examination were performed. Stephen is a normal-appearing male child with descending testes. I will send Stephen to a pediatric surgeon for further evaluation and probable surgery.

6. _____ A new patient is seen in the office for an itchy, red rash that has been present for 3 days. The physician performed an expanded problem focused history and a problem focused examination. The physician diagnoses the patient with contact dermatitis caused

by a change in laundry detergents. The physician recommends over-the-counter medications for symptomatic relief. Medical decision making for this case is of low complexity.

7. _____ A 5-year-old new patient is brought in for her preschool physical with no problems found. The mother is concerned about her lack of progress and noticeable inability to concentrate at nursery school and is considering holding the child back from kindergarten. The physician spends an additional 15 minutes reassuring the mother that this is normal at the child's age. Code the services rendered.

8. _____ A patient is seen in the office for follow-up for a repeat Pap smear. The last Pap smear was normal. An expanded problem focused history and examination are performed, including a Pap smear, and the specimen was sent to pathology. The patient will be contacted when the results are received. She will return for follow-up in 1 year.

9. _____ A 45-year-old man is sent by his family physician to an orthopaedic surgeon's office for evaluation of acute pain and stiffness in his right elbow. In the history, the physician notes that the man is a farmer and uses his right hand. The patient has no other complaints and reports being in otherwise excellent health. He describes the pain as severe and unrelenting, and it prevents him from using the arm. The physical examination shows the man's right elbow to be slightly swollen with increased pain on movement. No other problems are noted with his right upper extremity. The physician diagnoses the problem as tendinitis and bursitis, starts the patient on a regimen of warm compresses, and gives the patient a prescription for an anti-inflammatory. A letter is sent to the family physician indicating the diagnosis and recommendations for treatment.

True or False (use a current CPT® book to mark each of the following T or F)

_____ 10. The three key components that are used in defining the levels of E/M services are time, counseling, and coordination of care.

_____ 11. An established patient is defined as one who has received professional services from the physician or another physician of the same specialty who belongs to the same group practice, within the past 3 years.

_____ 12. Prolonged services are used when a physician provides prolonged services involving direct patient contact or services not involving direct care that is beyond the usual service; this service may be reported in addition to other physician services, such as E/M visits.

_____ 13. When a primary care physician transfers the care of his patient to a cardiologist for management of a known heart condition, the cardiologist should use a new patient code to describe the E/M service rendered at this patient's initial visit.

_____ 14. Time is used as a key or controlling factor only if more than 50% of the E/M visit is dominated by counseling and/or coordination of care.

_____ 15. Flora Dunn, an established patient, came into the office for her yearly physical examination. Flora is 27 and in good health. The visit included a comprehensive history, comprehensive examination, counseling/anticipatory guidance/risk factor reduction interventions, and the ordering of appropriate laboratory/diagnostic procedures. The correct code for this case is 99395.

chapter 5

COMPLIANCE IN THE MEDICAL PRACTICE

LEARNING OBJECTIVES

■ Understand civil monetary penalties for noncompliance

■ Review and understand the type of audit performed by a carrier

■ Review services targeted for postpayment review

■ Understand the importance of a compliance plan and the relationship between coding guidelines and continuous monitoring

■ Understand the elements of a compliance plan

COMPLIANCE

The Health Insurance Portability and Accountability Act (HIPAA) was signed into law on August 21, 1996. A product of the Clinton health care reform proposal, HIPAA's primary purpose is to provide access to health insurance; reduce fraud and abuse; and provide administrative simplification.

The implementation of HIPAA gave the government more power in the area of civil and criminal enforcement tools to fight fraud and abuse in the federal health care programs. Five programs emerged in 1998 to implement the fraud and abuse incentives. The Fraud and Abuse Control Program was developed to coordinate federal, state, and local efforts in investigating and assessing civil and criminal penalties. The Medicare Integrity Program was designed to allow local medical fiscal intermediaries and insurance carriers to begin auditing records as part of fraud and abuse detection, utilization review, provider education, and payment determination. The Beneficiary Incentive Program provides incentives for beneficiaries to report suspected fraud or abuse by offering to give the beneficiary a portion of recovery made on claims of $100.00 or more that were recovered. The Healthcare Fraud and Abuse Data Collection Program created a national health care fraud and abuse database to track all sanctioned providers for all adverse action taken by government agencies. The last phase of HIPAA legislation, which is due to be fully implemented during 2002, will be related to privacy regulations and the electronic storage of health care information; this phase is called administrative simplification.

FRAUD AND ABUSE

A major responsibility of any Medicare carrier is to identify cases of suspected fraud and abuse and to develop and refer them to the Office of Inspector General (OIG) for consideration and application of criminal or civil monetary penalty or administrative sanction actions.

Fraud is an intentional deception or misrepresentation that an individual knows to be false or does not believe to be true, and makes knowing that the deception could result in some unauthorized benefit to himself/herself or some other person.

The most common kind of fraud arises from a false statement or misrepresentation made, or caused to be made, that is material to entitlement or payment under the Medicare program. The violator may be a provider, a beneficiary, or some other person or business entity.

Fraud in the Medicare program takes such forms as, but is not limited to:

1. Billing for services or supplies that were not provided. This includes billings for "no-shows," ie, billing Medicare for services that were not actually furnished because the patients failed to keep their appointments.
2. Claim forms that have been altered to obtain a higher reimbursement amount.
3. Provider's deliberate application for duplicate reimbursement, eg, billing both Medicare and the beneficiary for the same service, or billing both Medicare and another insurer in an attempt to get paid twice.
4. Soliciting, offering, or receiving a kickback, bribe, or rebate.
5. False representation with respect to the nature of services rendered, charges for services rendered, identity of the person receiving the services, dates of services, etc.
6. Claims for noncovered services billed as covered services, eg, routine foot care billed as a more involved form of foot care to obtain reimbursement, or acupuncture billed as a chiropractic subluxation.
7. Use of another person's Medicare card in obtaining medical care.
8. Alteration of claims history records to generate fraudulent payments.
9. Repeated violations of the participation agreement, assignment agreement, or limiting charge.
10. Billings based on "gang visits," eg, a physician visits a nursing home, walks through the facility, and bills for 20 nursing home visits without rendering any specific service to individual patients.

The type of abuse to which Medicare is most vulnerable is overutilization of medical and health care services. Abuse takes such forms as, but is not limited to:

1. Excessive charges for services or supplies.
2. Claims for services not medically necessary or, if medically necessary, not to the extent rendered, eg, a battery of diagnostic tests is given where, on the basis of diagnosis, only a few are needed.

3. Breaches of assignment agreements, which result in beneficiaries being billed for an amount disallowed by the carrier on the basis that such charges exceeded the reasonable charge criteria.
4. Provider exceeding the limiting charge.
5. Provider billing Medicare at a higher and different fee schedule rate than for non-Medicare patients.
6. Improper billing practices, including submittal of bills to Medicare instead of third-party payers that are primary insurers for Medicare beneficiaries.
7. Violations of Medicare participation agreements by providers or suppliers.
8. Claims involving collusion between a provider and a beneficiary, resulting in higher costs or charges to the Medicare program.

Although these types of practices may initially be categorized as abusive, under certain circumstances, they may develop into fraud.

CIVIL MONETARY PENALTIES LAW

Under the Medicare program, civil monetary penalties may be imposed where it has been determined that a person presents, or causes to be presented, a claim for an item or service not provided as claimed; an item or service that is false or fraudulent; a physician's service provided by a person who was not a licensed physician, whose license had been obtained through misrepresentation, or who improperly represented to a patient that he or she was a certified specialist; and an item or service furnished by an excluded person.

Civil monetary penalties may also be imposed against a person who presents or causes to be presented a request for payment in violation of a Medicare assignment agreement or a Medicare participating provider agreement.

Other situations where civil monetary penalties may be applied include, but are not limited to:

- Violation of assignment requirement for certain diagnostic clinical lab tests.
- Violation of requirement of assignment for nurse anesthetist services.
- Nonparticipating physician violation of charge limitation provisions for radiology services.
- Violation of assignment requirement for physician assistant services.
- Medicare nonparticipating physician's violation of limiting charge.
- Nonparticipating physician's violation of charge limitation provision for services subject to inherent reasonableness provisions, specified overpriced procedures, specified cataract procedures, A-mode ophthalmic ultrasound procedures, medical direction on nurse anesthetists, and certain purchased diagnostic procedures where markup is prohibited.
- Nonparticipating physician's violation of refund provision for unassigned claims for elective surgery.

■ Physician charges in violation of assignment provision for certain purchased diagnostic procedures where markup is prohibited or where a payment is prohibited for these procedures because of failure to disclose required information.

Carriers conduct internal audits to detect abusive and possible fraudulent activities. If such practices are detected, the carriers must advise providers of their audit findings and inform them of the corrective actions needed. The Office of Inspector General's Regional Office has directed carriers to advise providers that if corrective actions are not taken, administrative sanctions will be taken against them. Providers who have been informed of noncovered services or practices, but continue to provide and/or bill for them, or physicians whose claims must consistently be reviewed because of repeated overutilization or other abusive practices, could be subjected to administrative actions.

These actions include suspension from participation in the Medicare program and assessment of a civil monetary penalty. Carriers are required to conduct reaudits to determine if corrective action has been taken. If the reaudit indicates that corrective action was not taken, they are required to send the case to the Office of Inspector General's Regional Office, to be reviewed for possible civil and criminal action. Protecting Medicare trust funds is the responsibility of all concerned, including providers, beneficiaries, and insurance companies.

FEDERAL FALSE CLAIMS ACT

The Federal False Claims Act, Section 3729, pertains to any person who "knowingly makes, uses or causes to be made or used, a false record or statement to get a false or fraudulent claim paid or approved by the government."

The Federal False Claims Act stipulates that "whistleblowers" be rewarded with a percentage of the money that the government recovers as a result of their *qui tam* lawsuits. This provision helps encourage people to assist the government in stopping Medicare fraud.

Under the False Claims Act, the government may recover up to three times the amount of money it lost as a result of the defendant's fraud. The whistleblower's share is calculated on the basis of the amount the government recovers, not the actual losses.

CARRIER AUDITS

Carriers frequently conduct audits (reviewing the practitioner's medical record documentation) to validate that the level of service the practitioner has reported on the HCFA-1500 form is correctly reported and the chart documentation supports the service billed. Medicare routinely conducts three types of audits. These are prepayment audits, postpayment audits, and fraud and abuse audits.

Prepayment Audits

The prepayment audit is performed after Medicare receives the claim from the practitioner, but before payment of the claim. The audits are normally random, but they may also be provider specific. When errors are discovered in the prepayment audit, the claims are paid on the basis of the local medical review policy (LMRP), and an educational letter is sent to the practitioner indicating the errors uncovered.

Postpayment Audits

The postpayment audit is done after Medicare has paid the claim. These audits result in requesting a return of the overpayment. See Table 5-1 for a list of services currently targeted for postpayment review. The three types of postpayment audits are electronic media claims verification, focused medical review, and comprehensive medical review. Review the descriptions of each type of audit that appear after Table 5-1.

Electronic Media Claims Verification
This type of audit is used to verify the accuracy of the electronic claim(s) sent to Medicare with existing chart documentation.

Focused Medical Review
Section 1 842(a)(2)(B) of the Social Security Act requires carriers to apply safeguards against unnecessary utilization of services furnished by providers. This is accomplished by conducting prepayment and postpayment reviews to identify inappropriate, medically unnecessary, or excessive services and take action where a questionable pattern of practice is found. This identification effort is termed *medical review.*

In 1993, Medicare carriers implemented a new program for medical review. This program is called focused medical review (FMR). FMR is the targeting and concentration of more in-depth medical review efforts of claims for items, services, or providers that present the greatest risk of inappropriate program payment. The objectives of FMR are to maximize program protection, avoid provider hassle, and conduct the most cost-effective method of MR.

Carriers develop components of their FMR program (ie, local medical review policy, internal guidelines, and local screens) by identifying aberrances and areas subject to potential abuse or overutilization.

Carriers are responsible for targeting specific aberrances, and the individual providers of service are responsible for excessive atypical billings. This helps to eliminate the use of generic medical review screens, which affects the entire physician population.

Physician education and policy development are the major components resulting from FMR. A physician whose aberrant pattern cannot be logically explained can be placed on prepayment claim monitoring if the physician fails to take corrective action.

TABLE 5-1

Services Currently Targeted for Postpayment Review

Absorptiometry

Anesthesia standby, especially with eye surgery

Ambulatory surgery centers where an uncovered service is misrepresented as a covered service; cataracts, including excessive preoperative visual acuity testing; colonoscopy not indicated; consistent use of a single code or level of care; consultations, including repetitive high levels of visits, visits to established patients, minor diagnosis, cross consultation from subspecialty

Consultation services

Cryosurgery exclusively coded as 3 cm; culture and sensitivity of urine repeated within a week after the organism is identified

Cystoscopy billed separately from other endoscopic procedures; dilation and curettage on the same date as a hysterectomy or other gynecologic procedures

Durable medical equipment in a participating skilled nursing facility

Echo M-scans as routine screening

Electrocardiographic interpretation of a computer-analyzed electrocardiogram without manual review of the readout

Endoscopy in lieu of x-ray

Facelifts billed as removal of fatty tumors

Injections when oral medication would not be contraindicated

Intermittent positive-pressure breathing (IPPB) occasional, when inconsistent with diagnosis, condition, and/or normal treatment

Keratosis

Kidney, ureter, and bladder study

Levels 4 and 5 evaluation and management services

Repeat laboratory tests

Excision of physically impossible lesions

Office visits involving up-coding and overutilization

Sharing of surgery patients involving surgery and medical physicians of like but different subspecialties

Place of services where all services are in one type of facility

Preoperative and postoperative care not included in the global fee

Pulmonary therapy involving multiple treatments per patient in a hospital setting

Rehabilitation and psychiatric therapy involving nonphysician services that do not meet "incident to" requirements

Renal dialysis involving standard orders for laboratory tests of questionable, continuing necessity

Respiratory therapy too frequent entailing kickbacks or questionalble necessity

Seat lift chairs

Standing orders

TURP (transurethral resection) where vasectomy is billed as a separate procedure on the same day

Noninvasive vascular testing of questionable medical necessity, too frequent or too poorly documented

X-rays involving fragmentation of services, eg, angiography with multiple vessel studies, brain scan, brain scan with flow study billed on the same day

Routine chest x-rays and repeated x-rays with the absence of previous abnormalities

Stress testing too frequently or without need

Portable x-rays involving billing for two but rendering one

Comprehensive Medical Review

This type of review is an audit of a specific practitioner or practice that has already been identified as having unusual billing or documentation practices by way of the FMR. This type of review is more serious than the two previous reviews because problem areas have previously been identified. If a significant problem is found, the case may be referred to the fraud and abuse unit for further investigation.

Fraud and Abuse Audits

These types of audits may be performed as a result of the practitioner not taking appropriate corrective action after a previous review is performed. A patient or another third party complaint may also trigger these audits. In many cases, criminal or civil investigation and potential prosecution are the result of a fraud and abuse audit.

BENEFITS OF A COMPLIANCE PROGRAM

The Office of Inspector General (OIG) is an agency within the Department of Health and Human Services (HHS). The OIG and other federal agencies are charged with the responsibility for enforcement of federal law. This effort has emphasized the importance of voluntary development and implementation of compliance plans.

This guidance is based on fraud investigations and the regulations and guidelines of the Centers for Medicare and Medicaid Services (CMS). The government, especially the OIG, has a zero-tolerance policy toward fraud and abuse and will use extensive statutory authorities to reduce fraud in Medicare and other federally funded health care programs. Compliance plans offer the health care provider an opportunity to participate in a nationwide effort to reduce fraud and abuse in our national health care programs. Coding, billing, and reimbursement errors can be significantly reduced by means of a compliance plan.

The OIG has developed a work plan for physician practices that includes the recommended elements of a written compliance plan. This plan is available on the Internet at www.hhh.gov/oig. Elements of these guidelines can be used by all physician practices, regardless of size, to establish a compliance program. The OIG is not suggesting that all practices must implement all of the compliance elements discussed in the document, nor does the OIG suggest that if a practice does not incorporate all of these elements, it will be at a disadvantage when under the scrutiny of the OIG or other governmental agency. Rather, the guidelines represent suggestions on how to correct and prevent fraudulent activity, and they can be tailored to fit the individual needs and financial realities of any practice, be it a small solo practitioner, hospital-based physician, or group practice.

Ultimately each practice bears the responsibility for determining the appropriate topic areas and measures to be included in its compliance program. All providers should be aware that the development and implementation of compliance programs could raise a host of sensitive and complex legal issues. Nothing stated herein should substitute for or be used in lieu of legal advice from competent experienced counsel. In addition, it should be noted that implementing a compliance program will not protect a medical practice from criminal, civil, or administrative prosecution, but it may be a relevant factor in negotiations with the OIG.

Advantages of a compliance plan are many. Among the legal and business incentives, a compliance plan minimizes personal liability for the organization and allows the practice to attract more highly trained and motivated employees. The plan will keep insurance in force and minimize the adverse financial impact of fines and judgments. Having a compliance plan also protects the reputation and goodwill of the organization and stakeholders. In addition, organizations doing business with the government have an obligation to make limited inquiries to ensure that the claims they submit are accurate. Correct coding is an important element of accurate claim submission.

Compliance plans help address the ongoing threat of fraud and abuse audits. The "ostrich defense" is not valid under CMS: the "constructive knowledge" definition of the act attempts to address situations in which an individual has "buried his head" in the sand and failed to make simple inquiries that would alert him that false claims or incorrect coding was submitted. The practice must receive relevant and timely information about business performance and law compliance to satisfy the oversight and monitoring role. The compliance plan also helps avoid organization-wide risk from inconsistent or different management decisions regarding employment discrimination and coding, billing, and record keeping.

COMPLIANCE PLAN ELEMENTS

Every practice or medical group adopting a compliance plan should develop a program and policies that ensure that the plan is implemented and enforced. Compliance plans that are merely cosmetic are not effective and, in the long run, could harm the practice if not carried out properly. While the degree of formality of the program may vary with the size and scope of the organization, the comprehensive compliance program should include, at a minimum, a seven-part system. These seven critical elements are (1) written policies and procedures; (2) data tracking; (3) billing; (4) auditing and monitoring (internal or external); (5) marketing; (6) compliance with applicable HHS OIG fraud alerts; and (7) retention of records.

Written Policies and Procedures

Written policies should be developed and distributed that promote the practice's commitment to compliance, addressing specific areas of potential fraud, such as billing, marketing, and claims processing. Company standards, policies, and procedures for employees aimed at reducing the prospect of illegal conduct should be implemented.

Physicians, managers, and organization executives must be responsible for overall compliance with the company standards. A chief compliance officer or other appropriate management-level official should be designated and charged with the responsibility of operating the compliance program.

Education and training programs should be developed and offered to all employees. Training can be conducted in-house or outside the scope of the practice. The organization must take steps to communicate its standards and procedures to all employees by required participation in training programs and by distribution of publications explaining requirements.

Audits and/or other evaluation techniques should be used to monitor compliance and ensure a reduction in identified problem areas. An auditing system (internal or external) should be implemented and monitored and a reporting system publicized.

To ensure compliance with the plan, a code of improper/illegal activities must be developed and disciplinary action taken against employees who have violated internal compliance policies and applicable laws or who have engaged in wrongdoing. If violations are detected, the organization must take steps to respond to the offense and take additional steps to prevent recurrence of similar offenses.

Systemic and personnel concerns should be investigated and any problems identified must be remediated. Standards must be consistently enforced through appropriate disciplinary action.

Compliance should be promoted and adhered to as an element in the evaluation of supervisors, managers, and/or physicians. A policy should be developed against the employment or retention of sanctioned individuals (consultants, accountants, attorneys, etc).

A procedure should be maintained to receive complaints, adopt procedures to protect the anonymity of complaints, and adopt requirements applicable to creation and retention of records.

Every compliance plan should ensure that claims are submitted only for services that the provider has reason to believe are medically necessary. Upon request, a provider should be able to provide documentation (superbills, encounter forms, chart documentation, lab reports, etc) containing diagnosis codes, supporting the medical necessity of the service provided and billed to the insurance carrier. The provider must ensure that it bills only for services that meet the reimbursement rules for each individual program.

As a preliminary matter, the OIG recognized that physicians must be able to order tests, supplies, and/or services that they believe are appropriate for the treatment of the patient. However, the provider must be made aware that insurance carriers will pay only for treatment that meets the carrier definition of medical necessity. Providers should order only tests, supplies, and/or services that they believe are medically necessary for the treatment of their patients.

It is recommended that each practice should standardize its superbill, encounter form, history and physical forms, laboratory and medicine records, etc. Laboratory requisition forms should also be standardized with noncustomized test offerings. They should emphasize physician choice and encourage doctors to order, to the extent possible, only those tests that they believe are appropriate for each patient. In addition, the requisition forms should require physicians to document the need for each test ordered by inserting a diagnosis code for each one. Requisition forms should be designed to require physicians to order tests individually.

In addition, a printed statement should appear on every requisition form reiterating that when ordering tests for which Medicare reimbursement will be sought, providers (or other individuals authorized by law to order tests) should only order tests that are medically necessary for the diagnosis and treatment of a patient, rather than for screening purposes.

All health care organizations should provide all patients with annual written notices that set forth the following information:

- The Medicare medical necessity policy
- The individual component of every service, supply, and/or test ordered
- The CPT® or HCPCS code used to bill the Medicare program for such services
- A description of how the provider will bill Medicare for services
- The telephone number of the provider or practice and information on his or her general availability
- Written notice that not all medical services will be covered (Medicare waiver form)

Data Tracking

Each organization should retain and analyze CPT®, HCPCS, and ICD-9-CM code utilization on a yearly basis, for the top 50 codes. This tracking can enable the organization to determine overutilization of coding. Providers can accomplish this by tracking the number of services provided by CPT® or HCPCS code and/or the number of claims submitted to Medicare for each service, supply, and/or test. The organization would then compute the percentage growth in claims submitted for each of the top 50 codes from one year to the next. It is believed that if utilization of a code grew more than 10%, the medical practice should undertake a reasonable inquiry to ascertain the cause of such growth. If the practice determines that the increase in utilization occurred for a benign reason, such as extensive patient growth, opening of a new practice, adding more providers to the staff, etc, the practice need not take any action. However, if the practice determines that overutilization was caused by some other reason on the part of the facility, it should take steps that it deems reasonably necessary to address the possible issue of fraud and abuse. An external audit of the medical record for one or more physicians may be indicated to determine the specific cause of overutilization.

Billing

Organization compliance policies should ensure that all claims for services submitted to Medicare or any other federally funded health care programs are accurate and correctly identify the services provided by the physician (or other individual authorized by law to provide services).

Selection of CPT® and HCPCS Codes

Providers should choose only the code that most accurately describes the service performed, test ordered, and/or supplies furnished. To ensure code accuracy, it is recommended that the organization require an individual with technical expertise in coding, billing, and reimbursement to review the codes before such codes are approved for claims submission. The OIG views intentional up-coding (ie, the selection of a code to maximize reimbursement when such code is not the most appropriate descriptor of the service) as raising false claim issues. If the organization continues to have questions regarding code selection, even after review by a technical expert, the facility should direct its questions to its Medicare carrier or intermediary. A minimum of one external coding audit is recommended to ensure correct coding compliance.

Selection of ICD-9-CM Codes

At the direction of the CMS, Medicare carriers and intermediaries have established diagnoses that link to the procedure (excluding evaluation and management services), tests, and/or supplies to establish medical necessity before Medicare coverage will be assumed. Such diagnostic information may be submitted through the use of either ICD-9-CM codes or a narrative description. Organizational compliance policies should direct that providers will submit only the diagnosis that accurately describes the patient's condition, reason for test(s) ordered, surgery performed, and/or supplies.

Providers and staff *should not* use diagnosis information provided from earlier dates of service; use "cheat sheets" that provide diagnosis information that has triggered reimbursement in the past; use computer programs that automatically insert diagnosis codes without receipt of diagnostic information from the provider; or make up diagnosis information for claim submission purposes.

Providers and staff *should* contact the provider to obtain accurate diagnostic information, in the event the provider has failed to provide such information, and accurately translate narrative diagnoses obtained from the physician to ICD-9-CM codes.

Services Covered by Claims for Reimbursement

Organizational compliance policies should ensure that the provider only submits claims for services that were both ordered and performed. The OIG considers claims for surgeries not performed, tests not ordered, and/or supplies not furnished to be potential false claims. Adequate documentation to support the claims submitted must be available for review.

Compliance with Applicable HHS OIG Fraud Alerts

The HHS OIG periodically issues fraud alerts setting forth activities believed to raise legal and enforcement issues. Organizational compliance plans should require that any and all fraud alerts issued by the OIG be carefully considered by an attorney, chief compliance officer, and any other appropriate personnel. Moreover, the compliance plan should require that the organization cease and correct any conduct criticized in such a fraud alert, if applicable to the facility, and take reasonable action to prevent such conduct from recurring in the future. If appropriate, the facility should take steps regarding reporting and correction of the identified problem.

Marketing

Organizational compliance plans should require honest, straightforward, fully informative, nondeceptive marketing. It is in the best interest of patients, providers, staff, and Medicare alike that all understand the services offered by the organization and the financial consequences for Medicare, as well as other payers, for the services provided. Accordingly, organizations that market their services should ensure that their marketing information is clear, correct, nondeceptive, and fully informative. Marketing includes brochures, handouts, pamphlets, postcards, advertising, and/or commercials.

Retention of Records

Compliance programs should ensure that all records required either by federal or state law or by the compliance plan are created and maintained. One of the best ways to confirm that a compliance plan is effective is through reports that reflect results. The creation of such documents will reach the goal, but may also raise a variety of legal issues, such as patient privacy and confidentiality. These issues are best discussed with legal counsel.

Individual states generally set a minimum of 7 to 10 years for keeping reports, but it is the policy of most physicians to retain medical records of patients indefinitely; see Chapter 1 for a schedule for retention of records. A federal regulation mandates that assigned claims for Medicaid and Medicare be kept for 7 years; the provider is subject to auditing during this period.

Compliance as an Element of a Performance Plan

To ensure that organizational integrity rises to the level of importance required of providers participating in Medicare or other federally funded health care programs, compliance programs should require that promotion of and adherence to compliance be an element in evaluating the performance of managers and supervisors. They, along with other employees, should be periodically trained in new compliance policies and procedures.

In addition, all managers and supervisors involved in the marketing, billing of services, procedures, tests, and/or supplies, and those who oversee personnel, should discuss with all supervised employees the compliance policies and legal requirements applicable to their job function. They should also inform all supervised employees that strict compliance with these policies and requirements is a condition of employment. In addition, all supervised personnel should be informed that the organization will take disciplinary action up to and including termination for violation of these policies and requirements. Besides making performance of these duties an element in evaluation, the compliance officer or practice administrator may also choose to include in the compliance plan a policy that supervisors and managers may be sanctioned for failure to adequately instruct their subordinates. These sanctions may be invoked for failing to detect noncompliance with applicable policies and legal requirements, where reasonable diligence on the part of the supervisor or manager would have led him or her to discover any problems or violations and given the organization an opportunity to correct them earlier.

DESIGNATION OF A COMPLIANCE OFFICER

Every organizational compliance plan should require the designation of a chief compliance officer or an equivalent (eg, a committee). This individual should be responsible for:

- Development of the compliance policies and standards
- Overseeing and monitoring the organization's compliance activities
- Achieving and maintaining compliance

The individual should be delegated sufficient authority by the organization's governing body to undertake and comply with these responsibilities and should have open access to the governing body. Further, the chief compliance officer should develop and distribute to appropriate individuals all written compliance policies and procedures. These should be readily understandable by all employees and at a minimum should address these issues:

- Medical record documentation requirements
- Uniform coding—correct coding initiatives
- Thorough job descriptions
- Laws, regulations, and guidelines governing federally funded health care programs
- Quality improvement plan
- Posting charges and payments
- Retention requirements
- Claims submissions and HCFA-1500 forms
- Electronic media claims (EMC) if applicable
- Security
- Plan of care
- Physician extenders (if applicable)
- OSHA
- CLIA
- Internal policies (terms of employment, vacations, sick days, etc)
- Management operating policies
- Training
- Continuing education

EDUCATION AND TRAINING

Organizational compliance programs should require training for all employees, especially personnel involved in billing (even the charge poster), sales, and marketing, as well as coders and/or providers. Such training should emphasize the organization's commitment to compliance with all laws, regulations, and guidelines of federal and state programs. Training should be conducted, at a minimum, annually and repeated at regularly scheduled times, with a variety of teaching methods used where appropriate. It is imperative that providers, coders, billers, and reimbursement specialists as well as practice administrators/managers keep current on changes in coding guidelines, billing requirements, and changes in insurance plans.

The training and education program should cover the organization's compliance policies or an annual review of policies and procedures, to ensure that all employees fully comprehend the implications of failing to comply with the compliance plan and all applicable health care program requirements. Employees should be informed that failure to report a potential violation by another employee, supervisor, manager, and/or outside contractor or provider can result in disciplinary action. Employees should also be fully informed that failure to comply might result in disciplinary action, suspension, and/or termination.

In addition to compliance and ethics training, we believe that the compliance plan should also address the need for periodic continuing education for all staff, which may be required by law or regulation for certain personnel. Continuing education programs of this type will help ensure a knowledgeable and more productive staff.

Some continuing education programs may include formal insurance courses, seminars (insurance, billing, reimbursement, legislative issues, etc), customized training sessions for the organization, subscriptions to bulletins and informational materials, activity with professional organizations, continuing education and training for clinical staff, and continuing education for administrative staff.

The organization's compliance program should leave no doubt in the minds of employees and others who are associated with the provider about the organization's commitment to compliance with all laws, regulations, and guidelines governing federally funded health care programs. Compliance should be one of the organization's most important priorities.

In addition to the compliance and continuing education training programs, a simple way to reemphasize this message is to post, in common work areas and other prominent places accessible to all employees, a notice clearly reminding employees of the organization's commitment to compliance with all laws and regulations.

COMMUNICATION

Access to the Compliance Officer

An open line of communication between the compliance officer and his or her staff is critical to the successful implementation and operation of a compliance program. If fraud and abuse are to be reduced, an open-door, complete-anonymity, nonretribution policy should be available to all employees to encourage communication. Working with or through legal counsel can clarify gray areas of interpretation of Medicare and Medicaid guidelines and regulations, but in all cases, the organization should encourage employees not to guess, but to ask if there is confusion or a question. Where appropriate, awards for reporting violations should be available.

Hotlines

Many vehicles exist for developing a line of communication between the employee and the compliance office. Hotlines may be an excellent vehicle for larger organizations; e-mail and written memoranda are other examples of lines of communication. We suggest that every organization have at least one vehicle for reporting violations to the compliance office. Organizations using hotlines should post in common work areas notices describing the hotline and providing the telephone number. Possible violations of compliance policies and/or legal requirements reported through the hotline should be investigated immediately to determine their veracity.

AUDITING AND MONITORING

The OIG will be critical of compliance plans and programs that exist on paper but are not earnestly implemented or enforced. In addition to education and training programs, policies, and notices, a successful compliance program should require thorough monitoring and implementation and regular reporting to medical directors, executive directors, senior executives, and/or members of the Board of Directors. Although monitoring techniques are available, an effective tool to ensure enforcement is the performance of regular, periodic audits of the organization's operations, with particular attention paid to the following areas:

- CPT®, HCPCS, and ICD-9-CM coding issues
- Billing
- Marketing notices and disclosures to physicians
- Forms (clinical and administrative)
- Superbills
- Pricing
- Reporting and recordkeeping
- Activities of all employees, including providers
- Contracts
- Competitive practices
- Marketing materials
- OSHA and CLIA

Such audits should be designed and implemented to ensure compliance with the organization's compliance policies, compliance plan, and all applicable federal and state laws.

Quality assurance and zero tolerance of fraud and abuse should be the goal of the compliance division, and auditing is believed to be a good tool to use to reach that goal. Compliance audits should be conducted in accordance with preestablished comprehensive audit procedures and should include, at a minimum, on-site visits; interviews with personnel involved in management, coding and reimbursement (billing), marketing, providers, clinical staff, and others (contractors, etc); review of written materials and documentation used by the organization; and trend analysis study.

Formal audit reports should be prepared and submitted to the chief compliance officer and/or other governing body to ensure that the organization's management is aware of the results and can take whatever steps are necessary to correct past problems and prevent them from recurring. The audit or other analytical reports should specifically identify areas where corrective actions are needed. In certain cases, subsequent audits or studies would be advisable to ensure that the recommended corrective actions have been implemented and are successful.

DISCIPLINARY ACTION

A viable compliance program must include the initiation of corrective and/or disciplinary action against individuals who have failed to comply with the organization's compliance policies and/or federal or state laws, or who have otherwise engaged in wrongdoing that has the potential of impairing the organization's status as a reliable, honest, and trustworthy provider. The compliance program should also include a written policy statement setting forth the degrees of disciplinary action that will be imposed on employees for failing to comply with the organization's code of conduct, company policies, and the law. Employees must be advised and convinced that disciplinary action will be taken and punishment enforced for a discipline policy to have the required deterrent effect.

CORRECTIVE ACTION

The organization's compliance program should require that, when the chief compliance officer or others involved in management of the organization learn of potential violations or misconduct, they promptly investigate the matter to determine whether a violation has in fact occurred, so that management can take corrective action. Depending on the nature of the allegations, the investigation into allegation of wrongdoing or misconduct will probably include interviews and review of relevant documents, which include submitted claims, superbills, chart documentation, explanation of benefits, requisition forms, lab reports, etc. Some organizations may wish to engage outside auditors or counsel to assist them with the investigation. If an investigation of an alleged violation is undertaken and the compliance officer believes the integrity of the investigation may be at stake because of the presence of employees under investigation, then the employees allegedly involved in the misconduct should probably be removed from their current work activity until the investigation is completed. In addition, the organization should take steps to prevent the destruction of documents or other evidence relevant to the investigation. Once the investigation is completed, if disciplinary action is warranted, it should be immediate and imposed in accordance with the organization's written standards of disciplinary action.

If management receives credible evidence of misconduct from any source and, after the appropriate investigative inquiry, has reasonable grounds to believe that the misconduct violates criminal law, constitutes a violation of civil law, or violates rules and regulations governing federally funded health care programs, the organization must take corrective action. When reporting misconduct within the organization, the chief compliance officer should include evidence disclosed to the organization from another source. The organization should continue to investigate the violation and, once finished, should notify the governing body of the outcome of the investigation, including a description of the violation on the operation of federally funded health care programs or their beneficiaries.

Corrective action must occur immediately. For instance, if the investigation reveals that the organization received overpayments, such sums should be promptly repaid to the appropriate federally funded health care program. Failure to repay the overpayment immediately could be interpreted as an intentional attempt to hide overpayment from the government. For that reason, organizational compliance and written policies and procedures should emphasize that money to which the organization has no legal entitlement in the first place may not be legally retained and must be returned immediately. In addition to making prompt restitution and taking corrective action, the organization should take any disciplinary action necessary to cure the problems identified by the investigation and prevent it from happening again.

NONEMPLOYMENT OR NONRETENTION OF SANCTIONED INDIVIDUALS

Compliance programs should prohibit the employment of individuals who have been convicted of a criminal offense related to health care or who are listed by a federal agency as debarred, excluded, or otherwise ineligible for participation in federally funded health care programs. In addition, under resolution of such criminal charges or proposed debarment or exclusion, individuals who are charged with criminal offenses related to health care or proposed for exclusion should be removed from direct responsibility for or involvement in any federally funded health care program. If resolution results in conviction, debarment, or exclusions of the individual, the organization should terminate its employment of that individual or company.

A SUCCESSFUL COMPLIANCE PROGRAM

These basic recommended elements coupled with other published regulations and guidelines are the foundation for a comprehensive compliance plan for a medical practice. On advice from counsel and senior management, the organization should add or modify these elements to better reflect the corporate structure of the organization, its mission, and its employee composition. By implementing an effective compliance plan, the organization will achieve better quality control of claim submission and reduce the risk of criminal and civil liabilities.

A successful compliance program will produce more informed, highly trained, and motivated employees; more effective operations; increased compliance with federal and state laws, organizational policies, and contracts; and reduced risk of civil penalties or criminal sanctions against the organization.

The next step is to develop and distribute a written code of conduct to all employees, begin formal training for all employees, continuously expand internal compliance auditing and reporting, engage an outside organization to perform chart audits on a yearly basis, and, most importantly, strengthen feedback loops for compliance questions.

KEY TERMS

Abuse—A practice that results in unnecessary costs to a government program, in which it is not possible to determine whether the error was committed knowingly or willingly. These incidents or practices are not considered fraudulent, but they are inconsistent with accepted medical business or fiscal practice.

Audit—Examination of the systems used to make sure a department or hospital is running correctly. These systems are sometimes called "monitors." For example, if a refrigerator is used to store medications, it is important that the refrigerator is working properly. Staff members monitor the refrigerator by checking the thermometer and recording the temperature. The monitor, in this case, is checking the thermometer. An audit checks the thermometer on a regular basis to make sure it is working properly.

Compliance—An effort to reduce fraud in a medical organization to reduce coding, billing, and reimbursement errors and improve quality and standards in the medical facility.

Compliance officer—A person designated by an organization to oversee compliance, address problematic areas, develop policies and standards, and oversee compliance activities.

Compliance plan—A plan that contains policies and procedures for the medical organization and includes seven key elements.

CPT® coding—Current Procedural Terminology; an alphanumeric coding system maintained and published by the American Medical Association to convert widely accepted uniform descriptions of medical, surgical, and diagnostic services rendered by health care providers.

Department of Justice—The government department that represents the citizens of the United States in enforcing the law in the public interest and plays a key role in protecting against criminals; ensuring healthy competition of business; safeguarding the consumer; enforcing drug, immigration, and naturalization laws; and protecting citizens through effective law enforcement. The Department conducts all suits in the Supreme Court in which the United States is concerned. It represents the government in legal matters rendering legal advice and opinions, upon request, to the President and to the heads of the executive departments. The affairs and activities of the Department are generally supervised and directed by the Attorney General.

False claim—An erroneous record or statement knowingly made, used, or caused to be made by a practitioner to get a claim paid by a government payer.

Fraud—Deliberate misrepresentation of facts to deceive or mislead another party.

HCPCS—The HCFA Common Procedural Coding System used for reporting outpatient health care services provided to government insurance carriers. This system contains alphanumeric codes for reporting physician and nonphysician services not included in the CPT® nomenclature.

Health Insurance Portability and Accountability Act (HIPAA)—Legislation passed by Congress in 1996 that contains provisions for insured persons enrolled in employer-sponsored insurance programs to retain the right to new health insurance when they change jobs without regard to their current health status. This law is also referred to as the Kennedy-Kassebaum bill.

ICD-9-CM—International Classification of Diseases, Ninth Revision, Clinical Modification; the coding nomenclature used for reporting medical diagnoses and procedures.

Insurance carrier—An insurance company that underwrites polices that cover health care services.

Medical record—Written or graphic information documenting facts and events during the rendering of patient care or services.

Medicaid—A federally aided, state-operated program that assists low-income persons in need of medical care.

Medicare—A nationwide government health insurance program for persons 65 years of age or older and certain disabled or blind persons regardless of income, administered by the Centers for Medicare and Medicaid Services (CMS).

Office of the Inspector General (OIG)—An agency within the Department of Health and Human Services (HHS) charged with the responsibility for enforcement of federal law.

Record retention—A recommended time period during which records in a medical organization should be kept.

Third-party payer—Insurance carrier that intervenes to pay hospital or medical bills.

Upcoding—Inappropriate practice of assigning a higher procedure code than what was actually performed, to imply a greater degree of complexity or longer time for the procedure. Medicare requires that all procedures performed on a patient be written in the patient's chart. What is written in the chart must match the procedure code level given.

TEST YOUR KNOWLEDGE

True or False

_____ 1. The government has a zero-tolerance policy toward fraud and abuse and will use extensive statutory authorities to reduce fraud in Medicare and other federally funded health care programs.

_____ 2. The "ostrich defense" is the type of situation where an individual has "buried his head in the sand" regarding false claims or incorrect coding being submitted.

_____ 3. The best way to confirm that a compliance plan is effective is through reports that reflect results.

_____ 4. Compliance programs should prohibit the employment of individuals who have been convicted of a criminal offense related to health care or who are listed by a federal agency as debarred, excluded, or otherwise ineligible for participation in federally funded health care programs.

_____ 5. A successful compliance program increases the risk of civil penalties or criminal sanctions against the provider.

_____ 6. The use of newsletters, Web sites, and e-mail is an effective way to establish lines of communication with employees regarding compliance.

_____ 7. The OIG recommends the organization keep appropriate records to withstand an audit every other year.

_____ 8. Corrective action includes investigating, reporting, and correcting the identified problems.

_____ 9. An investigation of the billing department may include submitted claims, superbills, chart documentation, explanation of benefits, requisition forms, and lab reports.

_____ 10. Employees should be informed that failure to report a potential violation by another employee, supervisor, manager, and/or outside contractor or provider can result in disciplinary action.

Complete the Following Statements With a Word or Phrase From the List

standards of conduct	medical necessity	compliance
fraud alert	retention of records	purpose of a compliance plan
compliance officer	corrective action	formal insurance course
hotline	continuing education	internal and external
compliance plan elements	OIG/HHS	HCFA
data tracking		

11. To comply with the established and understood standards is called

_____.

12. A _____ is a warning that sets forth activities believed to raise legal and enforcement issues.

13. The _____ is responsible for enforcement of federal law, thus emphasizing the importance of voluntary development and implementation of compliance plans.

14. _____ is the process of code utilization.

15. _____ are records required by federal, state, or local laws that are created and maintained for a certain period of time.

16. A _____ oversees and monitors the organization's activities.

17. Written policies and procedures, designation of a compliance officer, education and training, communication, auditing and monitoring, disciplinary action, corrective action, and retention of sanctioned individuals are _____.

18. _____ is a line of communication between the employee and the compliance officer.

19. One form of continuing education is a _____ _____.

20. Establishing _____ is when a physician must document the need for each service, test, or supply by linking to a diagnosis code.

Multiple Choice (choose the correct answer for the following questions)

21. Employees should be informed that failure to comply with the compliance plan and all applicable health care program requirements may result in:
    a. disciplinary action.
    b. suspension.
    c. termination.
    d. all of the above.

22. Providers/staff should:
    a. use diagnostic information provided from earlier dates of service.
    b. use "cheat sheets" that provide diagnostic information that has triggered reimbursement in the past.
    c. alter dates and procedures in the chart.
    d. none of the above.

23. Marketing materials may include brochures, handouts, pamphlets, postcards, and commercials. These materials should contain information that:
    a. is clear and fully informative.
    b. is deceptive.
    c. advertises that the provider knows the ins and outs of how to get the claim paid.
    d. both a and c.

24. All managers and supervisors involved in the marketing and billing of services, and those who oversee personnel, should:

    a. discuss with all supervised employees the compliance policies and legal requirements applicable to their job function.

    b. inform all supervised employees that they can ignore all policy regarding compliance.

    c. promote employees who are in violation with the regulations and standards.

    d. both b and c.

25. Training of all employees, management, and physicians should be:

    a. conducted, at a minimum, annually.

    b. repeated at regularly scheduled times, with a variety of teaching methods.

    c. an ongoing process that includes new personnel and retraining of current personnel.

    d. all of the above.

CHART AUDIT PROCESS— THE MEDICAL RECORD REVIEW

LEARNING OBJECTIVES

- Complete the steps in the chart audit process
- Utilize tools to complete the audit process
- Perform actual chart audit cases
- Successfully complete end-of-chapter application exercises

THE AUDIT PROCESS

The previous four chapters focused on documentation, evaluation and management (E/M) guidelines, and information regarding the medical record and compliance. It is now time to describe the audit process. Auditing can be an extremely broad topic, ranging from the basic encounter to determine whether the level of service was billed accurately, to a comprehensive audit that thoroughly examines all aspects of the medical record and medical practice. This chapter will focus on the basic audit for determining whether the E/M service is billed appropriately on the basis of documentation.

Before beginning the process of auditing medical record documentation for correct coding, review some of the most common coding and documentation errors.

TOP CODING AND DOCUMENTATION ERRORS

1. The service is upcoded one level.
   - Documentation in the chart does not support the level of service.
2. The service is downcoded.
   - Documentation in the chart supports a higher level of service.
3. Chief complaint or reason for the visit is missing from the note.
4. Assessment is not always clearly documented.
   - Coders cannot use rule out, probable, or suspected conditions for a diagnosis.
   - When diagnosis is unknown or unclear, document signs and symptoms.

5. Documentation is not initialed or signed.

6. Tests ordered are not always listed in the documentation but are billed on the encounter form/superbill.

    - When tests are ordered, document in the plan.

7. Documentation of medication is not always clear.

8. Diagnosis is not always referenced correctly.

9. Documentation is missing.

10. Dictation is lost.

11. Superbill/encounter form and/or charge (fee) ticket are not available.

12. Documentation was not completed, so there is no record that an action was taken.

13. Superbill/encounter form is incomplete or incorrect.

14. Documentation is hard to read.

    - The auditor will disallow the visit when he or she cannot read documentation.

AUDITING AND ANALYZING YOUR MEDICAL RECORDS

The medical record serves a variety of purposes and is essential to the proper functioning of the medical practice—especially in today's complicated regulatory health care environment. The medical record (chart) should detail information pertinent to the care of the patient, document the performance of billable services, and serve as a legal document that describes a course of treatment. Periodic audits, whether internal or external, ensure that the record adequately serves these purposes and meets federal and state regulations.

Physicians and other practitioners face the challenge of submitting correct coding information through the billing process. Ensuring accurate and timely reimbursement at the highest level for which services are provided and ensuring that no fraudulent activities are occurring is a big task for a health care organization. Performing a coding audit in conjunction with ongoing monitoring and education will assist the organization in meeting the goal of compliance. Careful planning and implementation of the audit process is worth the time and effort invested.

Why Perform the Audit?

Auditing your charts can be a valuable learning experience. Three of the most important reasons to audit your medical records are:

- To assess the completeness of the medical record
- To determine the accuracy of the physician's documentation
- To discover lost revenue

An auditor (internal or external) examines the documentation to determine whether it adequately substantiates the service billed and identifies medical necessity. If the quality of the medical record is not reviewed on an ongoing basis, incorrect or inappropriate documentation and coding practices may not be uncovered.

Besides identifying potential risks to the organization, an audit helps ensure compliance with organization policies and procedures, payer regulations, and coding guidelines. Since compliance with government and private payer guidelines is important, the audit or medical record review is critical in all medical practices.

An audit should not be undertaken without the full support of the organization, such as medical directors, board of directors, or other administrative entities. It is much more beneficial to uncover potential problems before the organization is surprised by a request from a third-party payer, fiscal intermediary, or the Office of Inspector General (OIG). The audit also helps to give the organization the option to correct problems before further damage occurs. A great deal of information can be gathered when the documentation is compared to the charge ticket and the actual claim as to the accurate assignment of codes and whether the practitioner is coding and documenting appropriately.

Auditing vs Monitoring

Auditing is the process of examining the medical record, verifying information, and gathering baseline information to identify risk areas. Monitoring is the ongoing process of reviewing coding practices and the adequacy of the documentation and code selection. Monitoring should be conducted on a regularly scheduled basis and should include such activities as auditing, reviewing utilization patterns, reviewing computerized reports, and reimbursement. A monitoring system is usually put in place because of findings from the baseline audit. For example, if the organization has a problem with coding and documenting consultation codes appropriately, it may decide to direct the focus of future audits to this area. There may be more than one problem area within an organization, so analysis and reporting after the audit are key to setting appropriate criteria for monitoring the coding, billing, and documentation. Analysis and reporting will be discussed in detail in a later chapter.

Audit Objectives

An audit helps facilitate the maintenance of an accurate and complete assessment of the organization's coding and reimbursement practices. The audit helps ensure compliance with external regulations and internal policies by accurately reporting correct coding to insurance carriers. Potential risk areas and areas for improvement that have an impact on the financial and clinical aspect of the practice may be identified. The audit is also conducted to ensure that documentation in the medical record supports the CPT®, HCPCS, and ICD-9-CM code(s) assigned.

Practitioners must get involved and support the coding and/or billing team. Physicians should routinely assign the code(s) for all services, and the coding and billing team is best utilized to keep track of the rules for the practitioners and make sure that they have the appropriate tools to code and document accurately. Documentation is key to the code selection, and physicians must have help to cope with the overwhelming demands of paperwork that they may believe adds little value to patient care. Physicians typically appreciate feedback in coding because they are interested in receiving the correct reimbursement. They also understand that they are responsible for coding correctly and that this directly affects payment for their services, and ultimately affects the patients they serve.

Once problem areas are identified, the focus can then turn to education where it's most needed. Training needs vary, and auditing allows the organization to design an education model to suit specific needs. Auditing will also provide information on patterns and trends that may affect the organization.

The Baseline Audit

A baseline audit gives the organization information about the quality of their medical records and helps identify errors. Most baseline audits are random and should include all coding practices, including medical and surgical coding. The audit should be a sampling of all records and services and should include all physicians and practitioners in the organization. Begin by auditing a random sample of records. A random sample is one in which each record has an equal probability of being chosen for review. If you select specific records or levels of service, the audit is not random, but a focused review. An example of selecting a random sample would be to select dates of service and a specific number of patient records for each practitioner. The records should also be recent (within the past 3 months) and be flagged for review on completion of the documentation and billing process.

Audit Sample Size

The audit sample should include a certain percentage of patient encounters to ensure a representative sample. Auditing too few records may distort results, and auditing too many records becomes too time consuming and labor intensive and is normally not any more effective. The compliance officer, office manager, and/or practitioner should help determine the appropriate number of medical records to review. A good rule of thumb is to audit 10 to 15 records selected randomly for each practitioner. Another standard is to be consistent when choosing a sampling of medical records to eliminate confusion.

Monitoring Guidelines

After the baseline audit is completed and deficiencies are identified, monitor any internal risk areas on an ongoing basis. The definition of a risk area is any area that falls below the threshold for accuracy. Determine the acceptable threshold before performing a baseline audit. While 100% accuracy should be a goal for the practitioner, reasonable and obtainable goals should be set. It is helpful to classify variances by source. Review some potential deficiencies, which are listed below.

- Violation of official coding guidelines
- Documentation inadequate to support level of service billed (code selection)
- Noncompliance with third-party payer directives
- Code assigned, but not billed on claim form
- Service billed to the wrong provider
- Incorrect place of service
- Incorrect category of service (hospital, office, consultation, etc)

- Signature requirements not met
- Incorrect modifier usage

DETERMINING THE TYPE OF AUDIT

The first step in the audit process is to determine the objective of the audit being performed. Review records to validate complete and accurate coding, in accordance with Official Coding Guidelines and the National Correct Coding Initiative. Several books are available to assist in the process, including CPT® coding books, ICD-9-CM, HCPCS, carrier bulletins, carrier policy manuals, and local medical review policy (LMRP), to name a few.

Audits can be divided into three basic groups: presubmission audits, postpayment audits, and focused audits. Prepayment audits are performed before services are billed to the insurance carrier. Postpayment audits are performed after the service(s) are billed to the insurance carrier; in many cases, the carrier has either paid or denied the claim. Focused audits target a particular type of service. For example, an auditor might review a sampling or all of the level 4 or level 5 visits for the practice within a 6-month period. The audit focuses on a specific area in the practice or group that may pose potential problems. Normally this type of audit will follow a prepayment or postpayment audit after a problem is identified.

Depending on the purpose or scope of the audit, reviewing insurance information, explanation of benefits, or remittance advice and financial information may also be necessary. After determining what type of audit to perform, further divide chart audit objectives into two main categories: revenue and compliance.

Revenue

An audit's revenue objectives involve examining coding practices for revenue lost because of the improper use of codes. This process may also disclose inappropriate billing for incorrectly high reimbursement—an open invitation to a payer audit. When considering revenue, look at:

- Underbilled services
- Overbilled services—frequency or upcoding
- Undocumented services
- Denied services
- Downcoded services

Unbilled Services
Compare the medical record to the billing to identify services that are documented in the medical record but for some reason are not coded. This is often caused by ineffective communication between the provider and the billing staff or lack of knowledge on the part of the coders.

Overbilled and/or Underbilled Services
As with unbilled services, the search for overbilled or underbilled services begins with comparing the chart documentation to the billed codes. All services, including evaluation and management and surgical procedures,

should be documented with sufficient detail to allow coders to select the proper CPT® and/or HCPCS and ICD-9-CM codes.

Undocumented Services

A good audit (review) will identify instances in which codes are billed without proper supporting documentation. When a payer, either Medicare, Medicaid, or a third-party payer, requests written proof of billed charges, the provider must be able to substantiate the service. Some examples of commonly misplaced information are laboratory test results, x-ray reports, problem lists, and medication lists.

Denied or Downcoded Services

Analyze those services that are denied or downcoded by payers to discover the cause of the denial. This information comes from comparing the billed services to the explanation of benefits (EOB) or explanation of Medicare benefits (remittance advice) portion of the payer statement.

Compliance

The second set of audit objectives involves evaluating the documentation for compliance with Medicare, Medicaid, and third-party payer standards. Not only are compliance issues important to the overall good management of patients, they are also important for expedient and accurate reimbursement.

When looking at compliance issues, consider:

- Current patient data (see Figure 6-1)
- Physician signatures
- Signed consent forms (Figure 6-2)
- Medicare limitation of liability waiver (Figure 6-3)
- Insurance forms or HCFA-1500 forms (see Figure 6-4)

Current Patient Data

Examine the patient information sheet to verify that it collects all important information regarding the patient, such as date of birth, address, nearest living relative, and complete insurance information including a copy of the card in the chart.

The patient information sheet (Figure 6-1) should be updated regularly. Request that the patient with insurance sign an assignment of benefits form to ensure direct payment of insurance benefits to the provider. Update this record yearly. Medicare offers a lifetime signature form, which must also be kept on file by the provider.

Physician Signatures

A thorough audit will verify that all services and procedures provided to a patient are signed or initialed by the provider. The signature of the provider acknowledges that he/she has performed or supervised the service or procedure. An unsigned entry in a medical record may be viewed by an insurance payer as nonperformance of that service. Some areas of the

FIGURE 6-1

Patient information sheet

Patient Information		
Last Name: Thompson First Name: Natalie		Middle Initial: J

Street Address: 9216 Anchor Mark Drive

City: Indianapolis   State: Indiana   Zip: 46220   Phone:(317) 578-1211

Soc. Sec. #: 555 - 55 - 5555   Date of Birth: 06 - 04 - 1955   Age: 46   Sex: ☐M ☒F   Marital Status: Single

Responsible Party Information

Responsible Party: ☒ Self_____ (If self, go to next section)

Soc. Sec. #: ___-___-___   Phone: ( ) _____   Relation to Patient: _____

Employer: _____   Occupation: _____   Work Phone: ( ) _____

Work Address: _____

Employer Information

Patient Occupation: Telephone Operator

☒Full Time ☐Part Time ☐Retired ☐Student

Patient Employer:☐N/A Ameritech

Employer: Ameritech

Address: 220 N. Meridian Street; Anytown, Indiana 46204

Employer Phone: (317) 545- 1234

School: ☐N/A _____

Spouse Name: ☐N/A None _____

Spouse Address: _____

_____ Phone: (___) ___ - ___

Spouse Soc. Sec. #: _____

Spouse Occupation: _____

Spouse Employer: _____

Employer Address: _____

_____

Employer Phone: (___) ___ - ___

Emergency Information

In case of Emergency, please provide information of person not living with patient.

Name: Marissa Thompson   Relation to Patient: Mother

Street Address: 4567 Spring Road

City: Cincinnati   State: OHIO   Zip: 45660   Phone: (___) ___ - ___

Insurance Information

Primary Insurance: Blue Cross Blue Shield

Address: 125 West Market Street, Anytown, Ohio 46110

Phone: (555) 455-6712

Group/Policy #: 555-55-5555IN

Soc. Sec./ID #: 555-55-5555

Policyholder's Name: Natalie Thompson

Secondary Insurance: _____

Address: _____

_____

Phone: (___) ___ - ___

Group/Policy #: _____

Soc. Sec./ID #: _____

Policyholder's Name: _____

Insurance Authorization for Assignment of Benefits/Information Release:

I, the undersigned authorize payment of medical benefits to Practice Name for any services furnished me by the physician. I understand that I am financially responsible for any amount not covered by my contract. I also authorize you to release to my insurance company or their agent information concerning health care, advice, treatment or supplies provided to me. This information will be used for the purpose of evaluating and administering claims of benefits.

Natalie Thompson   12 - 09 - 2001

Patient, Parent or Guardian Signature (if child is under 18 years old)   Date

country do not currently require an original signature or the initials of the provider of the service. It is a good idea to check with each local carrier in your area to determine the requirement. The attending physician should countersign chart entries that are not in the physician's handwriting. This includes medical services performed by nurses or medical assistants, physician assistants, nurse practitioners, or any other member of the provider's staff.

Signed Consent Forms

The medical record of each patient who undergoes a procedure involving significant risk should contain a written consent form. Always obtain consent before an invasive procedure is conducted. The consent should state that the patient has been informed about the procedure, its risks and benefits, and any alternatives. It should also indicate that the patient understood the issues discussed and has given consent to treatment. This information may be kept in a separate section or may accompany the documentation of the procedure (Figure 6-2).

Medicare Limitation of Liability

The government has published a list of services it classifies as medically unnecessary for the Medicare program. When these services are provided to a Medicare beneficiary, obtain a signed waiver known as the limitation of liability or Advance Beneficiary Notification (Figure 6-3). This notification informs the patient in advance that the service he/she seeks may be denied, and if denied, he/she is responsible for the bill. If this consent form is not signed, the patient will not be liable for any denied services (Figure 6-3).

Insurance Claim Forms

An auditor should review claim forms, whether submitted electronically or by hard copy, to see that they are completed correctly. Include all pertinent dates and diagnostic and procedural coding information necessary for insurance payers to generate reimbursement. An HCFA-1500 claim form, which is the form used for submitting outpatient/office and other services to many insurance carriers, is shown in Figure 6-4.

PREPARING FOR THE AUDIT

In beginning the chart audit process, a few tools and records will be needed. Select a combination of the following:

- Ten to 15 medical records
- New patient visits
- Established patient visits
- Consultations
- Other
- Charge ticket/superbill
- Insurance information
- Explanation of benefits (EOB) or remittance advice (RA) from Medicare
- HCFA-1500 claim form (paper or electronic) (optional)
- Evaluation and management guidelines, both 1995 and 1997, from the Centers for Medicare and Medicaid Services

The audit tool is an important element of the audit process. Many audit tools are available on the market, or one can be designed to fit the auditor's

FIGURE 6-2

Consent to treat form

CONSENT TO TREAT

The term "health care provider(s)" in this document means <u>Compliance Medical Group (CMG),</u> its agent and employees, members of the medical staff, their agents and employees, and other health care practitioners who provide care to patients.

I understand that as part of my health care, this organization originates and maintains health records describing my health history, symptoms, examination and test results, diagnoses, treatment, and any plan for care including future treatment. I understand that this information serves as:

    1.   Basis for planning my treatment and care
    2.   Information used to file my claim with the insurance company (procedure and diagnosis)
    3.   Means by which a third-party payer can verify that billed services were actually provided
    4.   A tool for routine health care operations including assessing quality and reviewing competency of your staff and/or other health care providers.

I understand that I have been provided with the Notice of Information Practices that provides more complete information of uses and disclosures. I understand that I have the right to review the notice prior to signing this consent. I understand that the organization reserves the right to change their notice and practices and prior to implementation will mail a copy of any revised notice to the address I have provided. I understand that I have the right to restrict how my health information may be used or disclosed to carry out payment, treatment, or health care operations and that the organization is not required to agree to the restrictions requested. I understand that I have the right to revoke this consent in writing, except to the extent that the organization has already taken action on my behalf.

Permission is hereby granted to all health care providers involved in my care to administer such examination, treatment, testing, and procedures as are deemed necessary in the course of my care.

James Doe _____   01/21/2002 _____
Patient Signature   **Release of Information**   Date

Information about me necessary to substantiate my insurance claims may be released by the health care provider involved in my care.

☒ I am requesting the following restriction to the use or disclosure of my health information

_____

James Doe _____   01/21/2002 _____
Signature   Date

Carrie Jones _____   *Medical Assistant*   01/21/2002 _____
Witness   Title   Date

---

needs and practice. Figure 6-5 is a sample audit tool that will be used to audit the patient encounters throughout this text. Two additional audit tools are located in Appendix B for the auditor's use. It is important to be comfortable with the tool used. In addition to auditing on paper, several software vendors offer auditing software for use in the process. Once you begin auditing patient encounters on a regular basis, research the options available to find the best method for you.

FIGURE 6-3
Medicare Advance Beneficiary Notice

Date: 01/21/2002   Patient's Name: Mamie Johnston   Medicare # (HICN):   555-55-5555A

ADVANCE BENEFICIARY NOTICE (ABN)

NOTE: You need to make a choice about receiving these health care items or services.

We expect that Medicare will not pay for the item(s) or service(s) that are described below. Medicare does not pay for all of your health care costs. Medicare only pays for covered items and services when Medicare rules are met. The fact that Medicare may not pay for a particular item or service does not mean that you should not receive it. There may be a good reason your doctor recommended it. Right now, in your case, Medicare probably will not pay for –

Items or Services:
G0001 Q0091
Because:
Screening Pap and pelvic exam performed 1 year ago; patient does not meet high-risk criteria

The purpose of this form is to help you make an informed choice about whether or not you want to receive these items or services, knowing that you might have to pay for them yourself. Before you make any decision about your options, you should:

- Read this entire notice carefully.
- Ask us to explain, if you don't understand why Medicare probably won't pay.
  - Ask us how much these items or services will cost you (Estimated Cost: $\_45.00_____$),
  in case you have to pay for them yourself or through other insurance.

PLEASE CHOOSE ONE OPTION. CHECK ONE BOX. SIGN & DATE YOUR CHOICE.

☐ Option 1. YES.   I want to receive these items or services.

I understand that Medicare will not decide whether to pay unless I receive these items or services. Please submit my claim to Medicare. I understand that you may bill me for items or services and that I may have to pay the bill while Medicare is making its decision. If Medicare does pay, you will refund to me any payments I made to you that are due to me. If Medicare denies payment, I agree to be personally and fully responsible for payment. That is, I will pay personally, either out of pocket or through any other insurance that I have. I understand I can appeal Medicare's decision.

☒ Option 2. NO.   I have decided not to receive these items or services.
I will not receive these items or services. I understand that you will not be able to submit a claim to Medicare and that I will not be able to appeal your opinion that Medicare won't pay.

Date   01/21/2002   Signature of patient or person acting on patient's behalf

Mamie Johnston

NOTE: Your health information will be kept confidential. Any information that we collect about you on this form will be kept confidential in our offices. If a claim is submitted to Medicare, your health information on this form may be shared with Medicare. Your health information that Medicare sees will be kept confidential by Medicare.

OMB Approval No. 0938-0566   Form No. HCFA-R-131-G

FIGURE 6-4

HCFA-1500 claim form

PLEASE
DO NOT
STAPLE
IN THIS
AREA

CARRIER

HEALTH INSURANCE CLAIM FORM

PICA | PICA

1. MEDICARE   MEDICAID   CHAMPUS   CHAMPVA   GROUP HEALTH PLAN   FECA BLK LUNG   OTHER
(Medicare #) (Medicaid #) (Sponsor's SSN) (VA File #) (SSN or ID) (SSN) (ID)

1a. INSURED'S I.D. NUMBER   (FOR PROGRAM IN ITEM 1)

2. PATIENT'S NAME (Last Name, First Name, Middle Initial)

3. PATIENT'S BIRTH DATE MM DD YY   SEX   M   F

4. INSURED'S NAME (Last Name, First Name, Middle Initial)

5. PATIENT'S ADDRESS (No., Street)

6. PATIENT RELATIONSHIP TO INSURED   Self Spouse Child Other

7. INSURED'S ADDRESS (No., Street)

CITY   STATE

8. PATIENT STATUS   Single Married Other

CITY   STATE

ZIP CODE   TELEPHONE (Include Area Code) (   )

Employed   Full-Time Student   Part-Time Student

ZIP CODE   TELEPHONE (INCLUDE AREA CODE) (   )

9. OTHER INSURED'S NAME (Last Name, First Name, Middle Initial)

10. IS PATIENT'S CONDITION RELATED TO:

11. INSURED'S POLICY GROUP OR FECA NUMBER

a. OTHER INSURED'S POLICY OR GROUP NUMBER

a. EMPLOYMENT? (CURRENT OR PREVIOUS)   YES   NO

a. INSURED'S DATE OF BIRTH MM DD YY   SEX   M   F

b. OTHER INSURED'S DATE OF BIRTH MM DD YY   SEX   M   F

b. AUTO ACCIDENT?   PLACE (State)   YES   NO

b. EMPLOYER'S NAME OR SCHOOL NAME

c. EMPLOYER'S NAME OR SCHOOL NAME

c. OTHER ACCIDENT?   YES   NO

c. INSURANCE PLAN NAME OR PROGRAM NAME

d. INSURANCE PLAN NAME OR PROGRAM NAME

10d. RESERVED FOR LOCAL USE

d. IS THERE ANOTHER HEALTH BENEFIT PLAN?   YES   NO   *If yes*, return to and complete item 9 a-d.

READ BACK OF FORM BEFORE COMPLETING & SIGNING THIS FORM.

12. PATIENT'S OR AUTHORIZED PERSON'S SIGNATURE I authorize the release of any medical or other information necessary to process this claim. I also request payment of government benefits either to myself or to the party who accepts assignment below.

SIGNED _____ DATE _____

13. INSURED'S OR AUTHORIZED PERSON'S SIGNATURE I authorize payment of medical benefits to the undersigned physician or supplier for services described below.

SIGNED _____

PATIENT AND INSURED INFORMATION

14. DATE OF CURRENT: MM DD YY   ILLNESS (First symptom) OR INJURY (Accident) OR PREGNANCY(LMP)

15. IF PATIENT HAS HAD SAME OR SIMILAR ILLNESS. GIVE FIRST DATE MM DD YY

16. DATES PATIENT UNABLE TO WORK IN CURRENT OCCUPATION MM DD YY   FROM   TO MM DD YY

17. NAME OF REFERRING PHYSICIAN OR OTHER SOURCE

17a. I.D. NUMBER OF REFERRING PHYSICIAN

18. HOSPITALIZATION DATES RELATED TO CURRENT SERVICES MM DD YY   FROM   TO MM DD YY

19. RESERVED FOR LOCAL USE

20. OUTSIDE LAB?   YES   NO $ CHARGES

21. DIAGNOSIS OR NATURE OF ILLNESS OR INJURY. (RELATE ITEMS 1,2,3 OR 4 TO ITEM 24E BY LINE)

1. ____.____   3. ____.____

2. ____.____   4. ____.____

22. MEDICAID RESUBMISSION CODE   ORIGINAL REF. NO.

23. PRIOR AUTHORIZATION NUMBER

24. A DATE(S) OF SERVICE From MM DD YY To MM DD YY	B Place of Service	C Type of Service	D PROCEDURES, SERVICES, OR SUPPLIES (Explain Unusual Circumstances) CPT/HCPCS MODIFIER	E DIAGNOSIS CODE	F $ CHARGES	G DAYS OR UNITS	H EPSDT Family Plan	I EMG	J COB	K RESERVED FOR LOCAL USE
1										
2										
3										
4										
5										
6										

25. FEDERAL TAX I.D. NUMBER   SSN EIN

26. PATIENT'S ACCOUNT NO.

27. ACCEPT ASSIGNMENT? (For govt. claims, see back)   YES   NO

28. TOTAL CHARGE $

29. AMOUNT PAID $

30. BALANCE DUE $

31. SIGNATURE OF PHYSICIAN OR SUPPLIER INCLUDING DEGREES OR CREDENTIALS (I certify that the statements on the reverse apply to this bill and are made a part thereof.)

SIGNED _____ DATE _____

32. NAME AND ADDRESS OF FACILITY WHERE SERVICES WERE RENDERED (If other than home or office)

33. PHYSICIAN'S, SUPPLIER'S BILLING NAME, ADDRESS, ZIP CODE & PHONE #

PIN#   GRP#

PHYSICIAN OR SUPPLIER INFORMATION

(APPROVED BY AMA COUNCIL ON MEDICAL SERVICE 8/88)   **PLEASE PRINT OR TYPE**   APPROVED OMB-0938-0008 FORM HCFA-1500 (12-90),   FORM RRB-1500,
APPROVED OMB-1215-0055 FORM OWCP-1500,   APPROVED OMB-0720-0001 (CHAMPUS)

PERFORMING THE CHART AUDIT

1.   Gather reference material for the audit and assemble the necessary materials for the analysis, which include the audit tool, CPT® code book (current edition), ICD-9-CM, and a HCPCS code book. It is also helpful to have a medical dictionary available for looking up terms that are unfamiliar. In order to audit effectively, the evaluation and management CMS documentation guidelines for both 1995 and 1997 should be available for reference, along with a current Correct Coding Initiative edit book. Insurance billing policies and guidelines are often referred to when medical records are reviewed, and this is helpful in determining specific coverage issues.

2.   Select the medical records (charts) to be reviewed. Start by reviewing 10 to 15 charts for each physician to get a good sample of each physician's services. Another method is to target specific services. In either case, the charts selected should contain examples of services performed by each physician. Since the focus should be on current coding, review only those services that are less than 6 months old.

3.   Obtain insurance information to review for each medical record. Understanding each insurance carrier's billing guidelines and/or having access to the information is critical in the audit process. Gather insurance information, and insurance forms (HCFA-1500) or computerized insurance data, for each date of service assessed. Review the insurance information for completeness.

4.   Obtain explanations of benefits (EOBs) or remittance advice (RA) when performing a postpayment review to determine what level(s) of service was submitted to the insurance carrier.

Reviewing the EOB or Medicare RA statements provided by payers can be a valuable way for providers to discover unacceptable code use or incorrect sequencing of codes. When a certain service results in consistent denial or substantial reduction in payment by more than one payer, the coding practice should be analyzed and corrected. The review may reveal a claim form with codes that are:

- Outdated;
- Transposed; or
- Improperly sequenced.

The EOB and RA can provide a method to track payers' usual, customary, and reasonable (UCR) amounts. Compare the UCRs of different insurance companies for insight into keeping fees current and in line with the market. Unfortunately, EOBs and RAs can be difficult to read because each payer may have its own format. Whenever possible, ask the insurance carrier to provide specific information or a breakdown of the charges paid. Ideally, the EOB statement provided by the payer identifies the date of service, charges submitted, procedure code billed (CPT® and/or HCPCS level II code), diagnosis code billed (ICD-9-CM), allowed amount determined by the insurance carrier, and/or any deductibles and copayments the patient is responsible for.

5.   Develop a tally sheet or audit tool. Many different audit tools and auditing products (paper and electronic) exist in the market today. Select the tool that is most comfortable and easy to use.

AUDIT TOOL

Physician _____   Date of Audit _____

Patient Name _____

Date of Service_____   Date of Birth_____   Insurance _____

Practice CPT code(s) selected _____

Documented Diagnose(s) _____

❏ New Patient   ❏ Established Patient   ❏ Office Visit   ❏ Consultation   ❏ Hospital

❏ Hospital subsequent   ❏ Critical Care   ❏ Preventive   ❏ Other Procedures _____

HISTORY (Elements: Chief complaint, history of presenting illness (HPI), review of systems (ROS),
past medical, family, social history (PFSH)

History of Presenting Illness (HPI) Elements	Review of Systems	History
HPI ELEMENTS	**ROS Elements**	❏ Past Medical ❏ Family History ❏ Social History
❏ Location ❏ Quality ❏ Severity ❏ Duration ❏ Timing ❏ Context ❏ Modifying factors ❏ Associated signs and symptoms ❏ Status of 3 or more chronic conditions	❏ Constitutional ❏ Eyes ❏ ENT/mouth ❏ CV ❏ Resp ❏ GI ❏ GU ❏ Musculoskeletal ❏ Integ/Skin/Breast ❏ Neurological ❏ Psych ❏ Endo ❏ Hem/lymph ❏ Allerg/Immuno	Problem Focused N/A
Problem Focused (Min-1) Expanded Problem Focused (Min-1) Detailed AT LEAST 4 or at least 3 Chronic DX Comprehensive AT LEAST 4 or at least 3 Chronic DX	Problem Focused N/A **Expanded Problem Focused (2–9 systems)** Detailed (2–9 systems) Comprehensive (Min-10 required)	Expanded Problem Focused N/A Detailed 1 Comprehensive 2-Established 3-New

History: ☐ Problem focused ☐ Expanded problem focused ☐ Detailed ☐ Comprehensive

FIGURE 6-5
Audit tool—*continued*

GENERAL MULTI-SYSTEM EXAMINATION

Exam	At least 1 element identified by a bullet from any system	6 items identified by a bullet from any system	2 items identified by a bullet from a minimum of 6 systems (12)	2 items identified by a bullet from a minimum of 9 systems (18)
Constitutional	❏ Any one of three vitals ❏ General Appearance of Patient			
Eyes	❏ Conjunctiva and Lids ❏ Pupils & Irises ❏ Optic Discs			
ENT	❏ External Ears & Nose ❏ Hearing ❏ EAC's & TM ❏ Nasal Mucosa Septum & Turbinates ❏ Exam of Oropharynx; oral mucosa, salivary glands, hard and soft palates, tongue, tonsils and posterior pharynx			
Neck	❏ Neck ❏ Thyroid			
Respiratory	❏ Respiratory Effort ❏ Percussion ❏ Palpation ❏ Auscultation			
Cardiovascular	❏ Palpation of heart ❏ Auscultation ❏ Carotids ❏ Abdominal Aorta ❏ Femoral ❏ Pedal Pulses ❏ Extremities for edema and varicosities			
Chest	❏ Inspection of Breasts ❏ Palpation of breast and axillae			
GI (Abdomen)	❏ Masses/tenderness ❏ Liver and Spleen ❏ Hernia ❏ Anus, perineum & rectum ❏ Occult test			
GU	Male: ❏ Scrotal Contents ❏ Penis ❏ Prostate Glands Female: ❏ External Genitalia ❏ Urethra ❏ Bladder ❏ Cervix ❏ Uterus ❏ Adnexa/parametria			
Lymph	❏ Lymph nodes in 2 or more areas ❏ Neck ❏ Axillae ❏ Groin ❏ Other			
Musculoskeletal	❏ Gait & Station ❏ Digits & Nails muscles of at least one area ❏ 1). head, neck 2). spine, ribs, pelvis 3) right upper extremity 4) left upper extremity 5) right lower extremity 6) left lower extremity; with exam including ❏ Inspection and/or palpation ❏ ROM ❏ Stability ❏ Strength & Tone			
Skin	❏ Inspection of skin and subcutaneous tissues ❏ Palpation of skin and subcutaneous tissues			
Neuro	❏ Cranial Nerves ❏ Reflexes ❏ Sensation ❏ Judgment & Insight ❏ Orientation to time and place and place/person			
Psychiatric	❏ Memory ❏ Mood ❏ Mental Status Exam Complete ❏ Orientation to time and place and place/person ❏ Recent and remote memory ❏ Attention Span and Concentration ❏ Language (naming objects, repeating phrases etc. ❏ Judgment & Insight			

❏Problem focused   ❏ Expanded problem focused   ❏ Detailed   ❏ Comprehensive

Level of Exam 1995 _____   Level of Exam 1997 _____

FIGURE 6-5
Audit tool—*continued*

Medical Decision Making Audit of Evaluation and Management Service

Number of Diagnoses and Management Options	Points Assigned	Points Per Category	Amount and Complexity of Data	Points Assigned	Points Per Category
Self Limiting or Minor Problems (stable, improved, or worsening) Maximum of 2 points can be given	1		Ordered and/or reviewed clinical lab	1	
Established Problem – Stable Improved	1		Ordered and/or reviewed radiology	1	
Established Problem – Worsening	2		Discussed tests with performing or interpreting physician.	1	
New Problem – No Additional Work-up Planned Maximum of 1 problem given credit	3		Ordered and/or reviewed test in the CPT Medicine Section	1	
New Problem – Additional Work-up Planned	4		Independent visualization and direct view of image, tracing, specimen	2	
Total Points:			Decision to obtain old records or additional HX from someone other than patient, eg family, caretaker, prev. phys.	1	
			Reviewed and summarized old records and/or obtained history from someone other than patient.	2	
			Total Points		

Table of Risk--------The Highest Level in ONE Area Determines the Overall Risk

Level of Risk	Presenting Problem(s) or	Diagnostic Procedure or	Management Options
Minimal	❏ One self-limited or minor problem, ie: cold, insect bite, tinea coporis	❏ Laboratory tests requiring venipuncture ❏ Chest X-Ray ❏ EKG/Eeg ❏ Urinalysis ❏ Ultrasound, eg, echocardiography ❏ KOH prep	❏ Rest ❏ Gargles ❏ Elastic Bandages ❏ Superficial Dressing
Low	❏ Two or more self-limited or minor Problems ❏ One stable chronic illness, eg, well controlled hypertension, non-insulin dependent diabetes, cataract, BPH ❏ Acute uncomplicated illness or injury, eg cystitis, allergic rhinitis, simple sprain.	❏ Physiological tests not under stress, eg, pulmonary, function test ❏ Non-cardiovascular imaging studies with contrast, eg, barium enema ❏ Superficial needle biopsies ❏ Clinical laboratory tests requiring arterial puncture ❏ Skin biopsies	❏ Over-the-counter drugs ❏ Minor surgery with no identified risk factors ❏ Physical therapy ❏ Occupational therapy ❏ IV Fluids without additives
Moderate	❏ One or more chronic illnesses with mild exacerbation, progression, or side effects of treatment. ❏ Two or more stable chronic illnesses ❏ Undiagnosed new problem with uncertain prognosis, eg lump in breast. ❏ Acute illness with systemic symptoms, eg, pyelonephritis, pneumonitis, colitis.	❏ Physiological tests under stress, eg, cardiac stress test, fetal contraction stress test. ❏ Diagnostic endoscopies with no identified risk factors. ❏ Deep needle or incisional biopsy ❏ Cardiovascular imaging studies with contrast and no identified risk factors eg, anteriogram, cardiac catheterization ❏ Obtain fluid from body cavity eg, lumbar puncture, thoracentesis, culdocentesis.	❏ Minor surgery with identified risk factors. ❏ Elective major surgery (open, percutaneous or endoscopic)with no identified risk factors. ❏ Prescription drug managemt. ❏ Therapeutic nuclear medicine ❏ IV fluids with additives ❏ Closed treatment of fracture or dislocation w/o manipulation.
High	❏ One or more chronic illnesses w/severe exacerbation, progression, or side effects of treatment. ❏ Acute or chronic illness or injuries that pose a threat to life or bodily function eg, multiple trauma, acute ML pulmonary embolus, severe respiratory distress, progressive severe rheumatoid arthritis, psychiatric illness w/potential threat to self or others, peritonitis, acute renal failure. ❏ An abrupt change in neurologic status, eg, seizure TIA, weakness, or sensory loss.	❏ Cardiovascular imaging studies with contrast with identified risk factors. ❏ Cardiac electrophysiological tests ❏ Diagnostic endoscopies with identified risk factors. ❏ Discography	❏ Elective major surgery (open, percutaneous or endoscopic) with identified risk factors. ❏ Emergency major surgery (open percutaneous or endoscopic) ❏ Parenteral control substances ❏ Drug therapy requiring intensive monitoring for toxicity. ❏ Decision not to resuscitate or to de-escalate care because of poor prognosis.

FIGURE 6-5

Audit tool—*concluded*

Decision Making Total: ----2 of 3 Must Meet

Points Assigned	1	2	3	4
Number of DX	❑ Minimal	❑ Limited	❑ Multiple	❑ Extensive
Amount of Data	❑ Minimal	❑ Limited	❑ Moderate	❑ Extensive
Risk of Complications	❑ Minimal	❑ Low	❑ Moderate	❑ High
Levels	❑ Straight Forward	❑ Low Complexity	❑ Moderate Complexity	❑ High Complexity

Level of Service: History _____ Exam _____ Medical Decision Making

Chart Note

☐ Dictated ☐ Handwritten _____ ☐ Form   ☐ Illegible ☐ Note signed

☐ Signature missing ☐ Diagnosis Code(s) supported

Diagnosis Code(s) billed_____

Other services billed _____

Comments:

Auditor's Signature _____

The auditor will need a form to record the frequency of correct and incorrect coding and documentation errors. The following is an overview of information that should be recorded on the tally sheet (audit tool or audit sheet):

- Date of service
- Patient chart number and physician name
- Type of insurance
- Correct, incorrect, and corrected CPT® codes
- CPT® codes coded, but not documented
- CPT® codes documented, but not coded
- Correct, incorrect, and corrected ICD-9-CM codes
- ICD-9-CM codes coded, but documentation does not substantiate medical necessity
- Patient's consent for invasive procedures or high risk
- Physician's signature
- Patient's signature (for release of medical information and assignment of benefits)

6. Analyze the audit and compare the documentation to the procedure and diagnosis code(s) billed. Upon completion of the chart review (audit), total and analyze the tally sheets to determine practices that need attention as well as practice areas that are being performed well. Develop percentages in the following areas:

Correct use of CPT® codes
- Levels of service
- Diagnostic procedures
- Surgical codes

Incorrect use of CPT® and/or HCPCS codes
- Inadequate documentation
- Fragmented billing (unbundling)

Correct use of ICD-9-CM codes
- Medical necessity documented

Incorrect use of ICD-9-CM codes
- Inadequate documentation
- Incomplete coding
- Incorrect coding
- Appropriate physician signatures
- Signatures or initials missing from documentation
- Appropriate patient signatures
- Signatures missing from consent forms, HCFA-1500s, etc

7. Prepare the summary of findings (summary report). The summary will be covered in Chapter 7. The summary report can be customized to the practice or group but should contain elements identifying the problematic areas, numbers or percentages of incorrect coding vs correct coding based on documentation, any other coding or documentation issued identified in the audit, and recommendations for improvement.

8.   Review the audit summary and findings with the practitioner. An audit is not beneficial if communication between the practitioner and auditor does not take place. Corrective action cannot be effective if the practitioner is unaware of problems with his/her documentation.

9.   Taking action based on findings in the chart audit process is a critical step in the audit process. An audit is useless if no action is taken on the findings, even if that action is just an acknowledgment that the documentation, coding, and billing practices are acceptable. The physicians and the practice administrator should review the ratio of correct and incorrect coding as well as compliance and noncompliance issues. Areas of incomplete or inaccurate documentation can be identified and corrective action taken.

10.   Ongoing training is the next step in the auditing process. Once the problematic areas are identified, ongoing training is helpful to keep the practitioner apprised of coding and documentation guidelines, coding updates, and changes in carrier and government requirements.

11.   Establish a time frame to make needed changes based on the physician's or practice administrator's determination of the issues that require immediate attention and those that can wait for long-term revision and implementation.

AFTER THE AUDIT

Compile results in an organized fashion and prepare a detailed analysis and a results summary for the practitioner. A detailed analysis is a method of recording using a table format with details as part of the audit report, which include the patient identification name or unique number, date of service, and the CPT® code selected by the provider.

Physician Medical Record Detailed Analysis and Review Summary Report

Review the example of the medical record review summary report (Figures 6-6 and 6-7). The summary report is a detailed report given to the provider that indicates documentation compliance, identifies problem areas, and offers suggestions for improvement. This is a valuable tool when meeting with the provider after the audit is completed. Instructions for completing the summary report will be included when you begin the case studies.

KEY TERMS

Advance Beneficiary Notice (ABN)—Waiver notice given to Medicare beneficiaries when there is genuine doubt that the outpatient service being provided will be covered by Medicare because of medical necessity requirements. The notice must be given to a beneficiary before the service is performed. If Medicare rejects the claim and an ABN was signed, then the beneficiary can be billed for the service. An ABN cannot be given to every Medicare patient, only when circumstances suggest Medicare may not cover the service.

FIGURE 6-6
Detailed review analysis

PHYSICIAN MEDICAL RECORD REVIEW
COMPLIANCE MEDICAL GROUP
DETAILED REVIEW ANALYSIS & SUMMARY REPORT

Physician: David Doe, MD   Date of Review: 02/23/2002

Reviewer: Deborah Grider, CMA, CPC, CPC-H, CCS-P, CCP

Number of Charts Reviewed: 10

Patient ID	Service Date	Practice CPT® Code	History	Exam	Medical Decision Making	Documented CPT® Code
1000782	11/16/01	99202 99393	D	D	Low	99203 Documentation does not support office visit and preventive medicine services
1000703	11/15/01	99213	D	EPF	MOD	99213—based on medical necessity; documentation indicates 99214
997170	11/13/01	99213	D	EPF	Low	99213
999473	11/15/01	99203	C	D	MOD	99214—billed new patient visit; appears to be an established patient
1001773	11/17/01	90471 G0008	N/A	N/A	N/A	90471 G0008 Flu shot with administration
1000784	11/16/01	99203	D	D	MOD	99203
999475	11/15/01	99213	D	EPF	LOW	99213
997141	11/13/01	99213 87880	D	EPF	LOW	99213
996504	11/13/01	99213	EPF	EPF	MOD	99213
1001742	11/17/01	99213 90471 90658	D	EPF	LOW	99213 90471 90658

FIGURE 6-7
Summary report

PHYSICIAN MEDICAL RECORD REVIEW
COMPLIANCE MEDICAL GROUP
DETAILED REVIEW ANALYSIS & SUMMARY REPORT

Physician: David Doe, MD

Date of Review: 02/23/2002

Reviewer: Deborah Grider, CMA, CPC, CPC-H, CCS-P, CCP

Number of Charts Reviewed: 10

One service date was reviewed for each chart reviewed for appropriate coding and supporting documentation. Each chart was reviewed in detail for completeness.

E/M documentation appears to support service billed	8
E/M documentation in the record appears to support a lower level of service than billed	1
E/M documentation in the record appears to support a higher level of service than billed	0
E/M documentation in the record appears to support a different category of service (new, established, consultation, etc).	1

Other documentation coding issues:

1. Consent for treatment was found in all but one of the medical records reviewed.
2. All reports/consultations appeared to be initialed and/or dated by the provider.
3. Completed problem lists appeared to be located in all of the medical records reviewed.
4. A completed medication sheet did not appear to be located in one of the medical records reviewed.
5. All medical records reviewed were handwritten, recorded on an encounter form, and easy to read.
6. On one patient encounter, the provider appeared to bill a preventive visit along with a new patient office visit. Supporting documentation did not appear to support both encounters.
7. The patient's date of birth did not appear to be recorded correctly on the patient encounter form, but was recorded correctly on the history form.
8. On one patient encounter the provider billed a new patient visit but appeared to have previously seen the patient within the past 3 years, which meets established patient criteria.

RECOMMENDATIONS

1. Review problem areas with provider.
2. Review billing requirements for billing an office visit with preventive medicine on the same day.
3. Review criteria for the selection of new patient vs established patient.
4. Do a follow-up review in six (6) months.

Audit—An examination of the systems used to make sure a practitioner is billing and coding correctly. These systems are sometimes called "monitors." An audit checks the thermometer on a regular basis to make sure it is working properly.

Audit tool—A document sometimes referred to as a tally sheet, used to perform a medical record review (chart audit) and document the findings of each individual medical record audited.

Balanced Budget Act of 1997 (BBA)—An act passed by Congress, similar to HIPAA, that allocated a great deal of money to prevent fraud and abuse in the health care industry.

Beneficiary—A patient enrolled in the Medicare program.

Category of service—Location of service (ie, home, office, hospital, consultation, etc) and determination if the patient is new or established.

Chart entries—Dated entries made in the patient medical record by a physician, practitioner, nurse, or office staff.

Chief complaint—The reason for the patient visit.

Corporate compliance—A program that ensures that a company is following both its own policies and the government's laws and regulations. A compliance program is a way for a company to monitor itself using a system of checks and balances.

CPT®—Current Procedural Terminology. CPT® codes refer to types of procedures that a patient might receive.

DME—Durable Medical Equipment—Equipment that has been ordered by a physician for use by the patient at home which includes walkers, wheelchairs, hospital beds, etc.

DOJ—Department of Justice, a federal agency that handles the investigation and enforcement of federal criminal laws, including proven cases of fraudulent health care claims.

Downcoding—Process that occurs when the coding system used on a claim submitted to an insurance carrier does not match the coding system used by the company receiving the claim. If they do not match, the claims examiner has an opportunity to substitute a code with a lower value, which means lower reimbursement.

E/M—Evaluation and management; refers to codes that physicians may use to tell the government how complex and time consuming their examination of a patient was. Codes usually range from 1 (lowest complexity) to 5 (highest complexity). Elements that go into determining an appropriate E/M code level include (1) taking a history from the patient, (2) examining the patient, and (3) developing a diagnosis or care plan (called medical decision making).

False Claims Act—A federal law that was enacted in 1863, when Abraham Lincoln was president, that allows the government to sue those who submit incorrect claims for reimbursement from the government. Often these claims are honest billing errors, but the government still considers them false claims. An intent to defraud is not required. There are steep fines for submitting a false claim to the government—between $5000 and $10,000 for each claim falsely submitted plus triple damages. Having an effective corporate compliance program in place can reduce these fines.

Federal Sentencing Guidelines—Set of criteria used by the government for sentencing individuals and organizations for any federal crime, including health care fraud. Organizations that have effective compliance programs in place can reduce fines and penalties under the Federal Sentencing Guidelines.

Fraud—Intentionally providing false information to the government with the purpose of defrauding the government.

HHS—Health and Human Services—A federal governmental agency given the responsibility to oversee the government insurance program(s).

HIPAA—Health Insurance Portability and Accountability Act of 1996, passed by Congress. The portability part of this act made headlines when it was first released, allowing employees to take their health insurance with them when they change jobs. The accountability aspect of HIPAA gives the government its power to pursue health care providers they believe are committing fraud. One of the most significant parts of this Act is that a fund was created that will continue to finance fraud investigations and additional staff members.

History of present illness—A description in the patient's own words of the current illness, injury, or complaint related to location, severity, context, modifying factors, duration, etc.

Home Health Agency—An agency which provides nursing services to patients in their home(s). The agency may be private or public.

ICD-9-CM—International Classification of Diseases, Ninth Revision (Clinical Modification), a type of diagnosis code that must be used on claims submitted to insurance companies. In order to document that a service is medically necessary, the ICD-9-CM code must match the *procedure* code (CPT®; see above) given. For example, if a leg x-ray procedure is performed on someone who has a heart attack *diagnosis,* the leg x-ray may not be considered medically necessary.

Intermediary (or fiscal intermediary)—An insurance company that contracts with Medicare and other government health care programs to pay the claims of health care providers with government funds.

Level of E/M service—The level of visit or service dependent on three key components: history, examination, and medical decision making. Counseling, coordination of care, and time are also contributory elements in the selection of the level of service.

LMRP (Local Medical Review Policy)—A policy that designates that certain ICD-9-CM (see above) codes be present on a medical order for the order to be considered medically necessary (see below) and reimbursed. If these codes are not present, then an ABN (see above) may be required.

Medicaid—A health care program for eligible low-income individuals that is jointly financed through state and federal governments.

Medical decision making—The plan of care the practitioner deems appropriate medical care based on the presenting problem, diagnosis, diagnostic test ordered, and risk.

Medically necessary (or medical necessity)—Needed to be done on the basis of the patient's current condition. This condition must be documented in the patient's chart. Medicare considers medically unnecessary procedures (when the reason for performing the procedure is not properly documented) to be an example of fraudulent billing.

Medicare—A federal health care program for the elderly and disabled that pays a portion of a beneficiary's medical costs. There are two parts of Medicare coverage: Part A and Part B, which refer to differing levels of coverage for physicians and hospitals.

Medicare secondary payer (MSP)—A designation that Medicare will pay remaining costs after another insurance company has paid the majority of the bill. The government requires that providers ask Medicare beneficiaries a series of questions to determine whether another insurance program should be billed first, before Medicare is billed. This other insurance program is considered primary and Medicare secondary.

OIG (Office of Inspector General)—The office within HHS (see above) responsible for auditing health care providers and providing sanctions when necessary. The OIG drafted the document, "The OIG's Compliance Program Guidance for Hospitals," to tell health care providers the elements they would like to see in corporate compliance programs.

Operation Restore Trust—An effort by the government to address specific abuses within the health care industry. Current investigations include home health (see above), DME (see above), and nursing homes (ensuring that claims submitted by the nursing home correspond to the type of care provided).

Review of systems—An inventory of body systems that is part of the history and indicates negative or positive responses to medical problems.

Risk table—The table published by the Centers for Medicare and Medicaid Services that identifies the presenting problem and/or diagnoses, amount of data ordered or reviewed, and management options.

Tally sheet—See Audit tool.

Unbundling/bundling—The practices of combining or separating charges for related services. Medicare pays for many tests and procedures as a group. For instance, for a particular diagnosis, all services related to that diagnosis will be "bundled" into one payment. "Unbundling" refers to the practice of charging for a service individually when it should have already been covered as part of a group payment. For lab services, the government now says that "panel" tests—lab tests that are grouped or bundled together—must be unbundled if any of the tests are not medically necessary (see above).

Upcoding—The inappropriate practice of assigning a higher procedure code than what was actually performed. Every procedure performed by a health care provider has a code that corresponds to it. If a procedure requires complex tasks or a large amount of time, it has a higher code number assigned to it. Medicare requires that all procedures performed on a patient be written in the patient's chart. What is written in the chart must match the procedure code level given.

TEST YOUR KNOWLEDGE

Fill in the Blanks

1. Review _____ charts to get a good sample of each physician's services.

2. The auditor will need a form to record the _____ of correct and incorrect coding and documentation _____.

3. Comparing the documentation with the procedure and diagnosis is referred to as _____ the audit.

4. Providing feedback to the provider includes discussing _____ of the review.

5. The auditor must use current _____ code books as well as other reference materials.

6. Chart entries not made by the provider should be _____ by the attending physician, which includes services performed by any member of the provider's staff.

7. The government has published a list of services it classifies as _____ unnecessary for the Medicare program.

8. When considering revenue, one of the auditor's objectives is to examine _____ practices for _____ use of codes.

9. Compare the chart _____ to the codes billed to uncover overbilled or underbilled services.

10. A good medical record review will identify instances where codes are billed _____ supporting documentation.

ANALYZING THE OFFICE MEDICAL RECORD

CHART AUDITING STEP BY STEP

Step 1: The Audit Tool

The first step in the chart audit process is to become familiar with the audit tool(s). An audit tool has been provided for use with the audit cases provided later in this chapter. You will be using the tool for all of the case studies and test cases that will be audited. In addition, there are two other sample audit tools in Appendix B you may opt to use. The other tool you will be using is the charge ticket (superbill, charge ticket, or fee ticket). An explanation of benefits (EOB) and/or remittance advice (RA) will normally be reviewed but will not be provided with each case reviewed. Make several copies of the audit tool in Appendix B. Review the Centers for Medicare and Medicaid Services (CMS) evaluation and management (E/M) documentation guidelines for 1995 and 1997 in Chapter 3 before auditing each medical record. These are the guidelines that will be used to complete the chart audit process. The General Multi-system Exam Table and the Single Organ System Exam Tables are found in Appendix A.

A Detailed Analysis and Summary Form is also included in Appendix B. Please review both of these forms before you begin the exercises.

Step 2: Gather Reference Materials

Always have your code books available: CPT®, ICD-9-CM, and HCPCS. You may wish to have a medical dictionary, surgical cross-coder, Correct Coding Initiative edits, and other reference material as well. Keep a copy of the 1995 and 1997 CMS guidelines with you when performing the chart audit.

Step 3: Perform the Chart Audit

Audit a minimum of 10 medical records for each provider. Identify problem areas such as:

- Improper use of CPT® codes
- E/M code(s) not supported by the documentation
- Diagnosis code that is incorrect or does not indicate medical necessity
- Missing modifiers and/or incorrect modifier usage

- Forms missing in the chart
- Other procedures or services improperly reported
- Incorrect diagnosis linkage

Step 4: Complete the Review Analysis and Summary Report

Complete the review analysis identifying correct and incorrect coding. Complete the summary report identifying the number of encounters documented correctly and incorrectly, other coding issues, and suggestions for improvement.

Step 5: Meet With the Provider

Schedule a meeting with the provider to review coding errors, offer suggestions, and answer questions. Allow enough time to review all the medical records in which you found incorrect coding based on documentation. Provide handouts to the provider that will help him or her maintain compliance. Suggest periodic audits to monitor and maintain compliance.

BEGINNING THE AUDIT PROCESS

For the purpose of the following audit exercises, 10 medical records from various physicians will be audited. The physician practice is Multiple Specialty Group Inc. Results from the 10 exercises will be compiled along with a summary report, which will be completed in Chapter 8. Both tools, the review analysis and the summary report, are useful when speaking with the provider regarding problematic encounters; they include recommendations for improvement, which are important to maintain compliance in the medical record.

The 1995 and 1997 CMS guidelines will be used to compare the results of the review. The General Multi-system Exam Table will be used for each exercise unless otherwise indicated for the 1997 guidelines. Begin with the first encounter. Make at least 10 copies of the audit tool from Appendix B. Also make copies of the charge ticket(s) in Appendix B for the first 10 cases Both the audit tool and the charge ticket will be used for each exercise. Each encounter includes a charge ticket (superbill) for the case. The General Multi-system Exam Table located in Appendix A will be needed for a reference to complete the audit. Read each case carefully.

Case 1

Cooper, Angela M.   Date of Service: 11/1/2001

Patient presents to the office with a history of waking up with her nose bleeding. This is the second occurrence of epistaxis that I have treated her for. The bleeding has occurred off and on for the past week. She states that the bleeding has resolved. She also has a mild headache. Denies that she takes any aspirin. Denies shortness of breath or chest pain. Normal tympanic membranes. The examination of the nares shows evidence of former bleeding site; it is now resolved. Oropharynx is normal. Neck is supple and lungs are clear.

Assessment and Plan: Recurrent nosebleed. The patient is to return if bleeding recurs.

Ima Caring, MD

Now that you have read the encounter, it is time to break apart the key components and the elements that are part of the key components when auditing the medical record. Begin by reviewing the history.

┤AUDITING TIP
Begin by defining the history components, exam component, and medical decision making, and audit each component separately.

History

Chief Complaint: Patient presents to office with history of waking up with nose bleeding. *Note:* This is the primary reason for the encounter. The chief complaint should *always* indicate the reason for the patient encounter.

History of Present Illness (HPI): Patient has been treated by physician for epistaxis at a prior visit.

She states that the bleeding has resolved. The bleeding has occurred off and on for the past week. She is also experiencing some dryness and itching that is related to the bleeding.

Look carefully at the history of present illness. The elements you are looking for are location, quality, severity, duration, timing, context, modifying factors, and associated signs and symptoms. In this case, the *location* is indicated by nosebleed; *quality,* resolved; *duration,* bleeding has occurred for the past week; and *modifying factor,* mild headache.

Review of Systems (ROS): The patient denies shortness of breath or chest pain. Two systems are involved. See if you can identify the systems from the list below:

- ❏ Constitutional
- ❏ Cardiovascular
- ❏ GU
- ❏ Neurological
- ❏ Hem/lymph

- ❏ Eyes
- ❏ Respiratory
- ❏ Musculoskeletal
- ❏ Psych
- ❏ Allergic/Immunology

- ❏ ENT/mouth
- ❏ GI
- ❏ Integumentary/Skin/Breast
- ❏ Endo

If you selected cardiovascular (chest pain) and respiratory (shortness of breath), you are correct. If you missed this one, go back and review the systems again. Pay attention to the coding tips.

┤AUDITING TIP
Remember that the review of systems (ROS) is a series of positive and negative responses based on questions asked related to the HPI.

Past, Family, and/or Social History (PFSH): Now look at past medical history, family history, and social history.

Is there a past medical, family, and/or social history? You should not have found a PFSH within this encounter.

┤AUDITING TIP
Past medical history includes
1. Current medications
2. Illnesses or injuries
3. Prior surgeries
4. Allergies

Now that the history level has been defined, we have determined the following: There is a definitive chief complaint, and the HPI contains four elements. Review the 1997 CMS guidelines again for clarification; the HPI is extended. In the ROS, two systems were reviewed, which, according to the 1997 guidelines, is extended. No history area is addressed with this encounter. Since a history area was not addressed, this would be an expanded problem focused history.

It is apparent from the statement in the encounter, "This is the second occurrence of epistaxis that I have treated her for," that this is an established patient. The level of service for history is expanded problem focused. Since a past, family, or social history was not addressed, there is not enough information for a detailed history level.

Examine Table 7-1 that follows.

When selecting the history type, criteria for all three elements (HPI, ROS, and PFSH) must be met or exceeded. Thus, in Case 1, the history is expanded problem focused.

Examination

Review the elements documented in the examination. Begin by reviewing the systems that the physician examined: ENT, neck, and lungs.

- ENT: Normal tympanic membranes. The examination of the nares shows evidence of a former bleeding site; it is now resolved. Oropharynx is normal.
- Neck: Supple.
- Lungs: Clear to auscultation and percussion.

Turn to the General Multi-system Exam Table in Appendix A and review the elements in the encounter identified by a bullet.

TABLE 7-1

Categories for determining type of history

Type of History	History of Present Illness (HPI)	Review of Systems (ROS)	Past, Family, and/or Social History (PFSH)
Problem focused (PF)	Brief (1–3 elements)	N/A	N/A
Expanded problem focused (EPF)	Brief (1–3 elements)	Problem pertinent (minimum, 1 system)	N/A
Detailed (D)	Extended (≥ 4 elements, 1995 and 1997; status of ≥ 3 multiple chronic or inactive conditions, 1997 guidelines only)	Extended (2–9 systems)	Pertinent (one history area)
Comprehensive (C)	Extended (≥ 4 elements, 1995 and 1997; status of ≥ 3 multiple chronic or inactive conditions, 1997 guidelines only)	Complete (10 systems or some systems with statement "all others negative")	Complete (2 history areas for established; 3 history areas for new patient)

ENT

■ Otoscopic examination of external auditory canals and tympanic membranes

■ Inspection of nasal mucosa, septum, and turbinates

■ Examination of oropharynx: oral mucosa, salivary glands, hard and soft palates, tongue, tonsils, and posterior pharynx

Neck

■ Examination of neck (eg, masses, overall appearance, symmetry, tracheal position, crepitus)

Respiratory

■ Percussion of chest (eg, dullness, flatness, hyperresonance)

■ Auscultation of lungs (eg, breath sounds, adventitious sounds, rubs)

Notice that six elements are identified by a bullet from the General Multi-system Exam Table. Make sure you have the CMS guidelines and exam table with you when auditing any medical record. According to the 1997 guidelines, six elements identified by a bullet is categorized as an expanded problem focused examination. Not enough was documented to reach the detailed level, which requires two elements identified by a bullet in each of six organ systems or body areas, for a total of 12 elements.

When a physician's or practitioner's medical records are audited, a review of the 1995 and 1997 E/M guidelines would be appropriate. See Table 7-2 for the exam element requirements for the 1995 guidelines to see if the provider would reach a higher level of service using these guidelines.

The three systems examined were ENT, neck, and lungs. For 1995, Table 7-2 indicates that two to four systems and/or body areas would make an expanded problem focused examination. The 1997 guidelines indicate that six elements identified by a bullet in the Multi-system Exam Table

TABLE 7-2

1995 vs 1997 CMS examination documentation guidelines

Documentation Requirement	Problem Focused	Expanded Problem Focused	Detailed	Comprehensive
1995 body areas or organ systems	1 body area or organ system	2–4 body areas or organ systems	5–7 body areas or organ systems	8 or more body areas or organ systems OR comprehensive single organ system
1997 performance and documentation of elements identified by a bullet	1–5 elements identified by a bullet from 1 or more body areas or organ systems	6 elements identified by a bullet from 1 or more body areas or organ systems	2 elements identified by a bullet from 6 body areas or organ systems OR 12 elements from 2 more body areas or organ systems	2 elements identified by a bullet from 9 body areas or organ systems

would also be expanded problem focused. According to the documentation in the medical record and both the 1995 and 1997 guidelines, the exam is expanded problem focused (99213).

Medical Decision Making

Medical decision making is the final key component. The assessment and plan in the case report indicate recurrent nosebleed; the patient is to return if bleeding recurs.

See the medical decision making grid for number of diagnoses in Table 7-3. There is one diagnosis; recurrent nosebleed is documented. On the medical decision making grid, the first element is number of diagnoses or management options. Since this is a minor problem, the correct selection should be a self-limited or a minor problem. This is an established problem that has not improved.

One point is given for the number of diagnoses or management options based on the documentation.

The next step in the medical decision making process is to determine the amount and/or complexity of data reviewed. Use Table 7-4 to determine the point value for this element.

Since there was no pertinent data to review, the amount and complexity of data to be reviewed is not applicable with this encounter. When this category is assessed, the amount and complexity of data to review are considered minimal.

The last element in medical decision making is risk. The Risk Table is used, which is divided into three categories:

■ Presenting problem(s)
■ Diagnostic procedures ordered
■ Management options

Within the categories of risk, you will find four levels:

■ Minimal
■ Low
■ Moderate
■ High

T A B L E   7-3

Medical decision making grid for number of management options

Number of Diagnoses/Management Options	Points
Self-limited or minor (stable, improved, or worsened) ➜ Maximum 2 points in this category	1 point
Established problem (to examining MD); stable or improved	1 point
Established problem (to examining MD); worsening	2 points
New problem (to examining MD); no additional workup planned ➜ Maximum 3 points in this category	3 points
New problem (to examining MD); additional workup (eg, admit/transfer)	4 points
Total	**1 point**

In reviewing the table, note that the fewer and less complicated problems a patient presents with, the less risk. The more complex the diagnostic tests and/or management options, the more risk. In order to determine overall risk, you must select the level from each category based on the documentation in the medical record. Normally this information is located in the assessment and plan in the medical record, but it could be located anywhere in the chart note.

Reread the assessment and plan for the encounter for Case 1: recurrent nosebleed; the patient is to return if bleeding recurs. Now review the Table of Risk (Table 7-5) and select a level for each category.

The highest level in any given category is the overall risk. Risk categories in Case 1 are as follows:

Presenting problem
■ One self-limited or minor problem (recurrent nosebleed)—Minimal

Diagnostic procedure(s) ordered
■ None—Minimal

Management options
■ Return if problem reoccurs—Minimal

Table 7-6 will help determine level of service for medical decision making. This grid uses the point system from Tables 7-3 and 7-4. Notice that all three categories indicate minimal medical decision making in this case. The highest level attained in two of the three categories determines the level of E/M code as it relates to medical decision making.

The correct level of service for medical decision making in Case 1 is straightforward. It is difficult for you as a nonclinician to determine the provider's thinking in regard to management of the patient, so this system was developed to help the auditor determine the third key component.

T A B L E 7-4

Medical decision making grid for amount and/or complexity of data reviewed

Amount and/or Complexity of Data Reviewed	Points
Lab ordered and/or reviewed (regardless of number ordered)	1 point
X-ray ordered and/or reviewed (regardless of number ordered)	1 point
Medicine section (90701–99199) ordered and/or reviewed	1 point
Discussion of test results with performing physician	1 point
Decision to obtain old record and/or obtain history from someone other than patient	1 point
Review and summary of old records and/or obtaining history from someone other than patient and/or discussion with other health provider	2 points
Independent visualization of image, tracing, or specimen (not simply review of report)	2 points
Total	**None Reviewed**

TABLE 7-5

Table of risk

Level of Risk	Presenting Problem(s)	Diagnostic Procedure(s) Ordered	Management Options Selected
Minimal	■ One self-limited or minor problem, eg, cold, insect bite, tinea corporis	■ Laboratory tests requiring venipuncture ■ Chest x-rays ■ EKG/EEG ■ Urinalysis ■ Ultrasound, eg, echocardiography ■ KOH prep	■ Rest ■ Gargles ■ Elastic bandages ■ Superficial dressings
Low	■ Two or more self-limited or minor problems ■ One stable chronic illness, eg, well-controlled hypertension, non-insulin-dependent diabetes, cataract, BPH ■ Acute uncomplicated illness or injury, eg, cystitis, allergic rhinitis, simple sprain	■ Physiologic tests not under stress, eg, pulmonary function tests ■ Noncardiovascular imaging studies with contrast, eg, barium enema ■ Superficial needle biopsies ■ Clinical laboratory tests requiring arterial puncture ■ Skin biopsies	■ Over-the-counter drugs ■ Minor surgery with no identified risk factors ■ Physical therapy ■ Occupational therapy ■ IV fluids without additives
Moderate	■ One or more chronic illnesses with mild exacerbation, progression, or side effects of treatment ■ Two or more stable chronic illnesses ■ Undiagnosed new problem with uncertain prognosis, eg, lump in breast ■ Acute illness with systemic symptoms, eg, pyelonephritis, pneumonitis, colitis ■ Acute complicated injury, eg, head injury with brief loss of consciousness	■ Physiologic tests under stress, eg, cardiac stress test, fetal contraction stress test ■ Diagnostic endoscopies with no identified risk factors ■ Deep needle or incisional biopsy ■ Cardiovascular imaging studies with contrast and no identified risk factors, eg, arteriogram, cardiac catheterization ■ Obtain fluid from body cavity, eg lumbar puncture, thoracentesis, culdocentesis	■ Minor surgery with identified risk factors ■ Elective major surgery (open, percutaneous, or endoscopic) with no identified risk factors ■ Prescription drug management ■ Therapeutic nuclear medicine ■ IV fluids with additives ■ Closed treatment of fracture or dislocation without manipulation
High	■ One or more chronic illnesses with severe exacerbation, progression, or side effects of treatment ■ Acute or chronic illnesses or injuries that pose a threat to life or bodily function, eg, multiple trauma, acute MI, pulmonary embolus, severe respiratory distress, progressive severe rheumatoid arthritis, psychiatric illness with potential threat to self or others, peritonitis, acute renal failure ■ An abrupt change in neurologic status, eg, seizure, TIA, weakness, sensory loss	■ Cardiovascular imaging studies with contrast with identified risk factors ■ Cardiac electrophysiological tests ■ Diagnostic endoscopies with identified risk factors ■ Discography	■ Elective major surgery (open, percutaneous, or endoscopic) with identified risk factors ■ Emergency major surgery (open, percutaneous, or endoscopic) ■ Parenteral controlled substances ■ Drug therapy requiring intensive monitoring for toxicity ■ Decision not to resuscitate or to de-escalate care because of poor prognosis

TABLE 7-6

Categories of medical decision making

	Straightforward	Low Complexity	Moderate Complexity	High Complexity
Number of diagnosis or treatment options	**1 (Minimal)**	2 (Limited)	3 (Multiple)	4 (Extensive)
Amount and/or complexity of data to be reviewed	**1 (Minimal)**	2 (Limited)	3 (Moderate)	4 (Extensive)
Risk of complications, morbidity, mortality (from Risk Table)	**Minimal**	Low	Moderate	High

The following features of the encounter are used to determine the correct code based on history, examination, and medical decision making.

Category of service:	Office and/or outpatient—established patient
History:	Expanded problem focused
Examination:	Expanded problem focused
Medical decision making:	Straightforward

On the basis of the 1995 and 1997 CMS guidelines, the level of service the physician should have selected is expanded problem focused (99213)—**two out of three key components** for an established patient.

The Audit Tool

Now see how the audit tool should look. Verify the services billed on the charge ticket (Figure 7-1) with the level of service documented to determine if the practitioner billed the level of service documented to the insurance carrier. See Figure 7-2.

FIGURE 7-1

Charge ticket for patient Angela Cooper

OFFICE VISITS	Code	Fee		PROCEDURES	Code	Fee		IMMUNIZATIONS	Code	Fee
NEW				Aerosol Tx – Initial	94664			PPD (intradermal)	86580	
Exam Problem Focused	99201			Aerosol Tx - Subsequent	94665			TB Tine	86586	
Exam Exp Prob Focused	99202			Anoscopy	46600			Admin of vaccine-single	90471	
Exam Detailed	99203			Catheterization	53670			Admin of vaccine-2+	90472	
Exam Comp/Mod Complexity	99204			Cerumen removal	69210			Hib, HbOC-4 dose	90645	
Exam Comp/High Complexity	99205			Endometrial Biopsy	58100			Hib, PRP-D booster only	90646	
				Excision, benign lesion				Hib, PRP-OMP-3 dose	90647	
ESTABLISHED				Size Loc				Hib, PRP-T-4-dose	90648	
Exam Minimal w/Supervision	99211			Excision, malignant lesion				Influenza/whole virus		
Exam Problem Focused	99212			Size Loc				G0008 V04.8	90659	
x Exam Exp Prob Focused	99213	**65**		Excision, Skin Tags	11200			DtaP V06.8	90700	
Exam Detailed	99214			EKG with Interp	93000			DPT V06.1	90701	
Exam Comprehensive	99215			EKG rhythm strip	93040			DT pediatric V06.5	90702	
				I & D (abscess)	10060			Rubella V04.3	90706	
PREVENTIVE MEDICINE				Laceration repair				MMR V06.4	90707	
NEW				Size Loc				OPV V04.0	90712	
Physical infant – 1 yr	99381			Spirometry	94010			IPOL V04.0	90713	
Physical 1 yr – 4 yr	99382			Wart destruction	17110			Varicella V05.4	90716	
Physical 5 yr – 11 yr	99383			Sigmoidoscopy (flex)	45330			Td adult V06.5	90718	
Physical 12 yr – 17 yr	99384			Sigmoidoscopy (flex) w/biopsy	45331			DPT/HIB V06.8	90720	
Physical 18 yr – 39 yr	99385			Laryngoscopy/Diagnostic	31575			DTaP/HIB V06.8	90721	
Physical 40 yr – 64 yr	99386							Pneumoccoccal:		
Physical 65 yr – over	99387							G0009 V03.82	90732	
				OFFICE LABS				HEP B, PED/ADOL, IM V03.82	90744	
PREVENTIVE MEDICINE ESTABLISHED				Blood glucose	82962			HEP B, ADOL/RISK, IM V05.3	90745	
Physical infant – 1 yr	99391			Hemoccult	82270			HEP B, ADULT, IM V05.3	90746	
Physical 1 yr – 4 yr	99392			Medicare Hemoccult	G0107			HEP B/HIB V06.8	90748	
Physical 5 yr – 11 yr	99393			Hemoglobin QW	85018			**INJECTIONS**		
Physical 12 yr – 17 yr	99394			Pregnancy test	81025			Allergy-1	95115	
Physical 18 yr – 39 yr	99395			Strep test (quick) QW	86588			Allergy-2 or more	95117	
Physical 40 yr – 64 yr	99396			Urine dip with micro	81000			Benadryl < 50 mg	J1200	
Physical 65 yr - over	99397			Urine dip only	81002			Compazine < 10 mg	J0780	
				Urine micro only	81015			DepoMedrol 40 mg	J1030	
				Wet mount Q0111	87210			DepoMedrol 80 mg	J1040	
				Venipuncture/fingerstick	36415			Dexamethasone < 4 mg	J1100	
				Medicare venipuncture	G0001					
				SUPPLIES	99070			**DIAGNOSIS**		
				Medicare	A4550					
								Epistaxis	784.7	
				FORMS						
				Special Reports						

Patient: Cooper, Angela   DOB: 07/20/56   Date of Service: 11/01/2001   Return Visit: PRN

Multi-Specialty Group
Ima Caring, MD
555 Constitutional Boulevard
Anytown, USA 14589

FIGURE 7-2

Audit tool for patient Angela Cooper

Patient Name: Angela Cooper   DOB: 07/20/56

Date of Service: 11/01/2001   Practice CPT code(s) selected: 99213

Practice Diagnosis code(s) selected: 784.7 Epistaxis   Documented Diagnosis: 784.7 Epistaxis

HISTORY ELEMENTS: Chief complaint, history of present illness (HPI), review of systems (ROS), past medical, family, social history (PFSH)

History of Presenting Illness (HPI) Elements	Review of Systems	History
HPI ELEMENTS ■ Location ■ Quality ❑ Severity ■ Duration ❑ Timing ❑ Context ■ Modifying Factors ❑ Associated Signs and Symptoms	**ROS Elements** ❑ Constitutional ❑ Eyes ❑ ENT/mouth ■ CV ■ Resp ❑ GI ❑ GU ❑ Musculoskeletal ❑ Integ/Skin/Breast ❑ Neurological ❑ Psych ❑ Endo ❑ Hem/lymph ❑ Allerg/Immuno	■ Past Medical ■ Family ■ Social ❑ Past Medical ❑ Family History ❑ Social History
Brief (Min-1) Extended-AT LEAST 4 or at least 3 Chronic DX (1997) guidelines	Problem Pertinent (1) Extended (2-9 systems) Comprehensive (Min-10 required)	Problem Focused N/A Expanded Problem Focused N/A Detailed- 1 Comprehensive-2 Established 3-New

Documented History

❑ Problem focused   ■ Expanded problem focused   ❑ Detailed   ❑ Comprehensive

GENERAL MULTI-SYSTEM EXAMINATION

Exam	At least 1 element identified by a bullet from any system	6 items identified by a bullet from any system	2 items identified by a bullet from a minimum of 6 systems (12)	2 items identified by a bullet from a minimum of 9 systems (18)
Constitutional	❑ Any one of three vitals	❑ General Appearance of Patient		
Eyes	❑ Conjunctiva and Lids	❑ Pupils & Irises	❑ Optic Discs	
ENT	■ External Ears & Nose	❑ Hearing	■ EACs & TM	■ Nasal Mucosa Septum & Turbinates
Neck	■ Exam of Oropharynx; oral mucosa, salivary glands, hard and soft palates, tongue, tonsils and posterior pharynx			
Respiratory	■ Neck ❑ Thyroid			
Cardiovascular	❑ Respiratory Effort	■ Percussion	❑ Palpation	■ Auscultation
Chest	❑ Palpation of heart ❑ Auscultation ❑ Carotids ❑ Abdominal Aorta ❑ Femoral ❑ Pedal Pulses ❑ Extremities for edema and varicosities			

FIGURE 7-2 *continued*

Audit tool for patient Angela Cooper

Exam	At least 1 element identified by a bullet from any system	6 items identified by a bullet from any system	2 items identified by a bullet from a minimum of 6 systems (12)	2 items identified by a bullet from a minimum of 9 systems (18)
GI (Abdomen)	❑ Inspection of breasts ❑ Palpation of breast and axillae			

GU	❑ Masses/tenderness ❑ Liver and spleen ❑ Hernia ❑ Anus, perineum, & rectum
	❑ Occult test
	    Male: ❑ Scrotal contents ❑ Penis ❑ Prostate Glands
	    Female: ❑ External genitalia ❑ Urethra ❑ Bladder ❑ Cervix ❑ Uterus
	    ❑ Adnexa/parametria			

Lymph	❑ Lymph nodes in 2 or more areas ❑ Neck ❑ Axillae ❑ Groin ❑ Other			
Musculoskeletal	❑ Gait & station ❑ Digits & Nails muscles of at least one area ❑ 1) head, neck 2) spine, ribs, pelvis 3) right upper extremity 4) left upper extremity 5) right lower extremity 6) left lower extremity; with exam including ❑ Inspection and/or palpation ❑ ROM ❑ Stability ❑ Strength & tone			
Skin	❑ Inspection of skin and subcutaneous tissues ❑ Palpation of skin and subcutaneous tissues			
Neuro	❑ Cranial nerves ❑ Reflexes ❑ Sensation ❑ Judgment & insight ❑ Orientation to time, place & person			
Psychiatric	❑ Memory ❑ Mood & affect			

Documented Exam

❑ Problem focused   ■ Expanded problem focused   ❑ Detailed   ❑ Comprehensive

Level of Exam 1995: <u>Expanded Problem Focused</u>

Level of Exam 1997: <u>Expanded Problem Focused</u>

Medical Decision Making

Audit of Evaluation and Management Service

Number of Diagnoses and Management Options	Points Assigned	Points Per Category	Amount and Complexity of Data	Points Assigned	Points Per Category
Self-Limiting or Minor Problems (stable, improved, or worsening) Maximum of 2 points can be given	1	1	Ordered and/or reviewed clinical lab	1	
Established Problem – Stable Improved	1		Ordered and/or reviewed radiology	1	
Established Problem – Worsening	2		Discussed tests with performing or interpreting physician	1	
New Problem – No Additional Workup Planned	3		Ordered and/or reviewed test in the CPT	1	
Maximum of 1 problem given credit			Medicine Section		
New Problem – Additional Workup Planned	4		Independent visualization and direct view of image, tracing, specimen	2	
			Decision to obtain old records or additional HX from someone other than patient, eg, family, caretaker, previous phys	1	
Total Points:		1	Reviewed and summarized old records and/or obtained history from someone other than patient	2	
			Total Points		0

FIGURE 7-2 *continued*

Audit tool for patient Angela Cooper

Level of Risk	Presenting Problem(s)	Diagnostic Procedure(s) Ordered	Management Options Selected
Minimal	■ One self-limited or minor problem, ie, cold, insect bite, tinea corporis	■ Laboratory tests requiring venipuncture ■ Chest x-ray ■ EKG/EEG ■ Urinalysis ■ Ultrasound, eg, echocardiography ■ KOH prep	■ Rest ■ Gargles ■ Elastic bandages ■ Superficial dressing
Low	■ Two or more self-limited or minor problems ■ One stable chronic illness, eg, well-controlled hypertension, non-insulin-dependent diabetes, cataract, BPH ■ Acute uncomplicated illness or injury, eg, cystitis, allergic rhinitis, simple sprain	■ Physiological tests not under stress, eg, pulmonary function test ■ Noncardiovascular imaging studies with contrast, eg, barium enema ■ Superficial needle biopsies ■ Clinical laboratory tests requiring arterial puncture ■ Skin biopsies	■ Over-the-counter drugs ■ Minor surgery with no identified risk factors ■ Physical therapy ■ Occupational therapy ■ IV fluids without additives
Moderate	■ One or more chronic illnesses with mild exacerbation, progression, or side effects of treatment ■ Two or more stable chronic illnesses ■ Undiagnosed new problem with uncertain prognosis, eg, lump in breast ■ Acute illness with systemic symptoms, eg, pyelonephritis, pneumonitis, colitis	■ Physiological tests under stress, eg, cardiac stress test, fetal contraction stress test ■ Diagnostic endoscopies with no identified risk factors ■ Deep needle or incisional biopsy ■ Cardiovascular imaging studies with contrast and no identified risk factors, eg, arteriogram, cardiac catheterization ■ Obtain fluid from body cavity, eg, lumbar puncture, thoracentesis, culdocentesis	■ Minor surgery with identified risk factors ■ Elective major surgery (open, percutaneous, or endoscopic) with no identified risk factors ■ Prescription drug management ■ Therapeutic nuclear medicine ■ IV fluids with additives ■ Closed treatment of fracture or dislocation w/o manipulation
High	■ One or more chronic illnesses with severe exacerbation, progression, or side effects of treatment ■ Acute or chronic illness or injuries that pose a threat to life or bodily function, eg, multiple trauma, acute MI, pulmonary embolus, severe respiratory distress, progressive severe rheumatoid arthritis, psychiatric illness with potential threat to self or others, peritonitis, acute renal failure ■ An abrupt change in neurologic status, eg, seizure, TIA, weakness, or sensory loss	■ Cardiovascular imaging studies with contrast with identified risk factors ■ Cardiac electrophysiological tests ■ Diagnostic endoscopies with identified risk factors ■ Discography	■ Elective major surgery (open, percutaneous, or endoscopic) with identified risk factors ■ Emergency major surgery (open, percutaneous, or endoscopic) ■ Parenteral controlled substances ■ Drug therapy requiring intensive monitoring for toxicity ■ Decision not to resuscitate or to de-escalate care because of poor prognosis

FIGURE **7-2** *continued*
Audit tool for patient Angela Cooper

Decision Making Total: 2 of 3 Must Meet

Points Assigned	1	2	3	4
Number of DX	❑ Minimal	❑ Limited	❑ Multiple	❑ Extensive
Amount of Data	■ Minimal	❑ Limited	❑ Moderate	❑ Extensive
Risk of Complications	■ Minimal	❑ Low	❑ Moderate	❑ High
Levels	■ Straightforward	❑ Low Complexity	❑ Moderate.Complexity	❑ High.Complexity

Level of Service: History   Expanded Problem Focused
                   Exam   Expanded Problem Focused
                   Medical Decision Making   Straightforward

Chart Note

☒ Dictated   ☐ Handwritten _____   ☐ Form   ☐ Illegible ☒ Note signed
☐ Signature missing ☒ Diagnosis code(s) supported

Other services billed: None _____

Comments:

Level of service supported on charge ticket. Physician billed 99213—expanded problem focused visit for an established patient.

Auditor Signature: *Mary Johnstone, CPC, CCS-P* _____ Date: 02/21/2001

TEST YOUR KNOWLEDGE

Make a copy of the audit tool (located in Appendix B) for each patient encounter (Cases 1 through 10). Review both the charge ticket, chart note, and diagnosis (medical necessity). Complete the audit tool for each encounter. Keep your audit tools handy. The analysis and summary report will be based on these 10 cases.

Case 1

Leghorn, Foghorn   Date of Service: 1/15/2002

S: Patient is here for recheck of extremity swelling. The patient states he has swelling of the right leg at all times. He takes Maxide, one tablet daily.

O: Age 77, weight 195, BP 136/76 by me.
    Lungs: clear
    Heart: sinus rhythm
    Extremities: 2+ pitting edema of the right ankle

A: Mild chronic edema improving on Maxide

FIGURE 7-3

Case 1, charge ticket

OFFICE VISITS NEW	Code	Fee
Exam Problem Focused	99201	
Exam Exp Prob Focused	99202	
Exam Detailed	99203	
Exam Comp/Mod Complexity	99204	
Exam Comp/High Complexity	99205	
ESTABLISHED		
Exam Minimal w/Supervision	99211	
x Exam Problem Focused	99212	45
Exam Exp Prob Focused	99213	
Exam Detailed	99214	
Exam Comprehensive	99215	
PREVENTIVE MEDICINE NEW		
Physical infant – 1 yr	99381	
Physical 1 yr – 4 yr	99382	
Physical 5 yr – 11 yr	99383	
Physical 12 yr – 17 yr	99384	
Physical 18 yr – 39 yr	99385	
Physical 40 yr – 64 yr	99386	
Physical 65 yr – over	99387	
PREVENTIVE MEDICINE ESTABLISHED		
Physical infant – 1 yr	99391	
Physical 1 yr – 4 yr	99392	
Physical 5 yr – 11 yr	99393	
Physical 12 yr – 17 yr	99394	
Physical 18 yr – 39 yr	99395	
Physical 40 yr – 64 yr	99396	
Physical 65 yr – over	99397	

PROCEDURES	Code	Fee
Aerosol Tx – Initial	94664	
Aerosol Tx – Subsequent	94665	
Anoscopy	46600	
Catheterization	53670	
Cerumen removal	69210	
Endometrial Biopsy	58100	
Excision, benign lesion		
Size Loc		
Excision, malignant lesion		
Size Loc		
Excision, Skin Tags	11200	
EKG with Interp	93000	
EKG rhythm strip	93040	
I & D (abscess)	10060	
Laceration repair		
Size Loc		
Spirometry	94010	
Wart destruction	17110	
Sigmoidoscopy (flex)	45330	
Sigmoidoscopy (flex) w/biopsy	45331	
Laryngoscopy/Diagnostic	31575	
OFFICE LABS		
Blood glucose	82962	
Hemoccult	82270	
Medicare Hemoccult	G0107	
Hemoglobin QW	85018	
Pregnancy test	81025	
Strep test (quick) QW	86588	
Urine dip with micro	81000	
Urine dip only	81002	
Urine micro only	81015	
Wet mount Q0111	87210	
Venipuncture/fingerstick	36415	
Medicare venipuncture	G0001	
SUPPLIES	99070	
Medicare	A4550	
FORMS		
Special Reports		

IMMUNIZATIONS	Code	Fee
PPD (intradermal)	86580	
TB Tine	86586	
Admin of vaccine-single	90471	
Admin of vaccine-2+	90472	
Hib, HbOC-4 dose	90645	
Hib, PRP-D booster only	90646	
Hib, PRP-OMP-3 dose	90647	
Hib, PRP-T-4-dose	90648	
Influenza/whole virus		
G0008 V04.8	90659	
DtaP V06.8	90700	
DPT V06.1	90701	
DT pediatric V06.5	90702	
Rubella V04.3	90706	
MMR V06.4	90707	
OPV V04.0	90712	
IPOL V04.0	90713	
Varicella V05.4	90716	
Td adult V06.5	90718	
DPT/HIB V06.8	90720	
DTaP/HIB V06.8	90721	
Pneumoccocal:		
G0009 V03.82	90732	
HEP B, PED/ADOL, IM V03.82	90744	
HEP B, ADOL/RISK, IM V05.3	90745	
HEP B, ADULT, IM V05.3	90746	
HEP B/HIB V06.8	90748	
INJECTIONS		
Allergy–1	95115	
Allergy–2 or more	95117	
Benadryl < 50 mg	J1200	
Compazine < 10 mg	J0780	
DepoMedrol 40 mg	J1030	
DepoMedrol 80 mg	J1040	
Dexamethasone < 4 mg	J1100	
X Vitamin B-12 < 1000 mcg	J3420	
DIAGNOSIS		
Edema	782.3	

Patient: Leghorn, Foghorn   DOB: 05/24/23   Date of Service: 01/15/2002   Return Visit: 2 months

Case 1

Multi-Specialty Group
Howard U. Feeling, MD
555 Constitutional Boulevard
Anytown, USA 14589

P: Continue Maxide daily. Patient also has pernicious anemia and is being given 1000 mcg vitamin B-12 IM today. Patient to follow up in 2 months and continue monthly vitamin B-12 injections for the anemia.

Howard U. Feeling, MD
Howard U. Feeling, MD

Case 2

Deere, Joan   Date of Service: 12/06/2001

CC: Burning on urination and wants pregnancy test.

S: 25-year-old female, who is a new patient, requests a pregnancy test because she stopped BC pills 3 months ago and has not had a period since. She also has burning on urination × 3 days. Patient denies vaginal discharge, fever, hematuria, or nocturia. Denies any nausea or vomiting.

O: Vital signs: T, 98.6; BP, 120/82; Wt, 120 lbs. Well-nourished, well-developed 25-year-old female, cooperative, nervous. Breasts no masses, lumps, or tenderness. Abdomen soft, nontender; no masses palpable. Pelvic exam revealed normal external genitalia and erythematous urethral meatus. Vaginal vault was clear and cervix normal. Fundus small, adnexa without masses or tenderness. Bladder negative for masses or tenderness. Rectal exam was negative for hemorrhoids or masses. Urine dip negative and urine pregnancy test negative.

A/P: 1. Dysuria: begin doxycycline 100 mg po bid × 7 days. She may have urethritis. Will send urine for culture. Encouraged to finish this medication no matter what the culture shows.

       2. Amenorrhea: apparently not due to pregnancy. May be post-pill phenomenon and explained this to her. Patient to return for reevaluation in 1 month or sooner if urinary symptoms have not improved.

Howard U. Feeling, MD
Howard U. Feeling, MD

FIGURE 7-4

Case 2, charge ticket

OFFICE VISITS NEW	Code	Fee		PROCEDURES	Code	Fee		IMMUNIZATIONS	Code	Fee
				Aerosol Tx – Initial	94664			PPD (intradermal)	86580	
Exam Problem Focused	99201			Aerosol Tx – Subsequent	94665			TB Tine	86586	
x Exam Exp Prob Focused	99202	75		Anoscopy	46600			Admin of vaccine-single	90471	
Exam Detailed	99203			Catheterization	53670			Admin of vaccine-2+	90472	
Exam Comp/Mod Complexity	99204			Cerumen removal	69210			Hib, HbOC-4 dose	90645	
Exam Comp/High Complexity	99205			Endometrial Biopsy	58100			Hib, PRP-D booster only	90646	
				Excision, benign lesion				Hib, PRP-OMP-3 dose	90647	
ESTABLISHED				Size ___ Loc ___				Hib, PRP-T-4-dose	90648	
Exam Minimal w/Supervision	99211			Excision, malignant lesion				Influenza/whole virus		
Exam Problem Focused	99212			Size ___ Loc ___				G0008 V04.8	90659	
Exam Exp Prob Focused	99213			Excision, Skin Tags	11200			DtaP V06.8	90700	
Exam Detailed	99214			EKG with Interp	93000			DPT V06.1	90701	
Exam Comprehensive	99215			EKG rhythm strip	93040			DT pediatric V06.5	90702	
				I & D (abscess)	10060			Rubella V04.3	90706	
PREVENTIVE MEDICINE				Laceration repair				MMR V06.4	90707	
NEW				Size ___ Loc ___				OPV V04.0	90712	
Physical infant – 1 yr	99381			Spirometry	94010			IPOL V04.0	90713	
Physical 1 yr – 4 yr	99382			Wart destruction	17110			Varicella V05.4	90716	
Physical 5 yr – 11 yr	99383			Sigmoidoscopy (flex)	45330			Td adult V06.5	90718	
Physical 12 yr – 17 yr	99384			Sigmoidoscopy (flex) w/biopsy	45331			DPT/HIB V06.8	90720	
Physical 18 yr – 39 yr	99385			Laryngoscopy/Diagnostic	31575			DTaP/HIB V06.8	90721	
Physical 40 yr – 64 yr	99386							Pneumoccocal:		
Physical 65 yr – over	99387							G0009 V03.82	90732	
				OFFICE LABS				HEP B, PED/ADOL, IM V03.82	90744	
PREVENTIVE MEDICINE ESTABLISHED				Blood glucose	82962			HEP B, ADOL/RISK, IM V05.3	90745	
Physical infant – 1 yr	99391			Hemoccult	82270			HEP B, ADULT, IM V05.3	90746	
Physical 1 yr – 4 yr	99392			Medicare Hemoccult	G0107			HEP B/HIB V06.8	90748	
Physical 5 yr – 11 yr	99393			Hemoglobin QW	85018			INJECTIONS		
Physical 12 yr – 17 yr	99394			Pregnancy test	81025			Allergy–1	95115	
Physical 18 yr – 39 yr	99395			Strep test (quick) QW	86588			Allergy–2 or more	95117	
Physical 40 yr – 64 yr	99396		X	Urine dip with micro	81000			Benadryl < 50 mg	J1200	
Physical 65 yr – over	99397			Urine dip only	81002	20		Compazine < 10 mg	J0780	
				Urine micro only	81015			DepoMedrol 40 mg	J1030	
				Wet mount Q0111	87210			DepoMedrol 80 mg	J1040	
				Venipuncture/fingerstick	36415			Dexamethasone < 4 mg	J1100	
				Medicare venipuncture	G0001					
				SUPPLIES	99070			DIAGNOSIS		
				Medicare	A4550			Dysuria	788.1	
				FORMS						
				Special Reports						

Patient: Deere, Joan   DOB 11/15/37   Date of Service 12/06/2001   Return Visit: 1 month

Case 2

Multi-Specialty Group
Howard U. Feeling, MD
555 Constitutional Boulevard
Anytown, USA 14589

Case 3

Lorenzo, Sophia   Date of Service: 01/12/2002

HISTORY: The patient is a 62-year-old female, who was referred to me for management of her cardiac problems of coronary artery disease and angina by Dr Olivia Hastings, who is also treating the patient for diabetes mellitus. This is her initial visit. Her current medications include Cardizem, Synthroid, and Micronase. Her most recent angina attack occurred a week ago when she was driving to work and the wheel came off the truck in front of her and flew toward her car, striking it but not causing her to have a loss of vehicle control. She pulled to the side and began to experience substernal chest pain associated with shortness of breath. The sheriff's department arrived. The patient was given some oxygen. She stated that she felt better. Then she went to work and the pain began again. This was associated with nausea and vomiting, diaphoresis, and radiation to both her arms. She states she has had pain before associated with exertion, but it has never lasted this long. She had nitroglycerin but did not have it with her to take when this pain occurred. The patient states that she has had two other anginal episodes that were relieved by nitroglycerin. The patient's past medical history is significant as stated above; she was noted to have had a thyroidectomy at age 47. Her family history is negative for heart disease, and the patient does not smoke or drink and exercises regularly. On ROS, other than symptoms noted above, there were no significant responses in CV and respiratory. All other systems were reviewed and no positive responses were noted.

PHYSICAL EXAMINATION: This is a female patient who appears mildly anxious. Blood pressure, 180/98; pulse, 100; temperature, 98.6; respiratory rate, 20. Blood pressure was repeated with reading of 164/88. HEENT: Atraumatic. Pink conjunctiva. Moist mucous membranes. Neck without jugular venous distention. Lungs clear. Chest with some palpable tenderness along the costochondral junction, but this does not reproduce the patient's pain. Heart regular rate and rhythm without murmur, rub, S3, or S4. Back with minimal thoracic paraspinous muscle tenderness. No edema, erythema, or ecchymoses. Abdomen: obese, nontender. Femoral pulses symmetrical. Extremities: no cyanosis, edema, or clubbing. Nervous system: other than the patient being anxious, unremarkable.

Electrocardiogram performed today revealed a normal sinus rhythm with some ectopy.

IMPRESSION: Angina that appears to be stable at the present time; CAD and type 2 diabetes, which Dr Hastings will continue to follow.

PLAN: Patient will be scheduled for appropriate cardiac workup including echocardiogram, chest x-ray, and laboratory studies. The possibility of cardiac catheterization was discussed with the patient; will wait for results of cardiac testing unless the patient's anginal symptoms worsen.

Howard U. Feeling, MD
_____
Howard U. Feeling, MD

FIGURE 7-5

Case 3, charge ticket

OFFICE VISITS NEW	Code	Fee		PROCEDURES	Code	Fee		IMMUNIZATIONS	Code	Fee
				Aerosol Tx – Initial	94664			PPD (intradermal)	86580	
Exam Problem Focused	99201			Aerosol Tx – Subsequent	94665			TB Tine	86586	
Exam Exp Prob Focused	99202			Anoscopy	46600			Admin of vaccine-single	90471	
Exam Detailed	99203			Catheterization	53670			Admin of vaccine-2+	90472	
X Exam Comp/Mod Complexity	99204	125		Cerumen removal	69210			Hib, HbOC-4 dose	90645	
Exam Comp/High Complexity	99205			Endometrial Biopsy	58100			Hib, PRP-D booster only	90646	
				Excision, benign lesion				Hib, PRP-OMP-3 dose	90647	
ESTABLISHED				Size Loc				Hib, PRP-T-4-dose	90648	
Exam Minimal w/Supervision	99211			Excision, malignant lesion				Influenza/whole virus		
Exam Problem Focused	99212			Size Loc				G0008 V04.8	90659	
Exam Exp Prob Focused	99213			Excision, Skin Tags	11200			DtaP V06.8	90700	
Exam Detailed	99214			X EKG with Interp	93000	45		DPT V06.1	90701	
Exam Comprehensive	99215			EKG rhythm strip	93040			DT pediatric V06.5	90702	
				I & D (abscess)	10060			Rubella V04.3	90706	
PREVENTIVE MEDICINE				Laceration repair				MMR V06.4	90707	
NEW				Size Loc				OPV V04.0	90712	
Physical infant – 1 yr	99381			Spirometry	94010			IPOL V04.0	90713	
Physical 1 yr – 4 yr	99382			Wart destruction	17110			Varicella V05.4	90716	
Physical 5 yr – 11 yr	99383			Sigmoidoscopy (flex)	45330			Td adult V06.5	90718	
Physical 12 yr – 17 yr	99384			Sigmoidoscopy (flex) w/biopsy	45331			DPT/HIB V06.8	90720	
Physical 18 yr – 39 yr	99385			Laryngoscopy/Diagnostic	31575			DTaP/HIB V06.8	90721	
Physical 40 yr – 64 yr	99386							Pneumoccocal:		
Physical 65 yr – over	99387							G0009 V03.82	90732	
				OFFICE LABS				HEP B, PED/ADOL, IM V03.82	90744	
PREVENTIVE MEDICINE ESTABLISHED				Blood glucose	82962			HEP B, ADOL/RISK, IM V05.3	90745	
Physical infant – 1 yr	99391			Hemoccult	82270			HEP B, ADULT, IM V05.3	90746	
Physical 1 yr – 4 yr	99392			Medicare Hemoccult	G0107			HEP B/HIB V06.8	90748	
Physical 5 yr – 11 yr	99393			Hemoglobin QW	85018			**INJECTIONS**		
Physical 12 yr – 17 yr	99394			Pregnancy test	81025			Allergy–1	95115	
Physical 18 yr – 39 yr	99395			Strep test (quick) QW	86588			Allergy–2 or more	95117	
Physical 40 yr – 64 yr	99396			Urine dip with micro	81000			Benadryl < 50 mg	J1200	
Physical 65 yr – over	99397			Urine dip only	81002			Compazine < 10 mg	J0780	
				Urine micro only	81015			DepoMedrol 40 mg	J1030	
				Wet mount Q0111	87210			DepoMedrol 80 mg	J1040	
				x Venipuncture/fingerstick	36415			Dexamethasone < 4 mg	J1100	
				Medicare venipuncture	G0001					
				SUPPLIES	99070			**DIAGNOSIS**		
				Medicare	A4550			Angina	413.9	
								Coronary Artery Disease	414.00	
								IDDM	250.00	
				FORMS						
				Special Reports						

Patient: Lorenzo, Sophia   DOB 11/15/37   Date of Service 01/12/2002   Return Visit: PRN

Case 3

Multi-Specialty Group
Howard U. Feeling, MD
555 Constitutional Boulevard
Anytown, USA 14589

Case 4

Marison, Jack   Date of Service: 01/12/2002

OFFICE VISIT

Reason for Visit f/u PVD, CAD, BPH, CHF

CAD — Very seldom TNG relieves

CHF — SOB only c̄ exertion On Toprol XL

PVD — No pain but swelling. On another diuretic

BPH — Stable

Insulin Dose
AM ___
PM ___
Oral ___
Agent ___

Had a Cataract Surg Three. July 24

BMI < 25

Physical Exam: BP 110/60 (L)   Wt. 159 #   T. 95.7
Tobacco Use   P 60   Ht 70 1/4"
Current
Former
(Never)

Eye ground — not well seen B eye
                          media cloudy
Chest Clear   Heart Reg Rhy   + early cataract

Ext th edema

Assessment/Plan

CAD ———→ Stable)
CHF ———→ Stable)   No changes in Rx presently
PVD ———→ Stable)
BPH ———→ Stable)   ✓ Mg ✓ d/c slow Mg if OK
                      Reduce allopurinol to 100 q4.

Follow-Up:

Rec 4 mo

Patient Billed for:

Howard U. Feeling, MD
Howard U. Feeling, MD

FIGURE 7-6

Case 4, charge ticket

OFFICE VISITS NEW	Code	Fee		PROCEDURES	Code	Fee		IMMUNIZATIONS	Code	Fee
				Aerosol Tx – Initial	94664			PPD (intradermal)	86580	
Exam Problem Focused	99201			Aerosol Tx – Subsequent	94665			TB Tine	86586	
Exam Exp Prob Focused	99202			Anoscopy	46600			Admin of vaccine-single	90471	
Exam Detailed	99203			Catheterization	53670			Admin of vaccine-2+	90472	
Exam Comp/Mod Complexity	99204			Cerumen removal	69210			Hib, HbOC-4 dose	90645	
Exam Comp/High Complexity	99205			Endometrial Biopsy	58100			Hib, PRP-D booster only	90646	
				Excision, benign lesion				Hib, PRP-OMP-3 dose	90647	
ESTABLISHED				Size Loc				Hib, PRP-T-4-dose	90648	
Exam Minimal w/Supervision	99211			Excision, malignant lesion				Influenza/whole virus		
X Exam Problem Focused	99212	65		Size Loc				G0008 V04.8	90659	
Exam Exp Prob Focused	99213			Excision, Skin Tags	11200			DtaP V06.8	90700	
Exam Detailed	99214			EKG with Interp	93000			DPT V06.1	90701	
Exam Comprehensive	99215			EKG rhythm strip	93040			DT pediatric V06.5	90702	
				I & D (abscess)	10060			Rubella V04.3	90706	
PREVENTIVE MEDICINE				Laceration repair				MMR V06.4	90707	
NEW				Size Loc				OPV V04.0	90712	
Physical infant – 1 yr	99381			Spirometry	94010			IPOL V04.0	90713	
Physical 1 yr – 4 yr	99382			Wart destruction	17110			Varicella V05.4	90716	
Physical 5 yr – 11 yr	99383			Sigmoidoscopy (flex)	45330			Td adult V06.5	90718	
Physical 12 yr – 17 yr	99384			Sigmoidoscopy (flex) w/biopsy	45331			DPT/HIB V06.8	90720	
Physical 18 yr – 39 yr	99385			Laryngoscopy/Diagnostic	31575			DTaP/HIB V06.8	90721	
Physical 40 yr – 64 yr	99386							Pneumoccocal:		
Physical 65 yr – over	99387							G0009 V03.82	90732	
				OFFICE LABS				HEP B, PED/ADOL, IM V03.82	90744	
PREVENTIVE MEDICINE ESTABLISHED				Blood glucose	82962			HEP B, ADOL/RISK, IM V05.3	90745	
Physical infant – 1 yr	99391			Hemoccult	82270			HEP B, ADULT, IM V05.3	90746	
Physical 1 yr – 4 yr	99392			Medicare Hemoccult	G0107			HEP B/HIB V06.8	90748	
Physical 5 yr – 11 yr	99393			Hemoglobin QW	85018			**INJECTIONS**		
Physical 12 yr – 17 yr	99394			Pregnancy test	81025			Allergy–1	95115	
Physical 18 yr – 39 yr	99395			Strep test (quick) QW	86588			Allergy–2 or more	95117	
Physical 40 yr – 64 yr	99396			Urine dip with micro	81000			Benadryl < 50 mg	J1200	
Physical 65 yr – over	99397			Urine dip only	81002			Compazine < 10 mg	J0780	
				Urine micro only	81015			DepoMedrol 40 mg	J1030	
				Wet mount Q0111	87210			DepoMedrol 80 mg	J1040	
			X	Venipuncture/fingerstick	36415	10		Dexamethasone < 4 mg	J1100	
				Medicare venipuncture	G0001					
				SUPPLIES	99070			**DIAGNOSIS**		
				Medicare	A4550			Coronary Artery Disease	414.00	
								CHF	428.0	
								Peripheral Vascular Disease	443.9	
				FORMS				Benign prostatic hypertrophy	600	
				Special Reports						

Patient: Marison, Jack   DOB: 04/11/27   Date of Service: 01/12/2002   Return Visit: 4 months

Case 4

Multi-Specialty Group
Howard U. Feeling, MD
555 Constitutional Boulevard
Anytown, USA 14589

Case 5

Mary Tyler   Date of Service: 02/01/2002

This is the third office visit for this 65-year-old female who for the past 4 to 5 weeks has been having significant sharp stabbing pains of her anterior chest, primarily with movement, especially when lying down or sitting up. She does not have any palpitations or any significant shortness of breath, cough, wheezing, fever, or chills. She does have a history of COPD with chronic mild exertional dyspnea.

ALLERGIES: NKA.

MEDICATIONS: Lanoxin q day, inhaler as needed

ROS: Eyes: No diplopia or new visual disturbance. Ears, Nose, and Throat: No tinnitus, otalgia, or sore throat. Cardiac: No sustained chest pain or palpitations. Pulmonary: COPD with chronic mild exertional dyspnea. Gastrointestinal: No melena, hematochezia, vomiting, or diarrhea. Musculoskeletal: As per history of present illness. The remaining systems are negative.

EXAM: Well-developed, well-nourished female in mild distress. Skin has no gross abnormalities. Pupils are equal, round, and reactive to light. Extraocular movements intact. Sclerae are clear. Conjunctivae are pink. Ears are normal. Pharynx is clear. Anterior chest wall tenderness, primarily from the mid and lower left sternal border, extending laterally across the costal chondral cartilage. No associated deformity, swelling, erythema. No gross abnormalities. Mildly diminished breath sounds bilaterally with no prominent rales, wheezing, rales, or rhonchi. No rubs. Heart regular rate and rhythm. No murmurs, clicks, or rubs. Abdomen is soft and nontender. Bowel sounds are normal. No masses. Extremities: Good color and warmth. EKG: dual-chamber pacemaker, rate of 60. Rhythm, sinus. No significant ectopy noted.

ASSESSMENT & PLAN: Chest wall pain. We will be placing her on anti-inflammatory drugs and will start her on the first dose of Motrin here. It is recommended that she go on regular Motrin, limit activities that exacerbate her discomfort, and will be back to see me in 2 weeks.

Howard U. Feeling, MD
Howard U. Feeling, MD

F I G U R E 7-7
F I G U R E 7-7

Case 5, charge ticket

OFFICE VISITS NEW	Code	Fee		PROCEDURES	Code	Fee		IMMUNIZATIONS	Code	Fee
				Aerosol Tx – Initial	94664			PPD (intradermal)	86580	
Exam Problem Focused	99201			Aerosol Tx – Subsequent	94665			TB Tine	86586	
Exam Exp Prob Focused	99202			Anoscopy	46600			Admin of vaccine-single	90471	
Exam Detailed	99203			Catheterization	53670			Admin of vaccine-2+	90472	
Exam Comp/Mod Complexity	99204			Cerumen removal	69210			Hib, HbOC-4 dose	90645	
Exam Comp/High Complexity	99205			Endometrial Biopsy	58100			Hib, PRP-D booster only	90646	
				Excision, benign lesion				Hib, PRP-OMP-3 dose	90647	
ESTABLISHED				Size Loc				Hib, PRP-T-4-dose	90648	
Exam Minimal w/Supervision	99211			Excision, malignant lesion				Influenza/whole virus		
Exam Problem Focused	99212			Size Loc				G0008 V04.8	90659	
X Exam Exp Prob Focused	99213	65		Excision, Skin Tags	11200			DtaP V06.8	90700	
Exam Detailed	99214		X	EKG with Interp	93000	45		DPT V06.1	90701	
Exam Comprehensive	99215			EKG rhythm strip	93040			DT pediatric V06.5	90702	
				I & D (abscess)	10060			Rubella V04.3	90706	
PREVENTIVE MEDICINE				Laceration repair				MMR V06.4	90707	
NEW				Size Loc				OPV V04.0	90712	
Physical infant – 1 yr	99381			Spirometry	94010			IPOL V04.0	90713	
Physical 1 yr – 4 yr	99382			Wart destruction	17110			Varicella V05.4	90716	
Physical 5 yr – 11 yr	99383			Sigmoidoscopy (flex)	45330			Td adult V06.5	90718	
Physical 12 yr – 17 yr	99384			Sigmoidoscopy (flex) w/biopsy	45331			DPT/HIB V06.8	90720	
Physical 18 yr – 39 yr	99385			Laryngoscopy/Diagnostic	31575			DTaP/HIB V06.8	90721	
Physical 40 yr – 64 yr	99386							Pneumoccoccal:		
Physical 65 yr – over	99387							G0009 V03.82	90732	
				OFFICE LABS				HEP B, PED/ADOL, IM V03.82	90744	
PREVENTIVE MEDICINE ESTABLISHED				Blood glucose	82962			HEP B, ADOL/RISK, IM V05.3	90745	
Physical infant – 1 yr	99391			Hemoccult	82270			HEP B, ADULT, IM V05.3	90746	
Physical 1 yr – 4 yr	99392			Medicare Hemocult	G0107			HEP B/HIB V06.8	90748	
Physical 5 yr – 11 yr	99393			Hemoglobin QW	85018			**INJECTIONS**		
Physical 12 yr – 17 yr	99394			Pregnancy test	81025			Allergy–1	95115	
Physical 18 yr – 39 yr	99395			Strep test (quick) QW	86588			Allergy–2 or more	95117	
Physical 40 yr – 64 yr	99396			Urine dip with micro	81000			Benadryl < 50 mg	J1200	
Physical 65 yr – over	99397			Urine dip only	81002			Compazine < 10 mg	J0780	
				Urine micro only	81015			DepoMedrol 40 mg	J1030	
				Wet mount Q0111	87210			DepoMedrol 80 mg	J1040	
				Venipuncture/fingerstick	36415			Dexamethasone < 4 mg	J1100	
				Medicare venipuncture	G0001					
				SUPPLIES	99070			**DIAGNOSIS**		
				Medicare	A4550			Chest wall pain	786.52	
				FORMS						
				Special Reports						

Patient: Tyler, Mary   DOB: 01/15/35   Date of Service: 02/01/2002   Return Visit: 2 weeks

Case 5

Multi-Specialty Group
Howard U. Feeling, MD
555 Constitutional Boulevard
Anytown, USA 14589

Case 6

Martin Sharp   Date of Service: 12/20/2001

CC: Diabetic ulcer left foot, elevated blood sugars.

HPI: This 65-year-old Medicare patient presented to the office because of high blood sugars. He also has a long history of insulin-dependent diabetes, chronic renal failure, and coronary artery disease. He had CABG surgery after suffering from a myocardial infarction in 1998. He has diabetic peripheral vascular disease with a history of below-the-knee amputation of his right leg. He presently has an open necrotic area on the left foot, most likely due to PVD. Patient is disabled due to his chronic illness. He denies hypertension, shortness of breath. Significant past history is detailed above. Current Medications: 70/30 insulin in the morning and 20 units in the evening, Cardizem CD 180mg once daily, Imdur 60 mg once a day, Lasix 80 mg one a day, Pepcid 20 mg twice a day, Paxil 10 mg three times a day, Nitrostat as needed

PHYSICAL EXAMINATION

Vital signs:	Temperature 97.7, pulse 77, respirations 20, blood pressure 146/62
HEENT:	Unremarkable
Neck:	Carotid bruit. The neck is supple.
Heart:	Regular rate and rhythm
Lungs:	Clinically clear
Abdomen:	Soft, nontender, no organomegaly
Extremities:	Right below-the-knee amputation. There is a necrotic area on the left heel and an open ulcer on the foot.

The patient's previous lab workup showed a hemoglobin of 9.4, hematocrit of 29.6, white blood count 8.6, platelet count 336,000. Urinalysis is abnormal with 25–50 RBCs, 50–100 WBCs, small amount of bacteria, glycosuria, and proteinuria. Chemistry: sodium 130, potassium 4.1, chloride 92, CO_2 31, anion gap 11, glucose 260. BUN 53 and creatinine 3.2. Blood cultures and urine cultures have been ordered. The patient has been started on Floxin 400 twice a day. He had a CT scan of the head, which is negative.

His EKG reveals right bundle-branch block with right axis deviation, bifascicular block, right bundle-branch block with left posterior fascicular block.

ASSESSMENT AND PLAN
1. Admit to hospital by Dr Brinklemyer
2. Uncontrolled diabetes
3. Atherosclerotic cardiovascular heart disease
4. Diabetic peripheral vascular disease with left heel and foot ulcer
5. Carotid stenosis
6. Status post right below-the-knee amputation
7. End-stage renal disease

Order:
1. CBC, WBC, Chem profile, CXR, EKG
2. IV antibiotics
3. Sliding scale insulin, Accuchecks q 2 hr
4. Whirlpool therapy for ulcers

Howard U. Feeling, MD
_____
Howard U. Feeling, MD

FIGURE 7-8

Case 6, charge ticket

OFFICE VISITS NEW	Code	Fee		PROCEDURES	Code	Fee		IMMUNIZATIONS	Code	Fee
				Aerosol Tx – Initial	94664			PPD (intradermal)	86580	
Exam Problem Focused	99201			Aerosol Tx - Subsequent	94665			TB Tine	86586	
Exam Exp Prob Focused	99202			Anoscopy	46600			Admin of vaccine-single	90471	
Exam Detailed	99203			Catheterization	53670			Admin of vaccine-2+	90472	
Exam Comp/Mod Complexity	99204			Cerumen removal	69210			Hib, HbOC-4 dose	90645	
Exam Comp/High Complexity	99205			Endometrial Biopsy	58100			Hib, PRP-D booster only	90646	
				Excision, benign lesion				Hib, PRP-OMP-3 dose	90647	
ESTABLISHED				Size Loc				Hib, PRP-T-4-dose	90648	
Exam Minimal w/Supervision	99211			Excision, malignant lesion				Influenza/whole virus		
Exam Problem Focused	99212			Size Loc				G0008 V04.8	90659	
X Exam Exp Prob Focused	99213	65		Excision, Skin Tags	11200			DtaP V06.8	90700	
Exam Detailed	99214			EKG with Interp	93000			DPT V06.1	90701	
Exam Comprehensive	99215			EKG rhythm strip	93040			DT pediatric V06.5	90702	
				I & D (abscess)	10060			Rubella V04.3	90706	
PREVENTIVE MEDICINE NEW				Laceration repair				MMR V06.4	90707	
				Size Loc				OPV V04.0	90712	
Physical infant – 1 yr	99381			Spirometry	94010			IPOL V04.0	90713	
Physical 1 yr – 4 yr	99382			Wart destruction	17110			Varicella V05.4	90716	
Physical 5 yr – 11 yr	99383			Sigmoidoscopy (flex)	45330			Td adult V06.5	90718	
Physical 12 yr – 17 yr	99384			Sigmoidoscopy (flex) w/biopsy	45331			DPT/HIB V06.8	90720	
Physical 18 yr – 39 yr	99385			Laryngoscopy/Diagnostic	31575			DTaP/HIB V06.8	90721	
Physical 40 yr – 64 yr	99386							Pneumoccocal:		
Physical 65 yr – over	99387							G0009 V03.82	90732	
				OFFICE LABS				HEP B, PED/ADOL, IM V03.82	90744	
PREVENTIVE MEDICINE ESTABLISHED				Blood glucose	82962			HEP B, ADOL/RISK, IM V05.3	90745	
Physical infant – 1 yr	99391			Hemoccult	82270			HEP B, ADULT, IM V05.3	90746	
Physical 1 yr – 4 yr	99392			Medicare Hemoccult	G0107			HEP B/HIB V06.8	90748	
Physical 5 yr – 11 yr	99393			Hemoglobin QW	85018			**INJECTIONS**		
Physical 12 yr – 17 yr	99394			Pregnancy test	81025			Allergy-1	95115	
Physical 18 yr – 39 yr	99395			Strep test (quick) QW	86588			Allergy-2 or more	95117	
Physical 40 yr – 64 yr	99396			Urine dip with micro	81000			Benadryl < 50 mg	J1200	
Physical 65 yr - over	99397			Urine dip only	81002			Compazine < 10 mg	J0780	
			X	Urine micro only	81015	25		DepoMedrol 40 mg	J1030	
				Wet mount Q0111	87210			DepoMedrol 80 mg	J1040	
				Venipuncture/fingerstick	36415			Dexamethasone < 4 mg	J1100	
			X	Medicare venipuncture	G0001	10				
				SUPPLIES	99070			**DIAGNOSIS**		
				Medicare	A4550			IDDM	250.73	
								Ulcer foot	707.1	
								Atherosclerosis heart	414.00	
				FORMS				Carotid stenosis	433.10	
				Special Reports				S/P below knee amputation	V49.75	
								ESRD	585	

Patient: Sharp, Martin   DOB: 10/20/34   Date of Service: 12/20/2001   Return Visit: Hospital Admission

Case 6

Multi-Specialty Group
Howard U. Feeling, MD
555 Constitutional Boulevard
Anytown, USA 14589

Case 7

Jimmy Dugan   Date of Service: 02/16/2002

Jimmy comes in today after not having been seen for 5 years. He has not been to any other physician. He is the son of James and Ronda Dugan. He called the office earlier this week and wanted to be seen because of unexplainable weight loss over the past year. He has lost some 20 pounds. He is presently divorced, lives alone at home, and is somewhat of a recluse. He is a two-pack-a-day smoker. He does have a chronic cough productive of clear to yellow mucus and did spit up blood on one occasion. He complains of chronic fatigue. He admits that he does not exercise much at all.

Findings today reveal a blood pressure of 130/80. Pulse 100 and regular. His weight is 128 pounds. He looks much older than his stated age. Somewhat haggard, apathetic in expression. Head, eyes, ears, nose, and throat otherwise within normal limits. His lungs aerate poorly throughout. He does have rales in his right base and bilateral rhonchi scattered. His heart tones are fair quality. Regular rate and rhythm are noted. A2 equals P2. No peripheral edema is noted. Abdomen is soft and nontender, no masses. Liver, kidney, and spleen are not palpable. Rectal examination reveals the prostate to be small, smooth, and symmetrical. I did have him get a chest x-ray prior to coming to the office and this was reported to show marked COPD. Dr Davidson, the radiologist, recommended that with the patient's clinical history he definitely advised that he get a chest CT to exclude underlying tumor with higher confidence. He also had a CBC and chem. –8 prior to coming to the office. The sodium and chloride were slightly low and 134 and 96, respectively. His blood sugar was 104. Calcium 8.8.

ASSESSMENT: COPD, rule out occult pulmonary neoplasm.

PLAN: For him to get a chest CT. I discussed the importance of his cessation of smoking at this time. I gave him a starter kit of Zyban protocol. Incidentally, he also had a sed rate, which was elevated at 41 mm per hour. He is to get a chest CT and will plan to see me back in 1 month for follow-up assessment. His appointment for his chest CT is Friday, April 28th, at 2:00 PM.

Howard U. Feeling, MD
Howard U. Feeling, MD

FIGURE 7-9

Case 7, charge ticket

OFFICE VISITS NEW	Code	Fee		PROCEDURES	Code	Fee		IMMUNIZATIONS	Code	Fee
				Aerosol Tx – Initial	94664			PPD (intradermal)	86580	
Exam Problem Focused	99201			Aerosol Tx – Subsequent	94665			TB Tine	86586	
Exam Exp Prob Focused	99202			Anoscopy	46600			Admin of vaccine-single	90471	
Exam Detailed	99203			Catheterization	53670			Admin of vaccine-2+	90472	
X Exam Comp/Mod Complexity	99204	155		Cerumen removal	69210			Hib, HbOC-4 dose	90645	
Exam Comp/High Complexity	99205			Endometrial Biopsy	58100			Hib, PRP-D booster only	90646	
				Excision, benign lesion				Hib, PRP-OMP-3 dose	90647	
ESTABLISHED				Size Loc				Hib, PRP-T-4-dose	90648	
Exam Minimal w/Supervision	99211			Excision, malignant lesion				Influenza/whole virus		
Exam Problem Focused	99212			Size Loc				G0008 V04.8	90659	
Exam Exp Prob Focused	99213			Excision, Skin Tags	11200			DtaP V06.8	90700	
Exam Detailed	99214			EKG with Interp	93000			DPT V06.1	90701	
Exam Comprehensive	99215			EKG rhythm strip	93040			DT pediatric V06.5	90702	
				I & D (abscess)	10060			Rubella V04.3	90706	
PREVENTIVE MEDICINE				Laceration repair				MMR V06.4	90707	
NEW				Size Loc				OPV V04.0	90712	
Physical infant – 1 yr	99381			Spirometry	94010			IPOL V04.0	90713	
Physical 1 yr – 4 yr	99382			Wart destruction	17110			Varicella V05.4	90716	
Physical 5 yr – 11 yr	99383			Sigmoidoscopy (flex)	45330			Td adult V06.5	90718	
Physical 12 yr – 17 yr	99384			Sigmoidoscopy (flex) w/biopsy	45331			DPT/HIB V06.8	90720	
Physical 18 yr – 39 yr	99385			Laryngoscopy/Diagnostic	31575			DTaP/HIB V06.8	90721	
Physical 40 yr – 64 yr	99386							Pneumoccocal:		
Physical 65 yr – over	99387							G0009 V03.82	90732	
				OFFICE LABS				HEP B, PED/ADOL, IM V03.82	90744	
PREVENTIVE MEDICINE ESTABLISHED				Blood glucose	82962			HEP B, ADOL/RISK, IM V05.3	90745	
Physical infant – 1 yr	99391			X Hemoccult	82270	15		HEP B, ADULT, IM V05.3	90746	
Physical 1 yr – 4 yr	99392			Medicare Hemoccult	G0107			HEP B/HIB V06.8	90748	
Physical 5 yr – 11 yr	99393			Hemoglobin QW	85018			**INJECTIONS**		
Physical 12 yr – 17 yr	99394			Pregnancy test	81025			Allergy–1	95115	
Physical 18 yr – 39 yr	99395			Strep test (quick) QW	86588			Allergy–2 or more	95117	
Physical 40 yr – 64 yr	99396			Urine dip with micro	81000			Benadryl < 50 mg	J1200	
Physical 65 yr – over	99397			Urine dip only	81002			Compazine < 10 mg	J0780	
				Urine micro only	81015			DepoMedrol 40 mg	J1030	
				Wet mount Q0111	87210			DepoMedrol 80 mg	J1040	
				Venipuncture/fingerstick	36415			Dexamethasone < 4 mg	J1100	
				Medicare venipuncture	G0001					
				SUPPLIES	99070			**DIAGNOSIS**		
				Medicare	A4550			COPD	496	
								Pulmonary Neoplasm	235.9	
				FORMS						
				Special Reports						

Patient: Dugan, Jimmy DOB: 1/14/49   Date of Service: 02/16/02   Return Visit: 1 month

Case 7

Multi-Specialty Group
Howard U. Feeling, MD
555 Constitutional Boulevard
Anytown, USA 14589

Case 8

Tom Smith   Date of Service: 12/14/2001

S: Tom, an established patient, is in the office today with concerns of a productive cough, which he's had for approximately 3 days. He says he is expectorating some dark yellow secretions. He does also have clear nasal secretions. No chills. No fever. Slight shortness of breath with exertion. No chest pain. No nausea, vomiting, diarrhea, or sore throat. Denies any peripheral edema. He has a long history of arteriosclerotic heart disease status post CABG, and he has been doing well with cardiac rehab.

O: Weight 183 and stable. Blood pressure 140/80. Temperature 96.7°. Pulse 60. Respirations 20. Ear canals are clear. Tympanic membranes are within normal limits. Nasal mucosa suffused with clear discharge. Turbinates slightly reddened and swollen. Posterior pharynx pink. No exudate. Tonsils nonvisualized. No lymphadenopathy present. Neck is supple. Thyroid not palpable. LUNGS: Aerate well throughout. He does have scattered rhonchi bilaterally, but no rales or consolidation or wheezes noted. CVS: Heart tones are clear and distinct. A2 equals P2. He does have a soft grade I-II/VI SEM over the entire precordial area. No peripheral edema is present.

A: 1. Acute bronchitis
    2. Hypertension
    3. CAD post CABG

P: Is to initiate Omnicef 600 mg daily for 10 days. A script was given. Also, Codiclear and Alupent liquid, equal parts, he may have 10 cc every 4-6 hours prn for coughing. Tom knows to let us know if he is no better or if symptoms worsen by Monday.

Howard U. Feeling, MD
Howard U. Feeling, MD

FIGURE 7-10

Case 8, charge ticket

OFFICE VISITS	Code	Fee		PROCEDURES	Code	Fee		IMMUNIZATIONS	Code	Fee
NEW				Aerosol Tx – Initial	94664			PPD (intradermal)	86580	
Exam Problem Focused	99201			Aerosol Tx – Subsequent	94665			TB Tine	86586	
Exam Exp Prob Focused	99202			Anoscopy	46600			Admin of vaccine-single	90471	
Exam Detailed	99203			Catheterization	53670			Admin of vaccine-2+	90472	
Exam Comp/Mod Complexity	99204			Cerumen removal	69210			Hib, HbOC-4 dose	90645	
Exam Comp/High Complexity	99205			Endometrial Biopsy	58100			Hib, PRP-D booster only	90646	
				Excision, benign lesion				Hib, PRP-OMP-3 dose	90647	
ESTABLISHED				Size Loc				Hib, PRP-T-4-dose	90648	
Exam Minimal w/Supervision	99211			Excision, malignant lesion				Influenza/whole virus		
Exam Problem Focused	99212			Size Loc				G0008 V04.8	90659	
X Exam Exp Prob Focused	99213	65		Excision, Skin Tags	11200			DtaP V06.8	90700	
Exam Detailed	99214			EKG with Interp	93000			DPT V06.1	90701	
Exam Comprehensive	99215			EKG rhythm strip	93040			DT pediatric V06.5	90702	
				I & D (abscess)	10060			Rubella V04.3	90706	
PREVENTIVE MEDICINE				Laceration repair				MMR V06.4	90707	
NEW				Size Loc				OPV V04.0	90712	
Physical infant – 1 yr	99381			Spirometry	94010			IPOL V04.0	90713	
Physical 1 yr – 4 yr	99382			Wart destruction	17110			Varicella V05.4	90716	
Physical 5 yr – 11 yr	99383			Sigmoidoscopy (flex)	45330			Td adult V06.5	90718	
Physical 12 yr – 17 yr	99384			Sigmoidoscopy (flex) w/biopsy	45331			DPT/HIB V06.8	90720	
Physical 18 yr – 39 yr	99385			Laryngoscopy/Diagnostic	31575			DTaP/HIB V06.8	90721	
Physical 40 yr – 64 yr	99386							Pneumoccoccal:		
Physical 65 yr – over	99387							G0009 V03.82	90732	
				OFFICE LABS				HEP B, PED/ADOL, IM V03.82	90744	
PREVENTIVE MEDICINE ESTABLISHED				Blood glucose	82962			HEP B, ADOL/RISK, IM V05.3	90745	
Physical infant – 1 yr	99391			Hemoccult	82270			HEP B, ADULT, IM V05.3	90746	
Physical 1 yr – 4 yr	99392			Medicare Hemoccult	G0107			HEP B/HIB V06.8	90748	
Physical 5 yr – 11 yr	99393			Hemoglobin QW	85018			**INJECTIONS**		
Physical 12 yr – 17 yr	99394			Pregnancy test	81025			Allergy–1	95115	
Physical 18 yr – 39 yr	99395			Strep test (quick) QW	86588			Allergy–2 or more	95117	
Physical 40 yr – 64 yr	99396			Urine dip with micro	81000			Benadryl < 50 mg	J1200	
Physical 65 yr – over	99397			Urine dip only	81002			Compazine < 10 mg	J0780	
				Urine micro only	81015			DepoMedrol 40 mg	J1030	
				Wet mount Q0111	87210			DepoMedrol 80 mg	J1040	
				Venipuncture/fingerstick	36415			Dexamethasone < 4 mg	J1100	
				Medicare venipuncture	G0001					
				SUPPLIES	99070			**DIAGNOSIS**		
				Medicare	A4550			Acute Bronchitis	466.0	
								Hypertension	401.9	
								ASHD	414.05	
				FORMS						
				Special Reports						

Patient: Smith, Tom DOB: 04/18/24   Date of Service: 12/14/01   Return Visit: PRN

Case 8

Multi-Specialty Group
Howard U. Feeling, MD
555 Constitutional Boulevard
Anytown, USA 14589

Case 9

Mary Smith   Date of Service: 11/20/2001

Mary comes in today as a new patient. She is the daughter of Joe and Nora Smith. She has been living out in Utah most of her adult life. She has recently gone through a rather nasty divorce and states that she has been harassed by her ex-husband and finally returned to Indiana to start a new life. This was her second marriage and she has been divorced for approximately a year. She moved here 6 months ago. She does have two children by a previous marriage. They are 27 and 21 years of age, both boys. They are not married but have girlfriends or fiancés or ongoing relationships and are still in Utah. Nancy states that she feels tired and extremely stressed. She is working third shift at X Brand Industries on US 31 North. She also states that she has a mole on her right upper arm. This is an irregular, deeply pigmented, but well-circumscribed lesion measuring approximately 8 × 9 mm. She states that she saw a physician at a convenience clinic just before coming out here. The doctor allegedly cut into the lesion and stated that it appeared to be benign and gave her some salve to put on this lesion, and she was instructed to return for follow-up. Ms Smith did not wish to do this but she is worried about the mole. We will schedule outpatient excisional biopsy of this lesion as soon as we can get it on our schedule. The only other health problem that she has is long-standing asthma, and she has an albuterol inhaler, which she used on a prn basis and apparently is getting good results with this.

OBJECTIVE: Ear canals are clean, drums intact. Nose and throat are benign. Neck supple. Thyroid not palpable. Trachea midline. Chest is symmetrical with equal excursions. Breasts are pendulous without mass or discharge. She is still menstruating and has some mastodynia, which is common for her just before her menses. Lungs have expiratory and inspiratory wheezy rhonchi but no rales or consolidation noted. Heart tones are good quality. Regular rate and rhythm are noted. A2 equals P2. Abdomen is soft and nontender. Liver, kidney, and spleen are not palpable.

ASSESSMENT: Situational anxiety depression; nevus of right upper arm; chronic fatigue syndrome.

PLAN: For her to get a chem.-13, lipid profile, and a T_4 and TSH as soon as possible. We will start her on Paxil 20 mg once daily. She is to return in 6-8 weeks for follow-up of the Paxil therapy, and we will also schedule a pelvic and Pap smear at that time.

Howard U. Feeling, MD
Howard U. Feeling, MD

FIGURE 7-11

Case 9, charge ticket

	OFFICE VISITS NEW	Code	Fee		PROCEDURES	Code	Fee		IMMUNIZATIONS	Code	Fee
					Aerosol Tx – Initial	94664			PPD (intradermal)	86580	
	Exam Problem Focused	99201			Aerosol Tx – Subsequent	94665			TB Tine	86586	
	Exam Exp Prob Focused	99202			Anoscopy	46600			Admin of vaccine-single	90471	
	Exam Detailed	99203			Catheterization	53670			Admin of vaccine-2+	90472	
	Exam Comp/Mod Complexity	99204			Cerumen removal	69210			Hib, HbOC-4 dose	90645	
X	Exam Comp/High Complexity	99205	100		Endometrial Biopsy	58100			Hib, PRP-D booster only	90646	
					Excision, benign lesion				Hib, PRP-OMP-3 dose	90647	
	ESTABLISHED				Size Loc				Hib, PRP-T-4-dose	90648	
	Exam Minimal w/Supervision	99211			Excision, malignant lesion				Influenza/whole virus		
	Exam Problem Focused	99212			Size Loc				G0008 V04.8	90659	
	Exam Exp Prob Focused	99213			Excision, Skin Tags	11200			DtaP V06.8	90700	
	Exam Detailed	99214			EKG with Interp	93000			DPT V06.1	90701	
	Exam Comprehensive	99215			EKG rhythm strip	93040			DT pediatric V06.5	90702	
					I & D (abscess)	10060			Rubella V04.3	90706	
	PREVENTIVE MEDICINE				Laceration repair				MMR V06.4	90707	
	NEW				Size Loc				OPV V04.0	90712	
	Physical infant – 1 yr	99381			Spirometry	94010			IPOL V04.0	90713	
	Physical 1 yr – 4 yr	99382			Wart destruction	17110			Varicella V05.4	90716	
	Physical 5 yr – 11 yr	99383			Sigmoidoscopy (flex)	45330			Td adult V06.5	90718	
	Physical 12 yr – 17 yr	99384			Sigmoidoscopy (flex) w/biopsy	45331			DPT/HIB V06.8	90720	
	Physical 18 yr – 39 yr	99385			Laryngoscopy/Diagnostic	31575			DTaP/HIB V06.8	90721	
	Physical 40 yr – 64 yr	99386							Pneumoccoccal:		
	Physical 65 yr – over	99387							G0009 V03.82	90732	
					OFFICE LABS				HEP B, PED/ADOL, IM V03.82	90744	
	PREVENTIVE MEDICINE ESTABLISHED				Blood glucose	82962			HEP B, ADOL/RISK, IM V05.3	90745	
	Physical infant – 1 yr	99391			Hemoccult	82270			HEP B, ADULT, IM V05.3	90746	
	Physical 1 yr – 4 yr	99392			Medicare Hemoccult	G0107			HEP B/HIB V06.8	90748	
	Physical 5 yr – 11 yr	99393			Hemoglobin QW	85018			INJECTIONS		
	Physical 12 yr – 17 yr	99394			Pregnancy test	81025			Allergy–1	95115	
	Physical 18 yr – 39 yr	99395			Strep test (quick) QW	86588			Allergy–2 or more	95117	
	Physical 40 yr – 64 yr	99396			Urine dip with micro	81000			Benadryl < 50 mg	J1200	
	Physical 65 yr – over	99397			Urine dip only	81002			Compazine < 10 mg	J0780	
					Urine micro only	81015			DepoMedrol 40 mg	J1030	
					Wet mount Q0111	87210			DepoMedrol 80 mg	J1040	
				X	Venipuncture/fingerstick	36415	20		Dexamethasone < 4 mg	J1100	
					Medicare venipuncture	G0001					
					SUPPLIES	99070			DIAGNOSIS		
					Medicare	A4550			Situational Anxiety depression	300.4	
									Chronic Fatigue syndrome	780.71	
									Nevus/right arm	216.6	
					FORMS						
					Special Reports						

Patient: Smith, Mary DOB: 09/02/56   Date of Service: 11/20/01   Return Visit: 6-8 weeks

Case 9

Multi-Specialty Group
Howard U. Feeling, MD
555 Constitutional Boulevard
Anytown, USA 14589

Case 10

Troy Dimly   Date of Service: 01/07/2002

Troy comes in today in follow-up of recently diagnosed type II diabetes. He had a hemoglobin A_{1c} on July 29th of 7.4%. He has lost 26 pounds since July and is feeling much better as a result. He also is having problems with erectile dysfunction. We discussed Viagra protocols and I gave him samples and video of same. I counseled him on the unlikely event of anginal type chest pains in proximity to taking Viagra therapy.

OBJECTIVE: Findings today reveal a blood pressure of 130/88. Pulse 80 and regular. His weight is 293 pounds; he weighed 319 pounds on November 7th. Color is good. Head, eyes, ears, nose, and throat within normal limits. Heart and lungs are clear and stable. No peripheral edema is noted.

ASSESSMENT: Type II diabetes; erectile dysfunction.

PLAN: For him to return in 4 months for follow-up assessment. If he has problems in the meantime he knows to get in touch sooner. We will have him get a hemoglobin A_{1c} today and notify him Monday of the result.

Howard U. Feeling, MD
Howard U. Feeling, MD

FIGURE 7-12

Case 10, charge ticket

OFFICE VISITS NEW	Code	Fee		PROCEDURES	Code	Fee		IMMUNIZATIONS	Code	Fee
				Aerosol Tx – Initial	94664			PPD (intradermal)	86580	
Exam Problem Focused	99201			Aerosol Tx – Subsequent	94665			TB Tine	86586	
Exam Exp Prob Focused	99202			Anoscopy	46600			Admin of vaccine-single	90471	
Exam Detailed	99203			Catheterization	53670			Admin of vaccine-2+	90472	
Exam Comp/Mod Complexity	99204			Cerumen removal	69210			Hib, HbOC-4 dose	90645	
Exam Comp/High Complexity	99205			Endometrial Biopsy	58100			Hib, PRP-D booster only	90646	
				Excision, benign lesion				Hib, PRP-OMP-3 dose	90647	
ESTABLISHED				Size Loc				Hib, PRP-T-4-dose	90648	
Exam Minimal w/Supervision	99211			Excision, malignant lesion				Influenza/whole virus		
Exam Problem Focused	99212			Size Loc				G0008 V04.8	90659	
Exam Exp Prob Focused	99213			Excision, Skin Tags	11200			DtaP V06.8	90700	
X Exam Detailed	99214	95		EKG with Interp	93000			DPT V06.1	90701	
Exam Comprehensive	99215			EKG rhythm strip	93040			DT pediatric V06.5	90702	
				I & D (abscess)	10060			Rubella V04.3	90706	
PREVENTIVE MEDICINE				Laceration repair				MMR V06.4	90707	
NEW				Size Loc				OPV V04.0	90712	
Physical infant – 1 yr	99381			Spirometry	94010			IPOL V04.0	90713	
Physical 1 yr – 4 yr	99382			Wart destruction	17110			Varicella V05.4	90716	
Physical 5 yr – 11 yr	99383			Sigmoidoscopy (flex)	45330			Td adult V06.5	90718	
Physical 12 yr – 17 yr	99384			Sigmoidoscopy (flex) w/biopsy	45331			DPT/HIB V06.8	90720	
Physical 18 yr – 39 yr	99385			Laryngoscopy/Diagnostic	31575			DTaP/HIB V06.8	90721	
Physical 40 yr – 64 yr	99386							Pneumoccocal:		
Physical 65 yr – over	99387							G0009 V03.82	90732	
				OFFICE LABS				HEP B, PED/ADOL, IM V03.82	90744	
PREVENTIVE MEDICINE ESTABLISHED				Blood glucose	82962			HEP B, ADOL/RISK, IM V05.3	90745	
Physical infant – 1 yr	99391			Hemoccult	82270			HEP B, ADULT, IM V05.3	90746	
Physical 1 yr – 4 yr	99392			Medicare Hemoccult	G0107			HEP B/HIB V06.8	90748	
Physical 5 yr – 11 yr	99393		X	Hemoglobin QW	85018	25		**INJECTIONS**		
Physical 12 yr – 17 yr	99394			Pregnancy test	81025			Allergy–1	95115	
Physical 18 yr – 39 yr	99395			Strep test (quick) QW	86588			Allergy–2 or more	95117	
Physical 40 yr – 64 yr	99396			Urine dip with micro	81000			Benadryl < 50 mg	J1200	
Physical 65 yr – over	99397			Urine dip only	81002			Compazine < 10 mg	J0780	
			X	Urine micro only	81015	20		DepoMedrol 40 mg	J1030	
				Wet mount Q0111	87210			DepoMedrol 80 mg	J1040	
			X	Venipuncture/fingerstick	36415	10		Dexamethasone < 4 mg	J1100	
				Medicare venipuncture	G0001					
				SUPPLIES	99070			**DIAGNOSIS**		
				Medicare	A4550			Diabetes Type II	250.00	
								Erectile Dysfunction	302.79	
				FORMS						
				Special Reports						

Patient: Dimly, Troy DOB: 03/03/66   Date of Service: 01/07/02   Return Visit: 4 months

Case 10

Multi-Specialty Group
Howard U. Feeling, MD
555 Constitutional Boulevard
Anytown, USA 14589

chapter 8

AUDIT REPORTING
MECHANISMS

LEARNING OBJECTIVES

■ Understand the purpose of a detailed review analysis
■ Understand the purpose of the summary report
■ Create a detailed analysis and summary report
■ Successfully complete end-of-chapter application exercises

ANALYSIS AND REPORTING

The next step of the audit process is to analyze and report the findings for each practitioner in the organization. Another tool necessary is an aggregate report to identify the health of the organization's coding and documentation practices as a whole. You may want to include the following items in the report:

■ Statistical analysis; include the total number of charts reviewed
■ The total number of medical records that support the level of service billed
■ The total number of medical records that support a higher level of service than billed
■ The total number of medical records that support a lower level of service than billed
■ Any other documentation or coding issues (ie, wrong surgical code, bundled code, etc)
■ Observations documenting specific findings
■ Recommendations to correct the problem
■ Identification of any persons responsible for correcting the problem if other than the practitioner

Detailed Review Analysis

Now that the audit is completed for the practitioner, a method of reporting the results should be created. Begin with the review analysis. Analysis is one of the most important steps in completing the audit process. The review analysis consists of the following:

- Patient identification
- Number or name
- Service date
- Practice CPT® codes
- The codes the provider selected to bill the carrier on the basis of documentation
- History
- Documented history
- Documented exam
- Documented medical decision making
- Based on presenting problem, diagnostic tests and data, and risk
- Documented CPT® codes
- Correct CPT® codes based on audit documentation (what level of service was actually documented)

The review analysis should display the findings in an organized format that allows the viewer to draw conclusions. Review the original purpose and objectives of the audit (type of audit). You should have prepared in advance the exact format (empty shell) of the table that the analysis will produce. Naturally, this table will be empty until the audit is complete and all information is gathered.

To prepare the analysis, review the cases audited for the physician. List all the pertinent data for each patient encounter (case number). This will be helpful for you and the provider to see at a glance what level of service was billed and what your audit results show. It will also help identify the charts that you will need to review for each provider audited. Review an example of a detailed analysis in Figure 8-1.

Now that the detailed review analysis is completed, it is time to complete the audit summary report. An example is located in Figure 8-2. This report is helpful when meeting with the provider to summarize the review of the medical records, and to identify any specific problems or recommendations. It is necessary to complete one summary report for each physician.

The summary report consists of the following:

Physician's name
- Physician: John Doe, MD

Date of review
- Date of review: 02/11/00

Reviewer (person who is auditing the medical records)
- Tanya Trickster, LPN, CPC

Number of charts reviewed
- The actual number of charts reviewed for each provider

The summary report should also contain brief statements about what you are looking for when performing the audit. For example, "one service date was reviewed for each chart audited for appropriate coding and supporting documentation. Each chart was reviewed in detail for completeness and the details of specific issues were documented."

FIGURE 8-1

Example of a detailed review analysis

PHYSICIAN MEDICAL RECORD REVIEW

DETAILED REVIEW ANALYSIS

Physician: John Doe, MD

Date of Review: 10/07/01

Reviewer: Tanya Trickster, LPN, CPC

Number of Charts Reviewed: 10

Patient ID	Service Date	Practice CPT® Code	History	Exam	Medical Decision Making	Documented CPT® Code
Terry Hodge	10/08/99	99202 90707	EPF	EPF	Low	99202 90707 90471 Did not bill administration code 90471
Michael Morris	11/09/99	99214	D	EPF-97 D-95	Low	99214-95 99213-97
Trina Lopez	10/14/99	99213	EPF	D	Low	99213
Mary Brennan	11/09/99	99212	PF	PF	SF	99212
Cathy Mark	10/14/99	99213 90659 G0008	EPF	EPF	Low	99213 90659 G0008
Harrison Ford	11/09/99	99396	D	EPF	Low	99213—documentation of history and exam does not appear to meet preventive medicine guidelines
Paul Bunyon	10/4/99	99212	D	PF	SF	99212
Mary Sparks	10/01/99	99213 J1030	PF	PF	Moderate	99212 J1030
Paula Pound	10/01/99	99393 17110	EPF	EPF	SF	99213— documentation of history and exam does not appear to meet preventive medicine guidelines
Thomas Goode	11/08/99	99213	EPF	D	SF	99213

The report may be customized on the basis of individual findings. These numbers may be presented as percentages or numbers, as you wish. Some providers prefer the use of numbers instead of percentages if the records are reviewed on an ongoing basis. Other helpful information includes:

- Evaluation and management (E/M) documentation appeared to support service billed.
- E/M documentation in the record appears to support a lower level of service than billed.
- E/M documentation in the record appears to support a higher level of service than billed.

FIGURE 8-2
Summary report

PHYSICIAN MEDICAL RECORD REVIEW
SUMMARY REPORT

Physician: John Doe, MD   Date of Review: 10/07/01

Reviewer: Tanya Trickster, LPN, CPC

Number of Charts Reviewed: 10

___

One service date was reviewed for each chart reviewed for appropriate coding and supporting documentation. Each chart was reviewed in detail for completeness.

E/M documentation appeared to support service billed.	70%
E/M documentation in the record appears to support a lower level of service than billed.	10%
E/M documentation in the record appears to support a higher level of service than billed.	0
E/M preventive medicine services appeared not to contain a comprehensive history and/or examination and did not qualify for preventive services.	20%

Other documentation coding issues:

1. Updated consent for treatment could not be located in two of the medical records reviewed.
2. All but one report/consultation appeared not to be initialed and/or dated by the provider.
3. Two preventive medicine visits did not appear to contain a comprehensive history based on CPT® guidelines for preventive medicine documentation.
4. Completed problem lists appeared to be located in all but one of the medical records reviewed.
5. A completed medication sheet did not appear to be located in two of the medical records reviewed.

RECOMMENDATIONS

1. Review problem areas with provider.
2. Review documentation guidelines for preventive medicine and documentation requirements for procedures.
3. Review compliance for dating and/or initialing documentation.
4. Review the organization's requirement for a completed medication sheet and complete problem list in each chart.
5. Reaudit medical records in 6 months for compliance.

- E/M documentation for consultation did not appear to support service billed.
- Surgical services appeared to support services billed.
- Surgical services did not appear to support services billed.

Also, other documentation and coding issues should be addressed that may or may not be part of the E/M service. These issues can be anything that is found in the medical record that may need improvement. Listed below are several examples of potential coding issues:

1. Updated consent for treatment could not be located in two of the medical records reviewed.
2. All but one report/consultation appeared not to be initialed and/or dated by the provider.
3. Two preventive medicine visits did not appear to contain a comprehensive history based on CPT® guidelines for preventive medicine documentation.
4. Completed problem lists appeared to be located in all but one of the medical records reviewed.
5. A completed medication sheet did not appear to be located in two of the medical records reviewed.

The last element of the summary report involves the auditor's (reviewer's) recommendations for improvement related to the audit findings. These issues will be discussed with the provider during the meeting.

Below are four examples of recommendations; however, the lists of recommendations vary depending on the specialty, type of practice, and individual coding and documentation issues with the provider.

1. Review problem areas with provider.
2. Review documentation requirements for consultation.
3. Review the 1997 E/M guidelines from the Centers for Medicare and Medicaid Services and the requirements.
4. Reaudit medical records in 6 months for compliance.

Compiling Results

Once the review analysis and summary report are completed for each practitioner, the next step is to schedule a meeting with the practitioner to discuss results of the medical record audit. Set a convenient time for the practitioner to allow for questions and time to review all the problematic medical record documentation. The focus of the meeting should be to explain the deficit areas related to the documentation and coding. Many times an audit discussion concentrates on errors, rather than highlighting the correct documentation and coding as well. Good results reinforce the best coding practices and show where the organization excels.

Target areas that need improvement. Look for trends and patterns that indicate coding and reimbursement variances or changes in procedures. This will help determine follow-up procedures. Review and analyze findings in a timely manner. Set priorities to address findings and take immediate action. It is always difficult to defend against accusations of fraud when you are aware of problems and do nothing to correct them.

It is a good idea to have a copy of the chart in front of you to show the provider specifically, on the basis of E/M and coding guidelines, where the problematic areas are so he/she will understand the areas that require improvement. As an auditor, it is also beneficial to have supporting carrier documentation available to back up what you are telling the practitioner. Some of these tools are as follows:

- Medicare carrier manual
- Medicaid carrier manual
- Third-party payer manual
- Reliable coding and billing publications

Once the practitioner receives the results of the review, this should not be the end. Ongoing audits and training should be standardized within the practice to maintain compliance. For example, if the problematic area is not enough documentation for a detailed level of service, the focus of the next review should be reviewing 10 to 15 detailed visits. If the problematic area is documentation of hospital visits, the next review should focus on hospital visits, and so on.

You might also identify lost revenue if, for example, the practitioner is consistently billing at a lower level than the documentation supports. However, make sure medical necessity supports billing at a higher level.

Once the practitioner understands in which area he or she needs to improve, offer suggestions for how you can help him or her achieve that goal. Coding training might be the next step in expediting change in the practitioner's documentation.

After the meeting, you might want to write a synopsis of the outcome of the meeting with the practitioner to help you with future audits and to document that you covered all deficit areas with the practitioner. Many times the practitioner will have unrelated coding and/or documentation questions. Then, the auditor will need to research the answers and provide supporting documentation and report back to him or her. The auditor must be certain to follow up with the practitioner on a timely basis.

In many cases, the auditor will review findings with a compliance officer, medical director, and/or others who are involved in the maintenance of compliance in the organization. Review Figure 8-3, which is an aggregate summary report for the Compliance Medical Group. This report is helpful in identifying the organization areas of concern and what areas to focus on for improvement.

Reaudit medical records in 6 months for compliance.

Aggregate Analysis

The aggregate analysis gives the organization an overview of the deficit areas at a glance.

FIGURE 8-3

Aggregate summary report

COMPLIANCE MEDICAL GROUP
PHYSICIAN MEDICAL RECORD REVIEW
AGGREGATE SUMMARY REPORT

Reviewer: Tanya Trickster, LPN, CPC   Date of Review: 10/07/01

Number of Charts Reviewed: 40

One service date was reviewed for each chart reviewed for appropriate coding and supporting documentation. Each chart was reviewed in detail for completeness.

E/M documentation appeared to support service billed.   21

E/M documentation in the record appears to support a lower level of service   6
than billed.

E/M documentation in the record appears to support a higher level of service   6
than billed.

E/M documentation appeared to be missing dictation and or a handwritten note.   2

E/M documentation appeared to bill the wrong category of service.   4

E/M documentation in the record appeared to be missing a key component: 3
history, examination, and/or medical decision making

Other documentation coding issues:

1. Updated consent for treatment could not be located in six of the medical records reviewed.
2. All but four reports/consultations appeared not to be initialed and/or dated by the provider.
3. Two dictations appeared to be missing for the date of service reviewed.
4. Three medical records appeared to be missing an E/M key component required to bill the level of service.
5. Completed problem lists appeared to be located in all but three of the medical records reviewed.
6. A completed medication sheet did not appear to be located in six of the medical records reviewed.

RECOMMENDATIONS

1. Review problem areas with provider.
2. Review documentation guidelines for preventive medicine and documentation requirements for procedures.
3. Review compliance for dating and/or initialing documentation.
4. Review the organization's requirement for a completed medication sheet and complete problem list in each chart.

FIGURE 8-4

Aggregate analysis

	E/M office visit documentation appeared to support service billed	E/M documentation in the record appears to support a lower level of service than billed	E/M documentation in the record appears to support a higher level of service than billed	E/M documentation appeared to be missing dictation and or a handwritten note	E/M documentation appeared to bill the wrong category of service	E/M documentation in the record appeared to be missing a key component; history, examination and/or medical decision making	Total Charts Reviewed
Caring, Ima, MD	6	0	2	0	1	1	10
Brinklemeyer, Harrison, MD	7	1	1	1	0	0	10
Doe, John, MD	5	2	1	1	1	0	10
Peterson, George, MD	3	0	2	1	2	2	10
Total	**21**	**6**	**6**	**2**	**4**	**3**	***40***

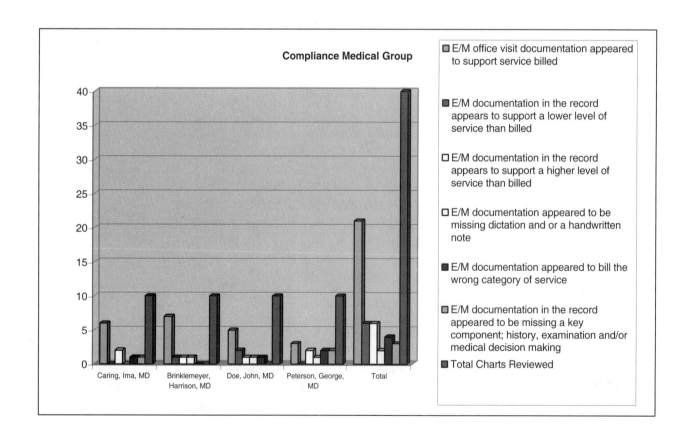

Take Action Based on Findings

A chart audit is useless if no action is taken to correct problematic areas or to acknowledge that the documentation, coding, and billing practices are acceptable. The practitioner, administrator, and/or compliance officer should review the ratio of correct and incorrect coding as well as compliance and non-compliance issues. Areas of incomplete or inaccurate documentation can be identified and corrective action taken.

Gather accuracy rates and trends on the total organization after the analysis and feedback with the practitioner. Encourage staff to discuss difficult coding issues. It may also be helpful to have a consultant or in-house coder to provide coding support to the entire organization on an ongoing basis.

Establish a time frame to make needed changes based on the practitioner's and/or compliance officer's determination of the issues that require immediate attention and those that can wait for long-term revision and implementation.

Determine whether it is necessary to submit a correct claim or refund any overpayments. Develop a policy to direct a course of action after an audit uncovers coding errors. Good communication is an important part of translating an audit into a positive endeavor. After an audit, it is a good time to reinforce compliance and to stress the importance of preventing coding and billing errors and correcting errors already made.

ONGOING MONITORING

It is important after the initial audit to continue to monitor for compliance and to ensure that improvements have been made. Develop a method or process to measure compliance and the effectiveness of the training that has been provided. To accomplish this goal, develop a schedule for subsequent audits. The frequency of the audits will depend on the number of problematic areas and the overall error rate of the organization. Normally audits are conducted monthly, quarterly, semi-annually, or annually. If you are auditing your medical records internally, perform an external audit at least once per year to ensure that the internal findings are objective. It is also important to maintain records or documentation of the follow-up monitoring activities to be able to report later on progress and findings.

EDUCATION AND TRAINING

Once problem areas are identified and a plan for improvement is outlined, a training plan should be implemented. The type and the focus of training is dependent on the problematic areas discovered during the baseline and subsequent audits. Some successful training programs include small groups and one-on-one training. Education should include all staff nurses and billing and coding staff, along with the practitioners. Attendance records should be maintained in addition to copies of the material used. An education schedule should be developed to ensure compliance. Some training suggestions include:

- Review topics where deficit areas are prevalent
- At monthly staff meetings, review coding changes, Medicare bulletins, fraud alerts, etc.
- Highlight quarterly correct coding initiative changes
- Discuss annual coding changes
- Review specific topics related to the specialty
- Present E/M documentation guideline update annually

When the problem is an area identified by a carrier or the Office of the Inspector General, OIG, schedule training immediately after the audit to ensure that compliance and the appropriate steps to resolve the problem areas are taken.

CORRECTIVE ACTION PLAN

Once problem areas have been addressed and training is scheduled, a corrective action plan should be implemented. A provider has a legal obligation to refund any overpayments made for improper coding and/or documentation. It is always a good policy to consult legal counsel before implementing corrective action and repayment. Policies and procedures should be established for reconciliation of audit findings before the baseline audit occurs. Ongoing auditing and monitoring may be conducted according to the established policies and procedures in the organization's compliance plan.

The OIG's self-disclosure protocol is published in the *Federal Register* and is designed "to address the concerns of practitioners by removing disincentives to participation." The OIG also emphasizes that providers have a legal and ethical obligation to identify and correct incidents of non-compliance. The OIG has stated, "while voluntary disclosure under the protocol does not guarantee provider protection from civil, criminal, or administrative actions, the fact that the provider voluntarily disclosed possible wrongdoing is a mitigating factor in OIG's recommendations to prosecuting agencies." Self-reporting offers providers the opportunity to minimize the potential cost and disruption of a full-scale audit and investigation to negotiate a fair monetary settlement, and to avoid an OIG permissive exclusion preventing the provider from doing business with federal health care programs. The OIG publication encourages providers to report suspected fraud, and will provide this information to determine action required after the audit.

The OIG also recommends that practitioners consult legal counsel before self-disclosing errors and/or overpayments to the OIG. Practitioners or organizations that discover errors that result in overpayment should initiate an attorney-client relationship with an attorney experienced in health care compliance and the law.

WHAT TRIGGERS A THIRD-PARTY PAYER AUDIT

Many of the factors that trigger an audit by a federal health care program or insurance carrier are based on specific criteria, which include:

- Ordering excessive tests
- Billing Medicare or another government program for care not provided

- Unbundling of procedures
- Waiving coinsurance and deductibles in absence of financial hardship
- Changing codes to get paid
- Coding based only on reimbursement and not medically necessary services
- Practitioner's profile does not meet the standards of the industry

KEY TERMS

Audit—Examination of the systems used to make sure a department or hospital is running correctly. These systems are sometimes called "monitors." For example, if a refrigerator is used to store medications, it's important that the refrigerator be working properly. An auditor will monitor the refrigerator by checking the thermometer and recording the temperature. The monitor, in this case, is checking the thermometer. An audit checks the thermometer regularly to make sure it is functioning properly.

Baseline audit—The first audit performed for an individual practicioner or group to determine the problematic areas in coding, billing, documentation, and/or compliance.

Correct Coding Initiative—A national policy implemented in 1996 by the Centers for Medicaid and Medicare Services (then the Health Care Financing Administration) aimed at controlling improper or incorrect practices in the filing of Medicare Part B claims.

Corrective action—Action taken to identify problem areas and implement a plan to change patterns and promote correct coding, documentation, and billing.

Detailed analysis report—A report, in table format, that summarizes the charts reviewed and the codes selected by the practicioner vs those documented.

Subsequent audits—Audits performed routinely to monitor coding and documentation practices.

Summary report—A report of audit findings in a simple, easy-to-read format that indicates incorrect coding and documentation and/or billing errors with recommendations for improvement.

Unbundling/bundling—The practices of combining or separating charges for related services. Medicare pays for many tests and procedures as a group. For instance, for a particular diagnosis, all services related to that diagnosis will be "bundled into one payment." "Unbundling" refers to the practice of charging for a service individually when it should have been already covered as part of a group payment. For lab services, the government now says that "panel" tests—lab tests that are grouped or bundled together—must be unbundled if any of the tests are not medically necessary.

Upcoding—The inappropriate practice of assigning a higher procedure code that reflects a higher procedure than what was actually performed. Every procedure performed by a health care provider has a code that corresponds to it. If a procedure requires complex tasks or a large amount of time, it has a higher code number assigned to it.

TEST YOUR KNOWLEDGE

Match the Following Terms:

Summary report	Evaluation and management guidelines	Audit
Training	Aggregate analysis report	Monitoring
Upcoding	Corrective action	Unbundling
	Detailed review analysis	

1. _____ Includes data such as patient ID, date of service, the CPT® code(s) the practice billed along with history, examination, medical decision making, and documented CPT® code(s).

2. _____ The frequency of conducting ongoing audits to maintain compliance.

3. _____ A plan to address deficit areas of compliance and to improve the documentation and coding in the organization.

4. _____ A method of examining the medical record to determine if the level of service billed/coded is supported by the documentation.

5. _____ Coding at a higher level than the documentation supports.

6. _____ A report that summarizes the overall results of an audit for the practitioner.

7. _____ Refers to the practice of charging for a service individually when it should have already been covered as part of a group payment.

8. _____ A report that summarizes the results of an audit for the entire organization.

9. _____ Guidelines that help determine the level of service based on three key components.

10. _____ A method of informing practitioners and/or staff of coding changes, instruction on guidelines, and other issues related to regulations by the insurance carrier.

Fill in the Blanks

11. Why is it important for the auditor to meet with the practitioner to review the audit findings? _____

12. After the auditor completes the audit, what is the next step in the reporting process? _____

13. What types of training are recommended to correct coding and/or documentation problems in the organization? _____
_____

14. Name seven of the criteria that may trigger a third-party or government audit.

_____

_____

_____

_____

_____

_____

_____

15. What step is appropriate for the organization as a course of action after coding errors are discovered during an audit? _____
_____

chapter 9

THE SURGICAL
MEDICAL RECORD

CHAPTER OBJECTIVES

■ Understand surgical terminology
■ Review modifiers used in surgery
■ Understand the general surgery coding guidelines
■ Understand how the Correct Coding Initiative affects coding of the
   surgical service
■ Understand how to review surgery records
■ Understand the reporting mechanisms of the audit
■ Successfully complete end-of-chapter application exercises

CODING BASED ON STANDARD OF SURGICAL PRACTICES

Accurately translating surgical and medical services into CPT® and
ICD-9-CM codes is challenging. Knowledge of procedural and
diagnostic coding rules, as well as a background in medical terminology,
is needed. In addition, specific knowledge of the procedure and services
performed by the physician is vital in assigning the proper CPT® codes.

In order to accurately audit the surgical medical record, the auditor must
have a good understanding of surgical terminology and anatomy. The
auditor must also understand the surgery coding guidelines, insurance
carrier rules, Correct Coding Initiative (CCI) edits, and how to code an
operative report.

Many insurance carriers monitor a physician's billing practices closely for
possible inappropriate billing and/or unbundling. It is essential that the
coding description accurately describe what actually transpired during the
patient encounter. Many activities are common to many or all procedures.

THE SURGICAL PACKAGE

The following are some examples of what is included in a surgical
procedure and cannot be billed separately:

■ Cleansing, shaving, and prepping of skin
■ Draping of patient

- Positioning the patient
- Insertion of intravenous access for medication (IV)
- Administration of sedative by the physician performing the procedure
- Local infiltration of medication—topical, or regional anesthetic administered by the physician performing the procedure
- Surgical approach, including identification of landmarks, incision, and evaluation of the surgical field
- Exploration of operative area
- Fulguration of bleeding points
- Simple debridement of traumatized tissue
- Lysis of a moderate amount of adhesions
- Isolation of neurovascular tissue or muscular, bony, or other structures limiting access to surgical field
- Surgical cultures
- Wound irrigation
- Insertion and removal of drains, suction devices, dressings, pumps into same site
- Surgical closure
- Application and removal of postoperative dressings including analgesic devices
- Application of splints with musculoskeletal procedures
- Institution of patient-controlled analgesia
- Photographs, drawings, dictation, transcription to document the services provided
- Surgical supplies

The area of greatest concern is inaccurately billing separately for procedures considered incidental to the major procedure. Many CPT® surgical narratives in the CPT® book include "with or without" or other language to include or exclude incidental services.

Numerous procedures are done in conjunction with other procedures, and often the CPT® code subsection notes and guidelines will indicate that one code includes a variety of the supporting procedures. It is imperative that new auditors begin the process by understanding the CPT® surgical coding rules and individual insurance carrier rules before auditing a surgical record.

SURGERY CODING RULES

The Surgery section is the largest in the CPT® book. Surgery is divided into 16 subsections. Most Surgery subsections are based on anatomic site (eg, integumentary or respiratory). Subheadings are further divided into category of procedure (eg, shaving or removal). Guidelines are found at the beginning of each of the six CPT® book sections. The guidelines define items that are necessary to appropriately interpret and report the procedures and services contained in that section. The surgery guidelines also contain many unlisted procedure codes presented by anatomic site. When an unlisted procedure code for surgery is used, a special report describing the procedure must accompany the claim. Common throughout the CPT® book are "notes." The information in the notes indicates special instructions

FIGURE 9-1

Note of instructions for grafts or implants

> **Grafts (or Implants)**
>
> Codes for obtaining autogenous bone,
> cartilage, tendon, fascia lata grafts, or other tissues,
> through separate incisions are to be used only when graft
> is not already listed as part of the procedure.

unique to the subheading. These notes should be reviewed before the
surgical procedure is audited. Review the example in Figure 9-1.

Global Surgery Package

Often, the time, effort, and services rendered when a procedure is
accomplished are bundled together to form a surgery package. Payment is
made for a package of services and not for each individual service provided
within the package. The CPT® book describes the surgery package as
including:

- The operation itself
- Local anesthesia: defined as local infiltration, metacarpal/digital block,
  or topical anesthesia
- Normal, uncomplicated follow-up care

The CPT® book further states that follow-up care for complications,
exacerbations, recurrence, and the presence of other diseases that require
additional services is not included in the surgery package. General
anesthesia for surgical procedures is not part of the surgery package, and
general anesthesia services are billed separately by the anesthesiologist

Third-party payers have varying definitions of what constitutes a surgery
package and varying policies about what is to be included in the surgery
package. Because surgery package rules define what is or is not included in
addition to the surgical procedure, the surgery package also defines the
services for which additional charges can or cannot be submitted. Included
in the definition for the surgery package are usually the preoperative care
and postoperative care, including complications up to a predefined number
of days before and after the surgery. The period of time after each surgery is
established by the third-party payer and is referred to as the global surgery
period, which is usually 0 to 90 days.

In order to determine global days, the auditor will need to obtain this
information from the insurance carrier or other sources. Many publications
and software packages on the market address global days for most carriers
and unbundling (Correct Coding Initiative edits).

Review the example below:

> Mary Smith is auditing surgical records for John Goodman, neurosurgeon. She
> must determine global days for this procedure. The patient is a Medicare patient.

TABLE 9-1

Medicare reimbursement tool

CPT® Code	Global Period	Global Split		Medicare Information
61120	90 days	Preoperative	0.11	Multiple surgery reduction
		Intraoperative	0.76	Assist at surgery with documentation
		Postoperative	0.13	
61154	90 days	Preoperative	0.11	Multiple surgery reduction
		Intraoperative	0.76	Assist at surgery with documentation
		Postoperative	0.13	Cosurgery with documentation
				Bilateral procedures allowed
61885	90 days	Preoperative	0.11	Multiple surgery reduction
		Intraoperative	0.76	Assist at surgery with documentation
		Postoperative	0.13	

Mary contacts the fiscal intermediary for Medicare and the following information is provided for the CPT® code(s) she has asked for. Review Table 9-1 above. The left-hand column indicates the CPT® code; the global period is the number of days the practitioner must provide uncomplicated follow-up care to the patient. The global split is the division of the preoperative reimbursement from the surgery and follow-up care. If the physician only provided a portion of the surgical service, reimbursement would be based on this table. The Medicare information is specific rules that apply to the code. This tool is helpful in determining if, for example, a cosurgeon is allowed to participate in the procedure for the payer. Notice that CPT® code 66154 does allow a cosurgeon for this procedure with appropriate documentation. Both the primary surgeon and cosurgeon may be required to provide their operative notes before being paid for the claim to determine how much work each physician provided.

Starred Procedures

Not all procedures include a surgical package. Many of these procedures that do not have a surgery package are identified by a star or asterisk (*) after the code number. Starred procedures have varying degrees of preoperative and postoperative services included with the operative procedure itself. Following the CPT® book guidelines for starred procedures, found at the beginning of the Surgery section, will ensure that the coder is aware of under which circumstances an E/M code may be billed with the procedure code. Review an example of a starred procedure (Figure 9-2) that appears in the CPT® book.

CORRECT CODING INITIATIVE (CCI)

In 1996, the Centers for Medicare and Medicaid Services (CMS) implemented a national policy aimed at controlling improper or incorrect practices in the filing of Medicare Part B claims. Many third-party payers and other insurance carriers now rely on the CCI when initiating policy for surgical procedural coding. The CCI replaced a variety of rebundling programs that were being used by local carriers. A comprehensive review of

FIGURE 9-2
Starred procedure code for simple repair

Repair Simple
Sum of lengths of repairs

12001*	Simple repair of superficial wounds of scalp, neck, axillae, external genitalia, trunk and/or extremities (including hands and feet); 2.5 cm or less
12002*	2.6 cm to 7.5 cm
12004*	7.6 cm to 12.5 cm
12005	12.6 cm to 20.0 cm

CPT® code descriptors, CPT® coding instructions, national and local coding edits, and Medicare billing history was followed by a comment period by specialty societies and the American Medical Association (AMA). After input from these groups and CMS's review of their comments, the code combinations became "correct coding edits."

As an ongoing process, the CCI constantly reviews code combinations and makes recommendations for addition and deletion of combinations from the correct coding edit list. After input is solicited and evaluated from specialty societies and the AMA, the edits are updated quarterly. The absence of a combination from the edit tables does not imply coverage. All changes are controlled and approved by CMS. Local carriers may not add or delete code combinations.

The code combinations fall into two categories and are listed on two tables, ie, Correct Coding (often referred to as rebundling) and Mutually Exclusive. Correct coding edits are established to deny component procedures that should not be separately reported with more comprehensive procedures. Mutually exclusive edits are established to deny one of a combination that would not or could not be performed at the same time on the basis of CPT® code description or standard medical practices. In those instances where it is proper and necessary to report a code combination performed on the same day that is normally prohibited by CCI, the CPT® modifier -59 should follow the procedure code.

UNBUNDLING

Unbundling a code is similar to coding an incidental procedure, but usually involves less subtle fragmenting of a bill. Never divide the components of a procedure when one code covers all the components.

Procedures should be reported with the CPT® and/or HCPCS codes that most comprehensively describe the services performed by the practitioner. Unbundling occurs when multiple procedures are billed separately when the services are covered by a single comprehensive code. Unbundling can result from two problems. The first is unintentional and results from not having a good understanding of coding, and the second is intentional, when practitioners manipulate the coding to maximize payment. Review the following examples of unbundling:

Example 1.   A physician performed a tenotomy with a radical resection of bone tumor on the phalanx of the toe on the left foot. The physician bills both 28175 and 28010. The CPT® definition for both codes is:

■ 28175   Radical resection of tumor, bone; phalanx of toe

■ 28010   Tenotomy, percutaneous, toe; single tendon

In this example, Figure 9-3, the physician has unbundled the codes based on the Correct Coding Initiative. Review the codes bundled into 28175.

Correct coding requires reporting a group of procedures with the appropriate comprehensive code.

FIGURE   9-3

List of codes bundled into code 28175, Correct Coding Initiative, October 2001

28175..............20000	20220	
20240	20550	
28001	28002	
28003	28005	
28008	28010	
28011	28024	
28030	28052	
28054	28072	
28080	28086	
28088	28092	
28108	28111	
28112	28113	
28124	28126	
28150	28153	
28160	28190	
28192	28193	
28234	28280	
28285	28286	
28312	28313	
29130	29131	
69990		

Example 2.   Dr Martin, a pulmonologist, performed a bronchoscopy with a transbronchial lung biopsy with fluoroscopic guidance. The physician billed:

■ 31628   Bronchoscopy (rigid or flexible); with transbronchial lung biopsy, with or without fluoroscopic guidance

■ 31622   Bronchoscopy (rigid or flexible); diagnostic, with or without cell washing (separate procedure)

■ 76000   Fluoroscopy (separate procedure), up to one hour physician time

According to the CCI and CPT® guidelines, the diagnostic bronchoscopy is a component of a therapeutic bronchoscopy, so it would be unbundling to bill 31622 with 31628. Also, 76000 is for 1 hour of fluoroscopy and the CPT® 31628 includes fluoroscopic guidance in the code definition. The correct way to code the encounter is by coding only 31628, because 31622 and 76000 are components of the code.

Reporting separate codes for related services when comprehensive code includes all services related to the comprehensive code is another form of unbundling or fragmentation of a code. See example 3 below.

Example 3.   Dr Smith performed a hysterectomy with severe endometriosis on October 21, 2001. The physician billed the follow CPT® code(s):

■ 58150   Total abdominal hysterectomy (corpus and cervix), with or without removal of tube(s), with or without removal of ovary(s)

■ 58940   Oophorectomy, partial or total, unilateral or bilateral

■ 58700   Salpingectomy, complete or partial, unilateral or bilateral (separate procedure)

Notice in the example above that 58150, the primary diagnosis code billed on the claim, includes the removal of the tubes (salpingectomy) and the ovaries (oophorectomy). By billing all three codes, the physician has fragmented the coding and unbundled the services into three separate services instead of one service, which is the appropriate method of coding the claim.

SEPARATE PROCEDURES

Separate procedures are defined in the CPT® nomenclature as services that are "commonly carried out as an integral component of a total service or procedure." These services are noted in the CPT® book with the parenthetical phrase "(separate procedure)" at the end of the description. When this phrase appears before the semicolon, all indented descriptions that follow are covered by it.

CPT® guidelines instruct that "the codes designated as 'separate procedure' should not be reported in addition to the code for the total procedure or service of which it is considered an integral component." The CPT® nomenclature further instructs that it is appropriate to report a separate procedure code by itself when the service is "carried out independently or considered to be unrelated or distinct from other procedures/services provided at that time." If a separate procedure code is to be reported in addition to other procedures/services, a modifier -59 should be appended. When used with a separate procedure code, modifier -59 indicates "that the procedure is not considered to be a component of another procedure, but is a distinct, independent procedure." Examples of a distinct, independent procedure include:

- Different session or patient encounter
- Different procedure or surgery
- Different site or organ system
- Separate incision or excision
- Separate lesion
- Separate injury (or area of injury in the case of extensive injuries)

Some procedures have the words "separate procedure" after the descriptor. Separate procedure does not mean that the procedure was the only procedure performed; rather, it is an indication of how the code can be used.

For example, the breast biopsy code 19100 has the words "separate procedure" after the description. Procedures followed by the words "separate procedure" are minor procedures that are coded only when they are the only service performed or when the procedure is on a different body area.

Modifier -59 is used with the procedure code to indicate that the procedure was not part of another procedure or service. When the same minor procedure is performed in conjunction with a related minor procedure, the minor procedure is considered incidental and bundled into the code with the major procedure.

Modifier -51 Exempt

Codes in the CPT® book with the symbol ⊘ indicate that the procedure is modifier -51 exempt. These surgical procedures have been determined to be

FIGURE 9-4

Code 44500: a code for a procedure that is modifier -51 exempt

⊘44500 Introduction of long gastrointestinal tube (eg, Miller-Abbott) (separate procedure)

either complex or labor intensive so that reimbursement is not normally reduced. When you find the ⊘ symbol, do not append -51 to the procedure. Review the example in Figure 9-4.

SCOPE PROCEDURES VS OPEN PROCEDURES

Scope procedures are a treatment for:

- Ulcers
- Endometriosis
- Lysis of adhesions
- Varices
- Gastrointestinal bleeding
- Other conditions

Surgical endoscopies include diagnostic endoscopies; do not code separately. Coding is based on the greatest depth reached. Do not code for a visit on the same day of service unless the patient is seen for an unrelated problem; use modifier -25 for the E/M service and the correct diagnosis (ICD-9-CM) code.

When multiple biopsies are obtained (same or different lesion), code only for the biopsies if the lesions are not excised. When multiple biopsies are obtained, code only once (single or multiple). When a biopsy and an excision are performed on different lesions, code both procedures and append a modifier.

Example: 45380   Colonoscopy, flexible, proximal to splenic flexure; with biopsy, single or multiple

DIAGNOSTIC SERVICES VS THERAPEUTIC SERVICES

Diagnostic services are not strictly global procedures. Code the care for the condition for which the diagnostic service was performed, or other concomitant conditions, separately. Diagnostic services may be performed with consultative services. However, the diagnostic services are then part of the overall assessment and should not be the treatment of the patient. The consultant does not assume the patient's medical management. It is important to understand the difference between diagnostic and therapeutic services.

Diagnostic services are performed to determine or establish a patient's diagnosis. This could be, for example, diagnostic arthroscopy or injection procedures for radiography. Diagnostic services include performance of the procedure and recovery of the patient after the procedure. Additional care of the underlying disease or injury may be coded separately. The follow-up period for diagnostic procedures is variable. Check with frequently used payers for their policies.

Therapeutic services are performed for treatment of a specific diagnosis. These services include performance of the procedure, various incidental elements, and normal follow-up care related to the procedure.

When a therapeutic procedure is performed at the same session as the diagnostic procedure, *only* the therapeutic procedure is reported.

> Example: 43235   Upper gastrointestinal endoscopy including esophagus, stomach, and either the duodenum and/or jejunum as appropriate; diagnostic, with or without collection of specimen(s) by brushing or washing (separate procedure)
>
>   43239   Upper gastrointestinal endoscopy including esophagus, stomach, and either the duodenum and/or jejunum as appropriate; with biopsy, single or multiple

When the EGD is performed and a biopsy specimen is obtained, it would be incorrect to code 43235 and 43239 because 43239 includes the diagnostic EGD. CPT® code 43235 is used for diagnostic purposes only.

ADD-ON CODES

Some procedures listed in the surgery section of the CPT® book are commonly carried out in addition to the primary procedure. These additional procedures are listed as "add-on" codes with the + symbol and are listed in Appendix E of the CPT® book. See Figure 9-5. Add-on codes can be identified with descriptors such as "each additional" or "list separately in addition to the primary procedure." An add-on code may not be used alone.

> Example: 44955   Appendectomy; when done for indicated purpose at time of other major procedure (not as separate procedure) (List separately in addition to code for primary procedure) (Principal Procedure Codes: 40490-58999)

FIGURE 9-5

Example of an add-on code

STAND-ALONE CODES AND INDENTED CODES

There are two types of codes: stand-alone codes and indented codes. Only the stand-alone codes have the full description. Descriptions for the indented codes include that portion of the stand-alone code description before the semicolon (;). The purpose of the semicolon is to save space. Review the following two examples of indented codes:

17260   Destruction, malignant lesion, any method, trunk, arms or legs; lesion diameter 0.5 cm or less
17261   lesion diameter 0.6 to 1.0 cm
17262   lesion diameter 1.1 to 2.0 cm

67208   Destruction of localized lesion of retina (eg, macular edema, tumors), one or more sessions; cryotherapy, diathermy
67210   photocoagulation
67218   radiation by implantation of source (includes removal of source)

BEGINNING THE SURGICAL AUDIT PROCESS

The four steps in auditing surgical medical records are as follows:

1. Determine what you are going to review (scope of review).
   - Type of services
   - Dates of services
2. Review operative note for the following information:
   - Preoperative information
   - Patient demographics
   - Surgery date
   - Preoperative anesthesia
   - Indication for procedure
   - Diagnostic reports
   - Intraoperative information
   - Preoperative diagnosis
   - Postoperative diagnosis
   - Surgeon/assistant surgeon/cosurgeons
   - Procedure title
   - Findings
   - Procedure details
   - Tissue/organ removed
   - Materials removed/inserted
   - Closure information
   - Blood loss/replacement
   - Wound status
   - Drainage
   - Complications noted
   - Postoperative condition of patient
   - IV infusion record
   - Signatures

- Legibility
- Support of procedure (CPT/HCPCS)
- Support of medical necessity (ICD-9-CM)

3. Report findings.
   - Complete a detailed analysis and/or summary report for the practitioner.
4. Educate.
   - Provide education on CCI edits, unbundling issues, problematic areas, and coding updates.

Before the auditor can begin auditing a surgical medical record, a tool for auditing should be developed. Following are a sample audit tool (Figure 9-6), a summary report (Figure 9-7), and a detailed analysis (Figure 9-8) that will be used to review the operative reports that will be audited later in the chapter.

Auditing the Surgical Medical Record

When beginning to review the operative report, it is important that you organize the tools you will need. The same types of tools are necessary as for auditing E/M visits and services for the physician. They are:

- Audit tool
- Charge ticket
- CPT® code book
- ICD-9-CM code book
- HCPCS code book
- National Correct Coding Initiative (NCCI) edits (book or software)
- Other pertinent coding publications
- Detailed analysis—for summarizing audit results
- Summary report—reporting audit results

Here are steps to take when auditing the note:

- Begin by making a copy of the operative report, if possible.
- Underline/highlight important information.
- Use medical references for unfamiliar terms.
- Cross out non–code-related documentation.
- Check bundling issues.
- Verify code sequencing when multiple procedures are performed.
- Apply necessary modifiers.

FIGURE   9-6

Sample surgery audit tool

Surgery Audit Tool

Patient Name: Paula Pekin   MR# 245678

Date of Birth: 04/10/32   Date of Procedure: 01/20/2001 Insurance Carrier: Medicare

Surgical Service (s) Billed: 31641   Bronchoscopy with destruction of tumor

Diagnosis Code (s) Billed: 162.4   Malignant neoplasm of middle lobe

Comments: Surgeon did not sign operative report; missing anesthesia on note

Documented	Y	N	N/A	Comments
Preoperative information	☒	☐	☐	
Patient demographics	☒	☐	☐	
Surgery date	☒	☐	☐	01/20/01
Preoperative anesthesia	☐	☒	☐	Not documented
Indication for procedure	☒	☐	☐	Malignant neoplasm of middle lobe
Diagnostic reports	☒	☐	☐	
Intraoperative information	☒	☐	☐	
Preoperative diagnosis	☒	☐	☐	Rule out malignancy
Postoperative diagnosis	☒	☐	☐	Malignant neoplasm of middle lobe
Surgeon/assistant/cosurgeons	☐	☐	☒	
Procedure title	☒	☐	☐	
Findings	☒	☐	☐	Sent to pathology
Procedure details	☒	☐	☐	
Tissue/organ removed	☒	☐	☐	Malignancy
Materials removed/inserted	☒	☐	☐	
Closure information	☒	☐	☐	
Blood loss/replacement	☒	☐	☐	1 pint blood
Wound status	☒	☐	☐	
Drainage	☒	☐	☐	
Complications noted	☐	☐	☒	No complications indicated
Postoperative condition of patient	☒	☐	☐	
IV infusion record	☒	☐	☐	
Signatures	☐	☒	☐	Signature missing on dictation
Legibility	☒	☐	☐	Dictated
Supports procedure (CPT/HCPCS)	☒	☐	☐	31641 Bronchoscopy
Supports medical necessity (ICD-9-CM)	☒	☐	☐	162.4 Malignant neoplasm of middle lobe

FIGURE 9-7
Sample surgery summary report

SURGERY SUMMARY REPORT

Physician: Steven Parkhurst II, MD   Date of Review:
                                                                      02/10/02

Reviewer: Stacy Elmhurst, CPC, CCS, CCS-P

Number of Operative Notes Reviewed: 10

Operative notes were reviewed for completeness and appropriateness of care along with coding documentation and medical necessity.

Documentation in the operative note appears to provide preoperative information	100%
Surgery date appears to be documented in the note	100%
Preoperative anesthesia appears to be documented in the note	80%
Indication for procedure appears to be documented in the operative report	100%
Preoperative diagnosis appears to be documented in the operative report	100%
Postoperative diagnosis appears to be documented in the note and supported by findings	100%
Surgeon/assistant/cosurgeons are listed in the operative note	70%
Findings appear to be indicated in the operative report	100%
Procedure details appear to be documented appropriately in the operative report	100%
Postoperative condition of patient appears to be indicated in the operative report	100%
The operative report appears to support procedure (CPT/HCPCS)	60%
The operative report appears to support medical necessity (ICD-9-CM)	100%

Other Documentation and Coding Issues:

1. Operative report 1—The service for the colonoscopy appeared to be unbundled. Only the therapeutic colonoscopy should be billed. The charge ticket indicated that a diagnostic and the therapeutic colonoscopy were billed together.
2. Two operative notes were not signed by the physician.
3. One operative report indicated multiple procedures, but the charge ticket did not appear to bill a modifier for multiple procedures (-51).

RECOMMENDATIONS
1. Review problem area(s) with provider.
2. Review unbundling guidelines.
3. Review use of modifiers when billing for surgery.
4. Review coding guidelines for therapeutic vs diagnostic procedures on same day.
5. Perform a follow-up audit review in 6 months.

FIGURE 9-8
Sample surgery detailed analysis

GENERAL SURGICAL GROUP
DETAILED ANALYSIS

Physician: Steven Parkhurst II, MD   Date of Review: 02/01/02

Reviewer: Mary R. Smith, CPC, CCS, CCS-P

Number of Operative Notes Reviewed: 10

| | Billed | | | Documented | | |
Patient	CPT ® Code	ICD-9-CM Code	MOD	CPT® Code	ICD-9-CM Code	MOD
Mary Doe	11301	173.6		11301	173.6	
John Renner	20600 20605	354.3 712.9		20600 20605-51	712.86 354.3	 -51
Marie Thomas	42820	474.02		42820	474.02	
Jake Rice	65436 65450 67250	370.55 370.55 370.55	 -51 -51	65436 65450-51	370.55 370.55	
Donna James	32020 33031	423.2 423.2	 -51	33031	423.2	
Susan Grimes	32110 32151 31622	861.32 861.32 861.32	 -51 -51	32110 32151	861.32 861.32	 -51
Renee Patterson	44110	230.3		44110	230.3	
Phil Miller	47425	574.30		47425	574.21	
Gayla Girvin	58661 58720	614.1 620.0	 -51	58661	614.1 620.0	
Norman Peeler	60505 60225	252.0 252.0		60505	252.0	

Begin by auditing exercises 1 through 3. Use the audit tool provided for surgical auditing in Appendix C. Check for correct CPT® coding, diagnostic coding, and codes that are unbundled. Verify what procedures are documented in the operative report vs reported and/or billed on the charge ticket.

Exercise 1

OPERATIVE REPORT 1

PATIENT: Marcus Willoughby   MR# 145678

DATE OF PROCEDURE: 01/04/02

PREOPERATIVE DIAGNOSIS: Refractory severe diarrhea with negative stool cultures

POSTOPERATIVE DIAGNOSIS: 1. No active colitis
2. No pseudomembranes noted
3. Normal terminal ileum that was visualized
4. Internal hemorrhoids

SURGEON: Steven Parkhurst II, MD

PROCEDURE: Colonoscopy to the terminal ileum with random biopsies

DESCRIPTION OF PROCEDURE: Following informed consent the patient was brought to the

endoscopy suite and given IV sedation. Colonoscope was inserted into the rectum and advanced to

the colon and beyond the splenic flexure, maneuvered through the hepatic flexure, and moved down

the ascending colon to the cecum. The appendiceal orifice was visualized and photographed and

was within normal limits. The scope was withdrawn from the right colon, pulled back to the

transverse, descending, sigmoid, and rectum; all adequately visualized and there was no active

colitis and no pseudomembranes noted. There were no masses palpable or mucosal abnormalities.

Random rectosigmoid biopsies were obtained and the scope was withdrawn.

PATHOLOGY REPORT:

Specimens: Tissue rectosigmoid biopsy.

Diagnosis: Histologically unremarkable fragments of superficial colonic mucosa. No evidence of

significant inflammation; no evidence of dysplasia.

Steven Parkhurst II, MD
_____
          Steven Parkhurst II, MD

(exercise continued on next page)

Exercise 1—*continued*

Surgical Coding Charge Ticket 1

Patient Name	Marcus Willoughby
Medical Record Number/Account Number	145678
Surgeon	Steven Parkhurst II, MD
Referring Physician	Thomas Jones, MD
Assistant Surgeon	None
Anesthesiologist	Local
Insurance Company	Medicare
Comments	Postoperative follow-up 2 weeks

Date of Surgery	Facility	Place of Service	CPT Code	Diagnosis Code(s)	Modifier	Quantity	Fee
01/04/02	Methodist Surg Cntr	OH	45380	455.0		1	900.00
01/04/02	Methodist Surg Cntr	OH	45378	787.91	-51	1	400.00

Legend:

Place of Service (POS): OP, outpatient hospital; IP, inpatient hospital; ER, emergency room; O, office

Outpatient hospital surgery centers: Memorial Hospital Surgery Center
Methodist Surgery Center
University Hospital Outpatient Center
Markham Memorial Surgery Center
Acme Hospital

Hospitals: University Hospital
Methodist Hospital
Johnson County Regional Medical Center
St Vincent Hospital Center
Acme Hospital

Surgery Case 1

General Surgical Group
Steven Parkhurst II, MD
4555 Constitutional Boulevard
Anytown, USA 14589

Exercise 1—concluded

Patient Name: Marcus Willoughby   MR# 145678

Date of Birth 02/14/37   Date of Procedure: 01/04/2002   Insurance Carrier: Medicare

Surgical Service(s) billed: 45378 and 45380

Diagnosis Code(s) billed: 455.0 and 787.91

Comments: Unbundled 45380—diagnostic colonoscopy included in therapeutic (45380) physician billed 45378 in addition to 45380 incorrectly

Documented	Y	N	N/A	Comments
Preoperative information	☒	☐	☐	
Patient demographics	☐	☐	☒	Not reviewed
Surgery date	☒	☐	☐	01/04/02
Preoperative anesthesia	☒	☐	☐	IV sedation
Indication for procedure	☒	☐	☐	Refractory severe diarrhea with negative stool cultures
Diagnostic reports	☒	☐	☐	Pathology following surgery
Intraoperative information	☒	☐	☐	OP note gives details of procedure
Preoperative diagnosis	☒	☐	☐	Refractory severe diarrhea with negative stool cultures
Postoperative diagnosis	☐	☐	☒	
Surgeon/assistant/cosurgeons	☐	☐	☒	
Procedure title	☒	☐	☐	Colonoscopy to terminal ileum with random biopsies
Findings	☒	☐	☐	Tissue biopsy negative
Procedure details	☒	☐	☐	
Tissue/organ removed	☒	☐	☐	Rectosigmoid biopsies
Materials removed/inserted	☒	☐	☐	Colonoscope inserted
Closure information	☐	☐	☒	
Blood loss/replacement	☐	☐	☒	
Wound status	☐	☐	☒	
Drainage	☐	☐	☒	
Complications noted	☐	☐	☒	
Postoperative condition of patient	☐	☒	☐	Not documented
IV infusion record	☐	☐	☒	Not available for review
Signatures	☒	☐	☐	
Legibility	☒	☐	☐	Dictated note
Supports procedure (CPT/HCPCS)	☐	☒	☐	Unbundled 45378 and 45380
Supports medical necessity (ICD-9-CM)	☒	☐	☐	

Did the physician (Steven Parkhurst II, MD) code the surgical encounter appropriately? According to CPT® guidelines for surgery coding and the CCI edits, the physician unbundled. Figure 9-9 verifies that CPT® 45378 is a component of 45380 and cannot be billed or charged separately. In some instances a modifier 0 will be appended next to the code pair, indicating that a procedure and/or service that is bundled may not be appended to the code(s) or paid separately. In the CCI edit manual, a modifier 1 indicates that modifier -58 or -59 is allowed and will bypass a carrier edit.

FIGURE 9-9

List of codes bundled into code 45380, Correct Coding Initiative, October 2001

CPT® 45380 ⟶

45380		
36000	36005	36010
36011	36012	36013
36014	36015	36410
45300	45305	45330
45331	45378	45382
45900	45905	45910
45915	46220	46600
46606	46940	46942
69990	90780	90781
90782	90783	90784
94760	94761	

Exercise 2

OPERATIVE REPORT 2

PATIENT: Patricia Beehive   MR# 145679

DATE OF PROCEDURE: 01/21/02

PREOPERATIVE DIAGNOSIS: 4.1-cm infected sebaceous cyst, back.
2.5-cm infected sebaceous cyst, posterior neck

ANESTHESIA: Local

POSTOPERATIVE DIAGNOSIS: Same.

OPERATION PERFORMED: 1. Excision of 4.1-cm benign cyst, back
                     2. Excision of 2.5-cm benign cyst, neck

PROCEDURE: The patient was placed in the prone position, after which
the back and posterior neck were prepped with Betadine scrub and
solution. Sterile towels were applied in the usual fashion, and 0.25%
Marcaine was injected subcutaneously in a linear fashion transversely
over each of the cysts asynchronously. Additional local anesthetic was
administered around the cysts. The lower cyst was excised. The cavity
was irrigated with copious amounts of Marcaine solution and then the
skin edges loosely reapproximated throughout with #3-0 nylon suture.
Following this, Marcaine was injected around the superior of the cyst and
an incision was made transversely across this and the cyst was completely
excised as well. Consequently, reexploration of the wound revealed scar
tissue in the base of the wound, and this was excised as well as possible
to ensure that the cyst was completely removed. The wound was irrigated
with Marcaine and packed with Iodoform, and sterile dressings were
applied. The patient was discharged with verbal and written instructions,
as well as Tylenol #3 for pain and a prescription for 30. Return visit in 3
days for packing removal.

Steven Parkhurst II, MD
Steven Parkhurst II, MD

(exercise continued on next page)

Exercise 2—*continued*

Surgical Coding Charge Ticket 2

Patient Name	Patricia Beehive
Medical Record Number/Account Number	145679
Surgeon	Steven Parkhurst II, MD
Referring Physician	None
Assistant Surgeon	None
Anesthesiologist	Local
Insurance Company	CIGNA
Comments	Follow up 3 days packing removal

Date of Surgery	Facility	Place of Service	CPT Code	Diagnosis Code(s)	Modifier	Quantity	Fee
01/21/02	Office	O	11406	706.2		1	225.00
01/21/02	Office	O	11423	706.2		1	125.00
01/21/02	Office	O	12002	706.2		1	75.00

Legend:

Place of Service (POS): OP, outpatient hospital; IP, inpatient hospital; ER, emergency room; O, office

Outpatient hospital surgery centers: Memorial Hospital Surgery Center
Methodist Surgery Center
University Hospital Outpatient Center
Markham Memorial Surgery Center
Acme Hospital

Hospitals: University Hospital
Methodist Hospital
Johnson County Regional Medical Center
St Vincent Hospital Center
Acme Hospital

Surgery Case 2

> General Surgical Group
> Steven Parkhurst II, MD
> 4555 Constitutional Boulevard
> Anytown, USA 14589

Exercise 2—*concluded*

Patient Name: Patricia Beehive   MR# <u>145679</u>

Date of Birth 02/14/37   Date of Procedure: 01/21/02   Insurance Carrier: CIGNA

Surgical Service(s) billed: <u>_11406, 11423, _12002</u>

Diagnosis Code(s) billed: 706.2

Comments: <u>A simple repair is included in the remove of a benign cyst. The physician billed a simple repair (12002) in addition to the cyst removals (11406 and 11423). Only 11406 and 11423 should be billed.</u>

Documented	Y	N	N/A	Comments
Preoperative information	☒	☐	☐	
Patient demographics	☐	☐	☒	Not reviewed
Surgery date	☒	☐	☐	01/21/02
Preoperative anesthesia	☒	☐	☐	Local anesthesia
Indication for procedure	☒	☐	☐	Infected sebaceous cyst
Diagnostic reports	☐	☐	☒	
Intraoperative information	☒	☐	☐	OP note gives details of procedure
Preoperative diagnosis	☒	☐	☐	Infected sebaceous cyst
Postoperative diagnosis	☒	☐	☐	Same as preoperative diagnosis
Surgeon/assistant/cosurgeons	☐	☐	☒	
Procedure title	☒	☐	☐	Excision 4.1-cm benign cyst, back Excision 2.5-cm benign cyst, neck
Findings	☒	☐	☐	Benign documented in note
Procedure details	☒	☐	☐	
Tissue/organ removed	☒	☐	☐	Cysts removed back and neck
Materials removed/inserted	☒	☐	☐	
Closure information	☒	☐	☐	Packed with Iodoform/sterile dressing applied
Blood loss/replacement	☐	☐	☒	
Wound status	☒	☐	☐	
Drainage	☐	☐	☒	
Complications noted	☐	☐	☒	
Postoperative condition of patient	☐	☒	☐	Not documented
IV infusion record	☐	☐	☒	Not applicable local
Signatures	☒	☐	☐	
Legibility	☒	☐	☐	Dictated note
Supports procedure (CPT/HCPCS)	☐	☒	☐	Billed for simple repair inappropriately
Supports medical necessity (ICD-9-CM	☒	☐	☐	

Did the physician (Steven Parkhurst II, MD) code the surgical encounter appropriately? The answer to the question is no. Dr Parkhurst indicated on the charge ticket that a simple repair (12002) was performed. Before you determine why it is incorrect, review the guidelines for excision of benign lesions in the CPT® book. The guidelines in the CPT® book indicate, "Excision of benign lesions of skin or subcutaneous tissues includes simple closure and local anesthesia." From the operative note, it is doubtful that a repair was even done; the note states, "The wound was irrigated with Marcaine and packed with Iodoform, and sterile dressings were applied." From this statement it appears the physician applied packing and sterile dressings and did not suture or use a material to close the wound. The CPT® codes 11406 and 11423 are correct for the excision of the benign cysts.

The next case that will be audited is an office surgical note. Pay special attention to the note; an office note is less formal and more of a narrative in general. You may need to determine if other services could be billed with the surgery. Remember to have your CPT®, ICD-9-CM, and HCPCS codebooks available along with the CCI edits for the current quarter.

Exercise 3

OFFICE PROCEDURE NOTE 3

PATIENT: Jerry Listen   MR 145785

DATE OF SERVICE: 02/02/02

This is an established patient who presents to the office with a new complaint of left elbow pain. The pain started about a month ago and has progressively gotten worse. It is exacerbated by rotation, flexion, and extension of the elbow. The patient is an avid tennis player and it seems that the pain is aggravated during play. He is in a tournament next week and is requesting help with pain relief. He has been on NSAIDs with very little effect. Denies any trauma, swelling, or warmth to the joint area. Examination revealed the left elbow has no swelling or ecchymosis. There is tenderness over the lateral epicondyle. The left shoulder and wrist are normal. The right upper extremity is normal. Neurological examination was unremarkable. After considering multiple diagnoses and determining the risk to the patient is moderate, the physician's impression is left lateral epicondylitis. The patient was given an injection of Aristospan (triamcinolone hexacetonide) 10 mg into the left elbow at the area of tenderness. He was told to use ibuprofen 600 mg and return for reevaluation in 2 weeks or sooner if the elbow gets worse.

Steven Parkhurst II, MD

Steven Parkhurst II, MD

Dictated: 02/04/02 not proofed

Exercise 3—*continued*

Surgical Coding Charge Ticket

Patient Name	Jerry Listen
Medical Record Number/Account Number	145785
Surgeon	Steven Parkhurst II, MD
Referring Physician	Howard Bruner, MD
Assistant Surgeon	None
Anesthesiologist	Local
Insurance Company	Continental Insurance
Comments	Postoperative follow-up 2 weeks

Date of Surgery	Facility	Place of Service	CPT® Code	Diagnosis Code(s)	Modifier	Quantity	Fee
02/02/02	Office	O	99213-25	726.32	-25	1	75.00
02/02/02	Office	O	20605	726.32		1	150.00
02/02/02	Office	O	J3303	726.32		2	65.00

Legend:

Place of Service (POS): OP, outpatient hospital; IP, inpatient hospital; ER, emergency room; O, office

Outpatient hospital surgery centers: Memorial Hospital Surgery Center
Methodist Surgery Center
University Hospital Outpatient Center
Markham Memorial Surgery Center
Acme Hospital

Hospitals: University Hospital
Methodist Hospital
Johnson County Regional Medical Center
St Vincent Hospital Center
Acme Hospital

Surgery Case 3

General Surgical Group
Steven Parkhurst II, MD
4555 Constitutional Boulevard
Anytown, USA 14589

Exercise 3—*continued*

Patient Name: Jerry Listen   MR# 145785

Date of Birth: 02/14/37   Date of Procedure: 02/02/02   Insurance Carrier: Continental
Insurance

Service(s) billed: 20605, J3303 and 99213-25

Diagnosis Code(s) billed: 726.32 Lateral epicondylitis of elbow

Comments: Billed 99213-25 appropriately; evaluated a new complaint prior to performing the
arthrocentesis (20605). The medication is billed appropriately with a J (HCPCS) code.

Documented	Y	N	N/A	Comments
Preoperative information	☒	☐	☐	
Patient demographics	☐	☐	☒	Not reviewed
Surgery date	☒	☐	☐	02/02/02
Preoperative anesthesia	☐	☐	☒	
Indication for procedure	☒	☐	☐	Left elbow pain
Diagnostic reports	☐	☐	☒	
Intraoperative information	☒	☐	☐	Joint injection
Preoperative diagnosis	☒	☐	☐	Left elbow pain
Postoperative diagnosis	☒	☐	☐	Lateral epicondylitis of elbow
Surgeon/assistant/cosurgeons	☐	☐	☒	
Procedure title	☐	☐	☒	
Findings	☐	☐	☒	
Procedure details	☐	☐	☒	
Tissue/organ removed	☐	☐	☒	
Materials removed/inserted	☒	☐	☐	Joint injection
Closure information	☐	☐	☒	
Blood loss/replacement	☐	☐	☒	
Wound status	☐	☐	☒	
Drainage	☐	☐	☒	
Complications noted	☐	☐	☒	
Postoperative condition of patient	☐	☐	☐	Not documented
IV infusion record	☐	☐	☒	
Signatures	☐	☒	☐	Signature missing on note
Legibility	☒	☐	☐	Dictated note
Supports procedure (CPT®/HCPCS)	☒	☐	☐	Yes
Supports medical necessity (ICD-9-CM	☒	☐	☐	Yes
Other services billed appropriately	☒	☐	☐	E/M evaluation billed with modifier -25 appropriate because physician evaluated new problem before performing procedure

Did the physician (Steven Parkhurst II, MD) code the surgical encounter appropriately? The physician billed an E/M office visit (99213) and appended modifier -25 (separately significant identifiable E/M service on the same day as a procedure or other service). The coding of this encounter is appropriate because the first line of the chart note indicates the patient came into the office with a new complaint of left elbow pain. Before the physician can perform the procedure, an evaluation is indicated to determine if the procedure would be medically beneficial.

KEY TERMS

Bilateral procedures—A unilateral procedure performed bilaterally, in which case the CPT® code is reported once and the modifier -50 is appended to the code. Modifier -50 identifies a procedure performed identically on the opposite side of the body. If the surgical code is bilateral, the CPT® code is reported once, even if the procedure is performed on both sides.

Complications following surgery—Any additional services requiring the intervention of the surgeon during the postoperative period of the surgery when additional trips to the operating room or abnormal medical intervention is necessary.

Excision/destruction—Procedures that remove or cut out a particular body area or part. All "-ectomy" (eg, excision or surgically cutting into) procedures are found under this subheading.

Fragmented or unbundled billing—The practice of separating charges for related services, an issue of great importance in today's health care reimbursement. Medicare, Medicaid, and other insurers carefully review charges and code applications because of this common practice. Often unbundling occurs because the office is submitting obsolete codes from outdated CPT® books. Very few offices intentionally fragment bills with the intent to commit fraud.

Global days—Period during which the carrier includes the follow-up care after the surgical service. Each individual insurance carrier defines the number of global days for each procedure.

Incision—A category of surgical services that involves cutting into the body. All "-otomy" (eg, cutting, making an incision into) procedures are located under this subheading. Incision codes include various drainage, exploration, piercing, puncture, and centesis procedures.

Intraoperative services—Those that are normally a usual and necessary part of a surgical procedure (eg, local, metacarpal, digital block, topical anesthesia, the operation itself).

Introduction or removal—A category of procedures that scope, irrigate, inject, insert, remove, or replace into various body areas.

Multiple procedures—Procedures rendered on the same date of service, at the same operative session, identified by modifier -51. When a procedure is performed with another separately identifiable procedure, the highest valued code is listed as the primary procedure and additional procedures are listed with -51. Operative reports should clearly indicate that the procedures were accomplished through separate incisions.

Other/miscellaneous procedures—Procedures that are unique and are not associated with other groupings. Some of these procedures include endoscopy, arthrodesis, manipulation, amputation, suture, fracture, dislocation, splints, strapping, casts, and unlisted procedures.

Postoperative visits—Follow-up visits after surgery during the postoperative period of the surgery (0–90 days, normally) related to recovery from the surgery. Each carrier defines global days individually.

Repair/reconstruction—Procedures that surgically improve and repair improperly functioning, deformed, or painful parts of the body. All "-orrhaphy" (suturing) or "-plasty" (surgical repair) procedures are found under this subheading.

Separate procedure—A component of a more complex service, usually not identified separately. When performed alone, it may be reported. A procedure that is carried out as an integral part of the total service does not warrant a separate identification. Separate procedure codes are often misread and coded with related cases. Related cases refer to procedures with the same diagnosis, same operative area, and same indication. Linking these procedures is referred to as fragmented billing.

Subsidiary codes/add-on codes—Any CPT® code that states "in addition to"; it does not require the use of modifier -50 or -51. If a subsidiary code indicates the surgical procedure could not be performed independently from the primary procedure, it is used as a supplementary code to the primary procedure and identifies the additional service.

TEST YOUR KNOWLEDGE

Fill in the Blanks

1. What tools are helpful when auditing surgical medical records? _____
    _____

2. Define unbundling: _____

3. Separate procedures are: _____

4. What is the CPT® symbol for new or revised text? _____

5. When diagnostic and therapeutic scope procedures are performed on the same day, how are they billed? _____
    _____

6. Name the four steps in auditing the surgical medical record.

    1. _____
    2. _____
    3. _____
    4. _____

7. What does global surgery package mean? _____

8. When the carrier indicates that the procedure has 60 global days, what does that mean? _____

9. Name at least five elements of the operative report (note).

    1. _____
    2. _____
    3. _____
    4. _____
    5. _____

10. Name the seven steps to take when auditing a surgical note.

    1. _____
    2. _____
    3. _____
    4. _____
    5. _____
    6. _____
    7. _____

chapter 10

TAKE THE
AUDITING CHALLENGE

Review the following 10 exam cases for Harrison Brinklemeyer, MD, at the
Principle Family Practice Group. Audit each medical record individually.
Use the CMS 1997 guidelines and exam tables. Make copies of the
audit tool you choose to audit with from Appendix C. Review the charge
ticket for the services rendered by Dr Brinklemeyer. You might want to
try using all three tools to find the one that works best for you. Once you
have finished auditing all 10 cases, complete the Detailed Analysis and
Summary Report.

FIGURE 10-1

Exam case 1 charge ticket

OFFICE VISITS NEW	Code	Fee	PROCEDURES	Code	Fee	IMMUNIZATIONS	Code	Fee
			Aerosol Tx – Initial	94664		PPD (intradermal)	86580	
Exam Problem Focused	99201		Aerosol Tx – Subsequent	94665		TB Tine	86586	
Exam Exp Prob Focused	99202		Anoscopy	46600		Admin of vaccine-single	90471	
Exam Detailed	99203		Catheterization	53670		Admin of vaccine-2+	90472	
Exam Comp/Mod Complexity	99204		Cerumen removal	69210		Hib, HbOC-4 dose	90645	
Exam Comp/High Complexity	99205		Endometrial Biopsy	58100		Hib, PRP-D booster only	90646	
			Excision, benign lesion			Hib, PRP-OMP-3 dose	90647	
ESTABLISHED			Size Loc			Hib, PRP-T-4-dose	90648	
Exam Minimal w/Supervision	99211		Excision, malignant lesion			Influenza/whole virus		
Exam Problem Focused	99212		Size Loc			G0008 V04.8	90659	
Exam Exp Prob Focused	99213		Excision, Skin Tags	11200		DtaP V06.8	90700	
Exam Detailed (x)	99214	100	EKG with Interp	93000		DPT V06.1	90701	
Exam Comprehensive	99215		EKG rhythm strip	93040		DT pediatric V06.5	90702	
			I & D (abscess)	10060		Rubella V04.3	90706	
PREVENTIVE MEDICINE			Laceration repair			MMR V06.4	90707	
NEW			Size Loc			OPV V04.0	90712	
Physical infant – 1 yr	99381		Spirometry	94010		IPOL V04.0	90713	
Physical 1 yr – 4 yr	99382		Wart destruction	17110		Varicella V05.4	90716	
Physical 5 yr – 11 yr	99383		Sigmoidoscopy (flex)	45330		Td adult V06.5	90718	
Physical 12 yr – 17 yr	99384		Sigmoidoscopy (flex) w/biopsy	45331		DPT/HIB V06.8	90720	
Physical 18 yr – 39 yr	99385		Laryngoscopy/Diagnostic	31575		DTaP/HIB V06.8	90721	
Physical 40 yr – 64 yr	99386					Pneumococcal:		
Physical 65 yr – over	99387					G0009 V03.82	90732	
			OFFICE LABS			HEP B, PED/ADOL, IM V03.82	90744	
PREVENTIVE MEDICINE ESTABLISHED			Blood glucose	82962		HEP B, ADOL/RISK, IM V05.3	90745	
Physical infant – 1 yr	99391		Hemoccult	82270		HEP B, ADULT, IM V05.3	90746	
Physical 1 yr – 4 yr	99392		Medicare Hemoccult	G0107		HEP B/HIB V06.8	90748	
Physical 5 yr – 11 yr	99393		Hemoglobin QW	85018		INJECTIONS		
Physical 12 yr – 17 yr	99394		Pregnancy test	81025		Allergy–1	95115	
Physical 18 yr – 39 yr	99395		Strep test (quick) QW	86588		Allergy–2 or more	95117	
Physical 40 yr – 64 yr	99396		Urine dip with micro	81000		Benadryl < 50 mg	J1200	
Physical 65 yr – over	99397		Urine dip only	81002		Compazine < 10 mg	J0780	
			Urine micro only	81015		DepoMedrol 40 mg	J1030	
			Wet mount Q0111	87210		DepoMedrol 80 mg	J1040	
			Venipuncture/fingerstick	36415		Dexamethasone < 4 mg	J1100	
			Medicare venipuncture	G0001				
			SUPPLIES	99070		DIAGNOSIS		
			Medicare	A4550				
						Carpal Tunnel	354.0	
			FORMS					
			Special Reports					

Patient: Brinkman, Brook   **DOB:** 04/10/72   **Date of Service:** 02/01/02   **Return Visit:** PRN

Exam case 1

Principle Family Practice Group
Harrison Brinklemeyer, MD
4555 Constitutional Boulevard
Anytown, USA 14589

Exam case 1

Patient: Brook Brinkman   Date of Service: 02/01/02   DOB: 04/10/72

HISTORY OF PRESENT ILLNESS: This is an established patient who has been complaining of left wrist pain for approximately 1 year. She has been receiving physical therapy for 6 months and it does not seem to be helping. She is a customer service rep and does repetitive computer work. She has been wearing bilateral wrist supports, which have helped to some extent.

PAST MEDICAL HISTORY: The patient has a history of T and A; hysterectomy 2 years ago; history of diabetes, hypertension. She does not complain of chest pain or shortness of breath or dizziness.

Allergies: No apparent allergies.

Medications: Patient takes Humulin 70/30 and Zestril.

PHYSICAL EXAMINATION:

General: This is a well-developed, well-nourished female in no acute distress. Head is normocephalic. Neck is supple with no masses. Carotid pulse is palpable and trachea is in midline. Chest is clear to auscultation and percussion. Examination of the heart shows no murmurs, gallops, or rubs. Abdomen is negative. Extremities: patient has left wrist weakness, unable to touch thumb and little finger together. There is a prominent mass on the palmar aspect of the left wrist.

PLAN: Patient will be seen at the ambulatory surgery center for carpal tunnel surgery in 2 weeks. In the meantime have placed the patient on pain management and she was placed on short-term disability.

Harrison Brinklemeyer, MD

FIGURE 10-2

Exam case 2 charge ticket

OFFICE VISITS NEW	Code	Fee		PROCEDURES	Code	Fee		IMMUNIZATIONS	Code	Fee
				Aerosol Tx – Initial	94664			PPD (intradermal)	86580	
Exam Problem Focused	99201			Aerosol Tx – Subsequent	94665			TB Tine	86586	
Exam Exp Prob Focused	99202			Anoscopy	46600			Admin of vaccine-single	90471	
Exam Detailed	99203			Catheterization	53670			Admin of vaccine-2+	90472	
Exam Comp/Mod Complexity	99204			Cerumen removal	69210			Hib, HbOC-4 dose	90645	
Exam Comp/High Complexity	99205			Endometrial Biopsy	58100			Hib, PRP-D booster only	90646	
				Excision, benign lesion				Hib, PRP-OMP-3 dose	90647	
ESTABLISHED				Size Loc				Hib, PRP-T-4-dose	90648	
Exam Minimal w/Supervision	99211			Excision, malignant lesion				Influenza/whole virus		
x Exam Problem Focused	99212	45.		Size Loc				G0008 V04.8	90659	
Exam Exp Prob Focused	99213			Excision, Skin Tags	11200			DtaP V06.8	90700	
Exam Detailed	99214			EKG with Interp	93000			DPT V06.1	90701	
Exam Comprehensive	99215			EKG rhythm strip	93040			DT pediatric V06.5	90702	
				I & D (abscess)	10060			Rubella V04.3	90706	
PREVENTIVE MEDICINE				Laceration repair				MMR V06.4	90707	
NEW				Size Loc				OPV V04.0	90712	
Physical infant – 1 yr	99381			Spirometry	94010			IPOL V04.0	90713	
Physical 1 yr – 4 yr	99382			Wart destruction	17110			Varicella V05.4	90716	
Physical 5 yr – 11 yr	99383			Sigmoidoscopy (flex)	45330			Td adult V06.5	90718	
Physical 12 yr – 17 yr	99384			Sigmoidoscopy (flex) w/biopsy	45331			DPT/HIB V06.8	90720	
Physical 18 yr – 39 yr	99385			Laryngoscopy/Diagnostic	31575			DTaP/HIB V06.8	90721	
Physical 40 yr – 64 yr	99386							Pneumococcal:		
Physical 65 yr – over	99387							G0009 V03.82	90732	
				OFFICE LABS				HEP B, PED/ADOL, IM V03.82	90744	
PREVENTIVE MEDICINE ESTABLISHED				Blood glucose	82962			HEP B, ADOL/RISK, IM V05.3	90745	
Physical infant – 1 yr	99391			Hemoccult	82270			HEP B, ADULT, IM V05.3	90746	
Physical 1 yr – 4 yr	99392			Medicare Hemoccult	G0107			HEP B/HIB V06.8	90748	
Physical 5 yr – 11 yr	99393			Hemoglobin QW	85018			**INJECTIONS**		
Physical 12 yr – 17 yr	99394			Pregnancy test	81025			Allergy–1	95115	
Physical 18 yr – 39 yr	99395			Strep test (quick) QW	86588			Allergy–2 or more	95117	
Physical 40 yr – 64 yr	99396			Urine dip with micro	81000			Benadryl < 50 mg	J1200	
Physical 65 yr – over	99397			Urine dip only	81002			Compazine < 10 mg	J0780	
				Urine micro only	81015			DepoMedrol 40 mg	J1030	
				Wet mount Q0111	87210			DepoMedrol 80 mg	J1040	
				Venipuncture/fingerstick	36415			Dexamethasone < 4 mg	J1100	
				Medicare venipuncture	G0001					
				SUPPLIES	99070			**DIAGNOSIS**		
				Medicare	A4550					
								Gastroenteritis resolved	558.9	
				FORMS						
				Special Reports						

Patient: Stoops, Martha   **DOB:** 03/20/25   **Date of Service:** 02/10/02   **Return Visit:** PRN

Exam case 2

Principle Family Practice Group
Harrison Brinklemeyer, MD
4555 Constitutional Boulevard
Anytown, USA 14589

Exam case 2

Patient: Martha Stoops   Date of Service: 02/10/02   DOB: 03/20/25

Patient is returning to our office for follow-up of her abdominal pain. The pain seems to have dissipated. There is some mild soreness that persists. No fever, chills, or development of guarding or rebound.

PHYSICAL EXAMINATION: Chest clear to auscultation and percussion. Heart: Regular rate and rhythm. Abdomen: Soft, nontender without distention. There is no rebound or guarding. Extremities negative for edema.

ASSESSMENT AND PLAN: Resolving gastroenteritis. Patient to continue on Zantac 300 mg tid and will return for follow-up prn.

Harrison Brinklemeyer, MD

FIGURE 10-3

Exam case 3 charge ticket

OFFICE VISITS NEW	Code	Fee		PROCEDURES	Code	Fee		IMMUNIZATIONS	Code	Fee
				Aerosol Tx – Initial	94664			PPD (intradermal)	86580	
Exam Problem Focused	99201			Aerosol Tx – Subsequent	94665			TB Tine	86586	
Exam Exp Prob Focused	99202			Anoscopy	46600			Admin of vaccine-single	90471	
Exam Detailed	99203			Catheterization	53670			Admin of vaccine-2+	90472	
Exam Comp/Mod Complexity	99204			Cerumen removal	69210			Hib, HbOC-4 dose	90645	
Exam Comp/High Complexity	99205			Endometrial Biopsy	58100			Hib, PRP-D booster only	90646	
				Excision, benign lesion				Hib, PRP-OMP-3 dose	90647	
ESTABLISHED				Size Loc				Hib, PRP-T-4-dose	90648	
Exam Minimal w/Supervision	99211			Excision, malignant lesion				Influenza/whole virus		
Exam Problem Focused	99212			Size Loc				G0008 V04.8	90659	
Exam Exp Prob Focused	99213			Excision, Skin Tags	11200			DtaP V06.8	90700	
Exam Detailed	99214			EKG with Interp	93000			DPT V06.1	90701	
Exam Comprehensive	99215			EKG rhythm strip	93040			DT pediatric V06.5	90702	
				I & D (abscess)	10060			Rubella V04.3	90706	
PREVENTIVE MEDICINE				Laceration repair				MMR V06.4	90707	
NEW				Size Loc				OPV V04.0	90712	
Physical infant – 1 yr	99381			Spirometry	94010			IPOL V04.0	90713	
Physical 1 yr – 4 yr	99382			Wart destruction	17110			Varicella V05.4	90716	
Physical 5 yr – 11 yr	99383			Sigmoidoscopy (flex)	45330			Td adult V06.5	90718	
Physical 12 yr – 17 yr	99384			Sigmoidoscopy (flex) w/biopsy	45331			DPT/HIB V06.8	90720	
Physical 18 yr – 39 yr	99385			Laryngoscopy/Diagnostic	31575			DTaP/HIB V06.8	90721	
Physical 40 yr – 64 yr	99386							Pneumococcal:		
Physical 65 yr – over	99387							G0009 V03.82	90732	
				OFFICE LABS				HEP B, PED/ADOL, IM V03.82	90744	
PREVENTIVE MEDICINE ESTABLISHED				Blood glucose	82962			HEP B, ADOL/RISK, IM V05.3	90745	
Physical infant – 1 yr	99391			Hemoccult	82270			HEP B, ADULT, IM V05.3	90746	
Physical 1 yr – 4 yr	99392			Medicare Hemoccult	G0107			HEP B/HIB V06.8	90748	
Physical 5 yr – 11 yr	99393			Hemoglobin QW	85018			**INJECTIONS**		
Physical 12 yr – 17 yr	99394			Pregnancy test	81025			Allergy–1	95115	
Physical 18 yr – 39 yr	99395			Strep test (quick) QW	86588			Allergy–2 or more	95117	
Physical 40 yr – 64 yr	99396			Urine dip with micro	81000			Benadryl < 50 mg	J1200	
Physical 65 yr – over	99397			Urine dip only	81002			Compazine < 10 mg	J0780	
				Urine micro only	81015			DepoMedrol 40 mg	J1030	
Hospital Consultation				Wet mount Q0111	87210			DepoMedrol 80 mg	J1040	
Initial problem focused	99251			Venipuncture/fingerstick	36415			Dexamethasone < 4 mg	J1100	
Iniital expanded PF	99252			Medicare venipuncture	G0001					
Initial detailed consult	99253									
Initial comp consult/mod	99254			**SUPPLIES**	99070			**DIAGNOSIS**		
x Initial comp consult/high	99255	350		Medicare	A4550					
								Depression	300.00	
				FORMS				Phantom leg syndrome	353.6	
				Special Reports						

Patient: Parker, Thomas   **DOB:** 01/02/65   **Date of Service:** 02/10/02   **Return Visit:** 6 months

Exam case 3

Principle Family Practice Group
Harrison Brinklemeyer, MD
4555 Constitutional Boulevard
Anytown, USA 14589

Exam case 3

Patient: Thomas Parker   Date of Service: 02/10/02   DOB: 01/02/65

This 37-year-old male patient is new to Manor Hospital. He was admitted
to this facility on 01/20/02 with the diagnoses of bilateral lower leg
amputation, ruptured spleen, lacerated liver, and fractured pelvis sustained
in a motor vehicle accident. Dr Lazro, his orthopedist, asked that I see
Mr Parker on consultation. The patient is admitted for therapy. Patient was
healthy prior to the accident. No history of diabetes, hypertension, cardiac,
or respiratory disease. Patient has had both legs amputated below the knee.
Splenectomy. Liver repair. Patient does not smoke or drink. Patient was an
avid runner prior to the accident.

REVIEW OF SYSTEMS:
HEENT: normal; respiratory: normal; cardiovascular: normal;
hematologic: normal except for splenectomy and repair of lacerated liver;
musculoskeletal: bilateral lower leg amputee. Healing pelvic fracture.
ROS otherwise normal.

PHYSICAL EXAMINATION:
General: Well-developed, well-nourished, depressed male in no acute
distress. BP 128/75. Pulse: 90, regular and strong. Temperature: normal.
Height: 5 foot 10 inches.
HEENT: Pupils are reactive to light and accommodations. No vessel
changes, exudates, or hemorrhages noted. Oral mucosa is normal.
No lesions noted.
Neck: Supple. No masses.
Respiratory: Normal. No wheezes or rubs appreciated. Clear to
auscultation.
Cardiovascular: Normal sinus rhythm. No murmurs.
Abdomen: Laparotomy scar is healing well. No signs of infection.
No evidence of masses or hernias.
Musculoskeletal: Patient is a bilateral lower leg amputee. Currently confined
to wheelchair. Pelvic fracture is healing according to x-rays. Lower leg
muscles have not been used since accident and are flaccid. Upper body is
within normal limits. Range of motion is good.
Neurological: Cranial nerves are intact. Moves all upper extremities on
command without difficulty. Hand grips strong bilaterally. Lower extremities
are flaccid and it is unclear whether patient is unable to move stumps or
will not move stumps.
Psychiatric: Patient is depressed, and this will be a concern that might
hinder him in therapy. Patient is oriented to person, place, and time.
Judgment is impaired because of depression. Patient does have phantom
leg syndrome.

PLAN: Patient will begin therapy to strengthen his lower stumps. He will
be fitted with prostheses and will begin rehabilitative therapy. Psychologist
will be obtained to help patient deal with depression and therapy. Patient
to continue same meds.

                                        Harrison Brinklemeyer, MD

FIGURE 10-4

Exam case 4 charge ticket

	OFFICE VISITS NEW	Code	Fee		PROCEDURES	Code	Fee		IMMUNIZATIONS	Code	Fee
			.		Aerosol Tx – Initial	94664			PPD (intradermal)	86580	
	Exam Problem Focused	99201			Aerosol Tx – Subsequent	94665			TB Tine	86586	
X	Exam Exp Prob Focused	99202	65		Anoscopy	46600			Admin of vaccine-single	90471	
	Exam Detailed	99203			Catheterization	53670			Admin of vaccine-2+	90472	
	Exam Comp/Mod Complexity	99204			Cerumen removal	69210			Hib, HbOC-4 dose	90645	
	Exam Comp/High Complexity	99205			Endometrial Biopsy	58100			Hib, PRP-D booster only	90646	
					Excision, benign lesion				Hib, PRP-OMP-3 dose	90647	
	ESTABLISHED				Size Loc				Hib, PRP-T-4-dose	90648	
	Exam Minimal w/Supervision	99211			Excision, malignant lesion				Influenza/whole virus		
	Exam Problem Focused	99212			Size Loc				G0008 V04.8	90659	
	Exam Exp Prob Focused	99213			Excision, Skin Tags	11200			DtaP V06.8	90700	
	Exam Detailed	99214			EKG with Interp	93000			DPT V06.1	90701	
	Exam Comprehensive	99215			EKG rhythm strip	93040			DT pediatric V06.5	90702	
					I & D (abscess)	10060			Rubella V04.3	90706	
	PREVENTIVE MEDICINE				Laceration repair				MMR V06.4	90707	
	NEW				Size Loc				OPV V04.0	90712	
	Physical infant – 1 yr	99381			Spirometry	94010			IPOL V04.0	90713	
	Physical 1 yr – 4 yr	99382			Wart destruction	17110			Varicella V05.4	90716	
	Physical 5 yr – 11 yr	99383			Sigmoidoscopy (flex)	45330			Td adult V06.5	90718	
	Physical 12 yr – 17 yr	99384			Sigmoidoscopy (flex) w/biopsy	45331			DPT/HIB V06.8	90720	
	Physical 18 yr – 39 yr	99385			Laryngoscopy/Diagnostic	31575			DTaP/HIB V06.8	90721	
	Physical 40 yr – 64 yr	99386							Pneumococcal:		
	Physical 65 yr – over	99387							G0009 V03.82	90732	
					OFFICE LABS				HEP B, PED/ADOL, IM V03.82	90744	
	PREVENTIVE MEDICINE ESTABLISHED				Blood glucose	82962			HEP B, ADOL/RISK, IM V05.3	90745	
	Physical infant – 1 yr	99391			Hemoccult	82270			HEP B, ADULT, IM V05.3	90746	
	Physical 1 yr – 4 yr	99392			Medicare Hemoccult	G0107			HEP B/HIB V06.8	90748	
	Physical 5 yr – 11 yr	99393			Hemoglobin QW	85018			INJECTIONS		
	Physical 12 yr – 17 yr	99394			Pregnancy test	81025			Allergy–1	95115	
	Physical 18 yr – 39 yr	99395	X		Strep test (quick) QW	86588			Allergy–2 or more	95117	
	Physical 40 yr – 64 yr	99396		X	Urine dip with micro	81000	15		Benadryl < 50 mg	J1200	
	Physical 65 yr – over	99397			Urine dip only	81002			Compazine < 10 mg	J0780	
					Urine micro only	81015			DepoMedrol 40 mg	J1030	
					Wet mount Q0111	87210			DepoMedrol 80 mg	J1040	
				X	Venipuncture/fingerstick	36415	10		Dexamethasone < 4 mg	J1100	
					Medicare venipuncture	G0001					
					SUPPLIES	99070			DIAGNOSIS		
					Medicare	A4550					
									Nausea with vomiting	787.01	
									E coli	041.4	
					FORMS				Acute pyelonephritis	590.10	
					Special Reports						

Patient: Thoroson, John   **DOB:** 06/12/94   **Date of Service:** 03/15/02   **Return Visit:** PRN

Exam case 4

Principle Family Practice Group
Harrison Brinklemeyer, MD
4555 Constitutional Boulevard
Anytown, USA 14589

Exam case 4

Patient: John Thoroson   Date of Service: 03/15/02   DOB: 06/12/94

This 7-year-old boy was brought to the office by his parents. This is the patient's first visit. He has been running an elevated temperature for the past 12 hours; the high was 102. He also complains of stomach pains and vomiting. The parents are very concerned.

No allergies or medications. Patient lives with his parents.

Well-developed, well-nourished child who is lethargic and pale. His temperature is 101. Pulse 110. Respirations 28. Eyes are normal. There is a minimal amount of inflammation of the tonsils. Ears, nose, and mouth are normal. Neck is supple. Skin examined—negative. Chest: Lung sounds are normal. Heart: Normal rhythm with no murmurs appreciated. Abdomen: Diffuse tenderness. No masses or organomegaly noted.

EXAMINATIONS: Labs normal except for UA dip which was positive. Urine culture is pending at this time.

ASSESSMENT AND PLAN: Ordered renal x-ray, UA, and labs. Urine culture is pending at this time. Acute pyelonephritis. Nausea with vomiting. Patient to return in 2 days.

ADDENDUM: Urine culture shows *E coli* >100,000. Renal x-ray indicates acute pyelonephritis. Patient's mother notified; begin antibiotic regimen and patient will return in 1 week unless condition worsens. Prescription called into Super K pharmacy.

Harrison Brinklemeyer, MD

FIGURE 10-5

Exam case 5 charge ticket

OFFICE VISITS	Code	Fee		PROCEDURES	Code	Fee		IMMUNIZATIONS	Code	Fee
NEW				Aerosol Tx – Initial	94664			PPD (intradermal)	86580	
Exam Problem Focused	99201			Aerosol Tx – Subsequent	94665			TB Tine	86586	
Exam Exp Prob Focused	99202			Anoscopy	46600			Admin of vaccine-single	90471	
Exam Detailed	99203			Catheterization	53670			Admin of vaccine-2+	90472	
Exam Comp/Mod Complexity	99204			Cerumen removal	69210			Hib, HbOC-4 dose	90645	
Exam Comp/High Complexity	99205			Endometrial Biopsy	58100			Hib, PRP-D booster only	90646	
				Excision, benign lesion				Hib, PRP-OMP-3 dose	90647	
ESTABLISHED				Size Loc				Hib, PRP-T-4-dose	90648	
Exam Minimal w/Supervision	99211			Excision, malignant lesion				Influenza/whole virus		
Exam Problem Focused	99212			Size Loc				G0008 V04.8	90659	
Exam Exp Prob Focused	99213			Excision, Skin Tags	11200			DtaP V06.8	90700	
Exam Detailed	99214			EKG with Interp	93000			DPT V06.1	90701	
Exam Comprehensive	99215			EKG rhythm strip	93040			DT pediatric V06.5	90702	
				I & D (abscess)	10060			Rubella V04.3	90706	
PREVENTIVE MEDICINE				Laceration repair				MMR V06.4	90707	
NEW				Size Loc				OPV V04.0	90712	
Physical infant – 1 yr	99381			Spirometry	94010			IPOL V04.0	90713	
Physical 1 yr – 4 yr	99382			Wart destruction	17110			Varicella V05.4	90716	
Physical 5 yr – 11 yr	99383			Sigmoidoscopy (flex)	45330			Td adult V06.5	90718	
Physical 12 yr – 17 yr	99384			Sigmoidoscopy (flex) w/biopsy	45331			DPT/HIB V06.8	90720	
Physical 18 yr – 39 yr	99385			Laryngoscopy/Diagnostic	31575			DTaP/HIB V06.8	90721	
Physical 40 yr – 64 yr	99386							Pneumococcal:		
Physical 65 yr – over	99387							G0009 V03.82	90732	
				OFFICE LABS				HEP B, PED/ADOL, IM V03.82	90744	
PREVENTIVE MEDICINE ESTABLISHED				Blood glucose	82962			HEP B, ADOL/RISK, IM V05.3	90745	
Physical infant – 1 yr	99391			Hemoccult	82270			HEP B, ADULT, IM V05.3	90746	
Physical 1 yr – 4 yr	99392			Medicare Hemoccult	G0107			HEP B/HIB V06.8	90748	
Physical 5 yr – 11 yr	99393			Hemoglobin QW	85018			**INJECTIONS**		
Physical 12 yr – 17 yr	99394			Pregnancy test	81025			Allergy–1	95115	
Physical 18 yr – 39 yr	99395			Strep test (quick) QW	86588			Allergy–2 or more	95117	
Physical 40 yr – 64 yr	99396			Urine dip with micro	81000			Benadryl < 50 mg	J1200	
Physical 65 yr – over	99397			Urine dip only	81002			Compazine < 10 mg	J0780	
				Urine micro only	81015			DepoMedrol 40 mg	J1030	
Nursing Home Initial				Wet mount Q0111	87210			DepoMedrol 80 mg	J1040	
Detailed	99301			Venipuncture/fingerstick	36415			Dexamethasone < 4 mg	J1100	
Comprehensive/mod/high	m			Medicare venipuncture	G0001					
Comprehensive intial	99303			**SUPPLIES**	99070			**DIAGNOSIS**		
				Medicare	A4550					
Nursing Home Subsequent								Hemiplegia	438.20	
Problem focused/interval	99311							Malnutrition	263.9	
X Expanded PF/interval	99312	125		FORMS				Psychosis	298.9	
Detailed/Interval	99313			Special Reports						

Patient: Gristmeyer, Nicholas   **DOB:** 09/07/19   **Date of Service:** 02/20/02   **Return Visit:** 3 months

Exam case 5

Principle Family Practice Group
Harrison Brinklemeyer, MD
4555 Constitutional Boulevard
Anytown, USA 14589

Exam case 5

Patient Name: Nicholas Gristmeyer   Date of Service: 02/20/02
                                          DOB: 09/07/19

This is an 82-year-old established patient who has been in the nursing
home for the past 2 months and is being evaluated on a monthly basis. He
has a previous history of left-sided cerebrovascular accident with right-sided
paralysis. The patient has been demented since his stroke and has been seen
by a psychiatrist, who diagnosed psychosis and placed him on risperidone
and lorazepam. Patient will open his eyes to name only. Does not answer
any questions. He has been having swallowing problems but has not
developed any signs of choking.

General: BP 125/78, P 78, weight 108 with a loss of 5 lbs since last month.
Laxity of the lower jaw; cataracts bilaterally.

Lungs: Clear to auscultation and percussion.

Heart: Normal sinus rhythm.

Abdomen: No masses or tenderness.

The patient responds to name only; right-sided paralysis due to old CVA.

ASSESSMENT AND PLAN: Right-sided paralysis; malnutrition with weight
loss; psychosis. Will have speech pathologist evaluate patient; begin calorie
enhanced diet and will follow up next P1. Continue same meds.

                                          Harrison Brinklemeyer, MD

F I G U R E 10-6

Exam case 6 charge ticket

OFFICE VISITS NEW	Code	Fee	PROCEDURES	Code	Fee	IMMUNIZATIONS	Code	Fee
			Aerosol Tx – Initial	94664		PPD (intradermal)	86580	
Exam Problem Focused	99201		Aerosol Tx – Subsequent	94665		TB Tine	86586	
Exam Exp Prob Focused	99202		Anoscopy	46600		Admin of vaccine-single	90471	
Exam Detailed	99203		Catheterization	53670		Admin of vaccine-2+	90472	
Exam Comp/Mod Complexity	99204		Cerumen removal	69210		Hib, HbOC-4 dose	90645	
Exam Comp/High Complexity	99205		Endometrial Biopsy	58100		Hib, PRP-D booster only	90646	
			Excision, benign lesion			Hib, PRP-OMP-3 dose	90647	
ESTABLISHED			Size Loc			Hib, PRP-T-4-dose	90648	
Exam Minimal w/Supervision	99211		Excision, malignant lesion			Influenza/whole virus		
Exam Problem Focused	99212		Size Loc			G0008 V04.8	90659	
Exam Exp Prob Focused	99213		Excision, Skin Tags	11200		DtaP V06.8	90700	
Exam Detailed	99214		EKG with Interp	93000		DPT V06.1	90701	
Exam Comprehensive	99215		EKG rhythm strip	93040		DT pediatric V06.5	90702	
			I & D (abscess)	10060		Rubella V04.3	90706	
PREVENTIVE MEDICINE			Laceration repair			MMR V06.4	90707	
NEW			Size Loc			OPV V04.0	90712	
Physical infant – 1 yr	99381		Spirometry	94010		IPOL V04.0	90713	
Physical 1 yr – 4 yr	99382		Wart destruction	17110		Varicella V05.4	90716	
Physical 5 yr – 11 yr	99383		Sigmoidoscopy (flex)	45330		Td adult V06.5	90718	
Physical 12 yr – 17 yr	99384		Sigmoidoscopy (flex) w/biopsy	45331		DPT/HIB V06.8	90720	
Physical 18 yr – 39 yr	99385		Laryngoscopy/Diagnostic	31575		DTaP/HIB V06.8	90721	
Physical 40 yr – 64 yr	99386					Pneumococcal:		
Physical 65 yr – over	99387					G0009 V03.82	90732	
			OFFICE LABS			HEP B, PED/ADOL, IM V03.82	90744	
PREVENTIVE MEDICINE ESTABLISHED			Blood glucose	82962		HEP B, ADOL/RISK, IM V05.3	90745	
Physical infant – 1 yr	99391		Hemoccult	82270		HEP B, ADULT, IM V05.3	90746	
Physical 1 yr – 4 yr	99392		Medicare Hemoccult	G0107		HEP B/HIB V06.8	90748	
Physical 5 yr – 11 yr	99393		Hemoglobin QW	85018		**INJECTIONS**		
Physical 12 yr – 17 yr	99394		Pregnancy test	81025		Allergy–1	95115	
Physical 18 yr – 39 yr	99395		Strep test (quick) QW	86588		Allergy–2 or more	95117	
Physical 40 yr – 64 yr	99396		Urine dip with micro	81000		Benadryl < 50 mg	J1200	
Physical 65 yr - over	99397		Urine dip only	81002		Compazine < 10 mg	J0780	
			Urine micro only	81015		DepoMedrol 40 mg	J1030	
			Wet mount Q0111	87210		DepoMedrol 80 mg	J1040	
Nursing Home Initial			Venipuncture/fingerstick	36415		Dexamethasone < 4 mg	J1100	
Detailed	99301		Medicare venipuncture	G0001				
Comprehensive/mod/high	99302							
Comprehensive intial	99303		**SUPPLIES**	99070		**DIAGNOSIS**		
			Medicare	A4550				
Nursing Home Subsequent						Cellulitis	682.7	
Problem focused/interval	99311					IDDM	250.01	
X Expanded PF/interval	99312	125	FORMS					
Detailed/Interval	99313		Special Reports					

Patient: Byers, Myrtle   **DOB:** 02/20/30   **Date of Service:** 02/12/02   **Return Visit:** 1 week

Exam case 6

Principle Family Practice Group
Harrison Brinklemeyer, MD
4555 Constitutional Boulevard
Anytown, USA 14589

Exam case 6

Patient: Myrtle Byers   Date of Service: 02/12/02   DOB: 02/20/30

S: This is a follow-up visit for this 71-year-old female. She was admitted to Manor Nursing Home 3 days ago with cellulitis of the left foot. She was placed in the nursing home for IV therapy for her cellulitis. She is recovering well and the infection is about gone. She has a history of IDDM (insulin dependent diabetes mellitus). She denies chest pain or shortness of breath. Patient is positive for pain in the left foot that is sometimes severe in nature.

Current medications: 70/30 insulin in the morning and 20 units in the evening, Cardizem CD 180 once daily, Imdur 60 mg once a day, Lasix 80 mg one a day, Pepcid 20 mg twice a day, Paxil 10 mg three times a day, Nitrostat as needed.

O: Well-developed, well-nourished female in no acute distress. BP: 128/75. Pulse: 80, regular and strong. Respirations: 12, unlabored and regular. Temperature: Normal. Height: 5 feet. Left foot shows slight reddening on the upper surface. Infection had decreased significantly. All other areas are normal.

A/P: Patient is doing well and will be taken off IV vancomycin. She will be discharged home tomorrow and will be given a prescription for penicillin. She is to follow up in my office in 1 week.

Harrison Brinklemeyer, MD

FIGURE 10-7

Exam case 7 charge ticket

OFFICE VISITS NEW	Code	Fee	PROCEDURES	Code	Fee	IMMUNIZATIONS	Code	Fee
			Aerosol Tx – Initial	94664		PPD (intradermal)	86580	
Exam Problem Focused	99201		Aerosol Tx – Subsequent	94665		TB Tine	86586	
Exam Exp Prob Focused	99202		Anoscopy	46600		Admin of vaccine-single	90471	
Exam Detailed	99203		Catheterization	53670		Admin of vaccine-2+	90472	
Exam Comp/Mod Complexity	99204		Cerumen removal	69210		Hib, HbOC-4 dose	90645	
Exam Comp/High Complexity	99205		Endometrial Biopsy	58100		Hib, PRP-D booster only	90646	
			Excision, benign lesion			Hib, PRP-OMP-3 dose	90647	
ESTABLISHED			Size Loc			Hib, PRP-T-4-dose	90648	
Exam Minimal w/Supervision	99211		Excision, malignant lesion			Influenza/whole virus		
Exam Problem Focused	99212		Size Loc			G0008 V04.8	90659	
X Exam Exp Prob Focused	99213	65	Excision, Skin Tags	11200		DtaP V06.8	90700	
Exam Detailed	99214		EKG with Interp	93000		DPT V06.1	90701	
Exam Comprehensive	99215		EKG rhythm strip	93040		DT pediatric V06.5	90702	
			I & D (abscess)	10060		Rubella V04.3	90706	
PREVENTIVE MEDICINE			Laceration repair			MMR V06.4	90707	
NEW			Size Loc			OPV V04.0	90712	
Physical infant – 1 yr	99381		Spirometry	94010		IPOL V04.0	90713	
Physical 1 yr – 4 yr	99382		Wart destruction	17110		Varicella V05.4	90716	
Physical 5 yr – 11 yr	99383		Sigmoidoscopy (flex)	45330		Td adult V06.5	90718	
Physical 12 yr – 17 yr	99384		Sigmoidoscopy (flex) w/biopsy	45331		DPT/HIB V06.8	90720	
Physical 18 yr – 39 yr	99385		Laryngoscopy/Diagnostic	31575		DTaP/HIB V06.8	90721	
Physical 40 yr – 64 yr	99386					Pneumococcal:		
Physical 65 yr – over	99387					G0009 V03.82	90732	
			OFFICE LABS			HEP B, PED/ADOL, IM V03.82	90744	
PREVENTIVE MEDICINE ESTABLISHED			Blood glucose	82962		HEP B, ADOL/RISK, IM V05.3	90745	
Physical infant – 1 yr	99391		Hemoccult	82270		HEP B, ADULT, IM V05.3	90746	
Physical 1 yr – 4 yr	99392		Medicare Hemoccult	G0107		HEP B/HIB V06.8	90748	
Physical 5 yr – 11 yr	99393		Hemoglobin QW	85018		**INJECTIONS**		
Physical 12 yr – 17 yr	99394		Pregnancy test	81025		Allergy-1	95115	
Physical 18 yr – 39 yr	99395		Strep test (quick) QW	86588		Allergy-2 or more	95117	
Physical 40 yr – 64 yr	99396		Urine dip with micro	81000		Benadryl < 50 mg	J1200	
Physical 65 yr – over	99397		Urine dip only	81002		Compazine < 10 mg	J0780	
			Urine micro only	81015		DepoMedrol 40 mg	J1030	
			Wet mount Q0111	87210		DepoMedrol 80 mg	J1040	
			Venipuncture/fingerstick	36415		Dexamethasone < 4 mg	J1100	
			Medicare venipuncture	G0001				
			SUPPLIES	99070		**DIAGNOSIS**		
			Medicare	A4550				
						Knee pain	719.48	
			FORMS					
			Special Reports					

Patient: Maple, Carlotta   **DOB:** 09/14/42   **Date of Service:** 02/10/02   **Return Visit:** 1 month

Exam case 7

Principle Family Practice Group
Harrison Brinklemeyer, MD
4555 Constitutional Boulevard
Anytown, USA 14589

Exam case 7

Patient: Carlotta Maple   Date of Service: 02/10/02   DOB: 09/14/42

This well-groomed established patient presents to renew her BP medication and have blood work done. The patient has no complaints. The patient has bilateral knee pain, tender and swollen. The patient was doing yard work and states she was on her knees too long. Patient denies shortness of breath or chest pain.

Height is 5'2", weight 125 lbs; BP is 140/70; heart rate is 72. Head and neck are within-normal limits. Chest is clear. CVS is normal. Knee pain bilaterally which appears swollen.

PLAN: Hydrochlorothiazide, 50 mg, once a day, #100; and Calan SR 240 mg, once a day, sample was given. The patient will return for EKG next week. Also, Voltaren, 75 mg once bid, sample given. The patient is noncompliant. She is not exercising and not dieting. Advised patient to continue low-fat diet and return in 1 month.

Harrison Brinklemeyer, MD

FIGURE 10-8

Exam case 8 charge ticket

OFFICE VISITS NEW	Code	Fee
Exam Problem Focused	99201	
Exam Exp Prob Focused	99202	
Exam Detailed	99203	
Exam Comp/Mod Complexity	99204	
Exam Comp/High Complexity	99205	
ESTABLISHED		
Exam Minimal w/Supervision	99211	
Exam Problem Focused	99212	
Exam Exp Prob Focused	99213	
x Exam Detailed	99214	100
Exam Comprehensive	99215	
PREVENTIVE MEDICINE NEW		
Physical infant – 1 yr	99381	
Physical 1 yr – 4 yr	99382	
Physical 5 yr – 11 yr	99383	
Physical 12 yr – 17 yr	99384	
Physical 18 yr – 39 yr	99385	
Physical 40 yr – 64 yr	99386	
Physical 65 yr – over	99387	
PREVENTIVE MEDICINE ESTABLISHED		
Physical infant – 1 yr	99391	
Physical 1 yr – 4 yr	99392	
Physical 5 yr – 11 yr	99393	
Physical 12 yr – 17 yr	99394	
Physical 18 yr – 39 yr	99395	
Physical 40 yr – 64 yr	99396	
Physical 65 yr – over	99397	

PROCEDURES	Code	Fee
Aerosol Tx – Initial	94664	
Aerosol Tx – Subsequent	94665	
Anoscopy	46600	
Catheterization	53670	
Cerumen removal	69210	
Endometrial Biopsy	58100	
Excision, benign lesion		
Size Loc		
Excision, malignant lesion		
Size Loc		
Excision, Skin Tags	11200	
EKG with Interp	93000	
EKG rhythm strip	93040	
I & D (abscess)	10060	
Laceration repair		
Size Loc		
Spirometry	94010	
Wart destruction	17110	
Sigmoidoscopy (flex)	45330	
Sigmoidoscopy (flex) w/biopsy	45331	
Laryngoscopy/Diagnostic	31575	

OFFICE LABS	Code	Fee
Blood glucose	82962	
Hemoccult	82270	
Medicare Hemoccult	G0107	
Hemoglobin QW	85018	
Pregnancy test	81025	
Strep test (quick) QW	86588	
Urine dip with micro	81000	
Urine dip only	81002	
Urine micro only	81015	
Wet mount Q0111	87210	
Venipuncture/fingerstick	36415	
Medicare venipuncture	G0001	

SUPPLIES	99070	
Medicare	A4550	
FORMS		
Special Reports		

IMMUNIZATIONS	Code	Fee
PPD (intradermal)	86580	
TB Tine	86586	
Admin of vaccine-single	90471	
Admin of vaccine-2+	90472	
Hib, HbOC-4 dose	90645	
Hib, PRP-D booster only	90646	
Hib, PRP-OMP-3 dose	90647	
Hib, PRP-T-4-dose	90648	
Influenza/whole virus		
G0008 V04.8	90659	
DtaP V06.8	90700	
DPT V06.1	90701	
DT pediatric V06.5	90702	
Rubella V04.3	90706	
MMR V06.4	90707	
OPV V04.0	90712	
IPOL V04.0	90713	
Varicella V05.4	90716	
Td adult V06.5	90718	
DPT/HIB V06.8	90720	
DTaP/HIB V06.8	90721	
Pneumococcal:		
G0009 V03.82	90732	
HEP B, PED/ADOL, IM V03.82	90744	
HEP B, ADOL/RISK, IM V05.3	90745	
HEP B, ADULT, IM V05.3	90746	
HEP B/HIB V06.8	90748	

INJECTIONS	Code	Fee
Allergy–1	95115	
Allergy–2 or more	95117	
Benadryl < 50 mg	J1200	
Compazine < 10 mg	J0780	
DepoMedrol 40 mg	J1030	
DepoMedrol 80 mg	J1040	
Dexamethasone < 4 mg	J1100	

DIAGNOSIS	Code	Fee
Hypertension	401.9	
Headaches	784.0	

Patient: Steiner, Martin   **DOB:** 04/10/55   **Date of Service:** 02/10/02   **Return Visit:** 1 month

Exam case 8

Principle Family Practice Group
Harrison Brinklemeyer, MD
4555 Constitutional Boulevard
Anytown, USA 14589

Exam case 8

Patient: Martin Steiner   Date of Service: 02/10/02   DOB: 4/10/55

CC: Check up on hypertension

HPI: Follow-up visit; using relaxation and atenolol. Still with severe headache pain. Feeling more steady on his feet. No chest pain or shortness of breath. Still with severe head and face pain. Still stating symptoms change with weather, today a particularly bad day. In hospital earlier this month with CT negative, MRI with periventricular changes with ischemia.

PE: Neck: Carotids without bruits
     Lungs: Clear to A&P
     Heart: RRR
     Ext: No edema

A/P: HTN-BP elevated, but much improved, controlled compared to initially. Pt took last meds 4 pm yesterday—elevation may be trough effect. Continue atenolol 50 mg OD. Check BP in am; if better controlled will change dosage to 25 mg BID. Headaches persistent. EEG without photon pattern. Refer to specialist. Follow up in 1 month.

Harrison Brinklemeyer, MD

FIGURE 10-9

Exam case 9 charge ticket

OFFICE VISITS NEW	Code	Fee	PROCEDURES	Code	Fee	IMMUNIZATIONS	Code	Fee
			Aerosol Tx – Initial	94664		PPD (intradermal)	86580	
Exam Problem Focused	99201		Aerosol Tx – Subsequent	94665		TB Tine	86586	
Exam Exp Prob Focused	99202		Anoscopy	46600		Admin of vaccine-single	90471	
Exam Detailed	99203		Catheterization	53670		Admin of vaccine-2+	90472	
Exam Comp/Mod Complexity	99204		Cerumen removal	69210		Hib, HbOC-4 dose	90645	
Exam Comp/High Complexity	99205		Endometrial Biopsy	58100		Hib, PRP-D booster only	90646	
			Excision, benign lesion			Hib, PRP-OMP-3 dose	90647	
ESTABLISHED			Size Loc			Hib, PRP-T-4-dose	90648	
Exam Minimal w/Supervision	99211		Excision, malignant lesion			Influenza/whole virus		
Exam Problem Focused	99212		Size Loc			G0008 V04.8	90659	
x Exam Exp Prob Focused	99213	65	Excision, Skin Tags	11200		DtaP V06.8	90700	
Exam Detailed	99214		EKG with Interp	93000		DPT V06.1	90701	
Exam Comprehensive	99215		EKG rhythm strip	93040		DT pediatric V06.5	90702	
			I & D (abscess)	10060		Rubella V04.3	90706	
PREVENTIVE MEDICINE			Laceration repair			MMR V06.4	90707	
NEW			Size Loc			OPV V04.0	90712	
Physical infant – 1 yr	99381		Spirometry	94010		IPOL V04.0	90713	
Physical 1 yr – 4 yr	99382		Wart destruction	17110		Varicella V05.4	90716	
Physical 5 yr – 11 yr	99383		Sigmoidoscopy (flex)	45330		Td adult V06.5	90718	
Physical 12 yr – 17 yr	99384		Sigmoidoscopy (flex) w/biopsy	45331		DPT/HIB V06.8	90720	
Physical 18 yr – 39 yr	99385		Laryngoscopy/Diagnostic	31575		DTaP/HIB V06.8	90721	
Physical 40 yr – 64 yr	99386					Pneumococcal:		
Physical 65 yr – over	99387					G0009 V03.82	90732	
			OFFICE LABS			HEP B, PED/ADOL, IM V03.82	90744	
PREVENTIVE MEDICINE ESTABLISHED			Blood glucose	82962		HEP B, ADOL/RISK, IM V05.3	90745	
Physical infant – 1 yr	99391		Hemoccult	82270		HEP B, ADULT, IM V05.3	90746	
Physical 1 yr – 4 yr	99392		Medicare Hemoccult	G0107		HEP B/HIB V06.8	90748	
Physical 5 yr – 11 yr	99393		Hemoglobin QW	85018		INJECTIONS		
Physical 12 yr – 17 yr	99394		Pregnancy test	81025		Allergy–1	95115	
Physical 18 yr – 39 yr	99395		Strep test (quick) QW	86588		Allergy–2 or more	95117	
Physical 40 yr – 64 yr	99396		Urine dip with micro	81000		Benadryl < 50 mg	J1200	
Physical 65 yr – over	99397		Urine dip only	81002		Compazine < 10 mg	J0780	
			Urine micro only	81015		DepoMedrol 40 mg	J1030	
			Wet mount Q0111	87210		DepoMedrol 80 mg	J1040	
			Venipuncture/fingerstick	36415		Dexamethasone < 4 mg	J1100	
			Medicare venipuncture	G0001				
			SUPPLIES	99070		DIAGNOSIS		
			Medicare	A4550				
						Otitis Externa	380.10	
			FORMS					
			Special Reports					

Patient: Paulern, Rebecca   **DOB:** 11/01/00   **Date of Service:** 02/10/02   **Return Visit:** 3 months

Exam case 9

Principle Family Practice Group
Harrison Brinklemeyer, MD
4555 Constitutional Boulevard
Anytown, USA 14589

Exam case 9

PEDIATRIC ACUTE VISIT

Patient Name: *Rebecca Paulern*   Date of Birth: *11/01/01*   Date of Service: *02/10/02*

Age: *6 months*   Sex *female*   Weight: *14lbs*   Length: *27inches*   Temp: *96.9*   ☒ Allergies reviewed

CC: *Here for ear pain. Rebecca pulling on ears constantly; unable to sleep x 3 days. Fever 101.*	❑ New ☒ Established

REVIEW OF SYSTEMS

	-	+	Abnormal Findings	Current Medications
fever	❑	❑		*None*
eye discharge/redness	❑	❑		
ear pulling/discharge	❑	☒	*Pulling on ears; crying; seems to be in pain*	
skin rashes	❑	❑		
perfusion/cyanosis	❑	❑		**PFSH** see form front of chart ❑ New pt - form completed ☒ Reviewed, no change ❑ Reviewed, updated
cough/trouble breathing	❑	❑		
temperament	❑		*Irritable; crabby and unable to sleep well*	

EXAM FINDINGS NOTED

AREA/SYSTEM	NORMAL			FINDINGS
Appearance	☒			
Eyes	☒ pupils	❑ red reflex	❑ sclera	
HENT	☒ fontanelles	❑ TMs ☒ nose	☒ pharynx	*Both Ears red; TM's red*
Neck	☒ supple	☒ nodes		
Respiratory	☒ effort	❑ auscultation	❑ percussion	
Cardiovascular	☒ sounds	☒ rate	☒ rhythm	
Abdomen	☒ soft	☒ nontender	❑ liver/spleen	
Skin	☒ color	❑ turgor		
Musculoskeletal	❑ tone	❑ hips	❑ lower extremities	
GU	❑ penis	❑ testicles	❑ labia	
Neuro	☒ alert	❑ activity		

ASSESSMENT/PLAN	PARENT/PATIENT EDUCATION
Otitis externa; both ears begin regimen of antibiotics; mom will call in 3 days with progress report. If not better will return in 10 days; will defer vaccinations until otitis clears up	☒ **Medication education/side effects** reviewed with parent/guardian

PHYSICIAN SIGNATURE: *Harrison Brinklemeyer*   **RETURN VISIT:** *10 days*

FIGURE 10-10

Exam case 10 charge ticket

OFFICE VISITS NEW		Code	Fee	PROCEDURES		Code	Fee	IMMUNIZATIONS		Code	Fee
				Aerosol Tx – Initial		94664		PPD (intradermal)		86580	
	Exam Problem Focused	99201		Aerosol Tx – Subsequent		94665		TB Tine		86586	
X	Exam Exp Prob Focused	99202	75	Anoscopy		46600		Admin of vaccine-single		90471	
	Exam Detailed	99203		Catheterization		53670		Admin of vaccine-2+		90472	
	Exam Comp/Mod Complexity	99204		Cerumen removal		69210		Hib, HbOC-4 dose		90645	
	Exam Comp/High Complexity	99205		Endometrial Biopsy		58100		Hib, PRP-D booster only		90646	
				Excision, benign lesion				Hib, PRP-OMP-3 dose		90647	
	ESTABLISHED			Size Loc				Hib, PRP-T-4-dose		90648	
	Exam Minimal w/Supervision	99211		Excision, malignant lesion				Influenza/whole virus			
	Exam Problem Focused	99212		Size Loc				G0008 V04.8		90659	
	Exam Exp Prob Focused	99213		Excision, Skin Tags		11200		DtaP V06.8		90700	
	Exam Detailed	99214		EKG with Interp		93000		DPT V06.1		90701	
	Exam Comprehensive	99215		EKG rhythm strip		93040		DT pediatric V06.5		90702	
				I & D (abscess)		10060		Rubella V04.3		90706	
	PREVENTIVE MEDICINE			Laceration repair				MMR V06.4		90707	
	NEW			Size Loc				OPV V04.0		90712	
	Physical infant – 1 yr	99381		Spirometry		94010		IPOL V04.0		90713	
	Physical 1 yr – 4 yr	99382		Wart destruction		17110		Varicella V05.4		90716	
	Physical 5 yr – 11 yr	99383		Sigmoidoscopy (flex)		45330		Td adult V06.5		90718	
	Physical 12 yr – 17 yr	99384		Sigmoidoscopy (flex) w/biopsy		45331		DPT/HIB V06.8		90720	
	Physical 18 yr – 39 yr	99385		Laryngoscopy/Diagnostic		31575		DTaP/HIB V06.8		90721	
	Physical 40 yr – 64 yr	99386						Pneumococcal:			
	Physical 65 yr – over	99387						G0009 V03.82		90732	
				OFFICE LABS				HEP B, PED/ADOL, IM V03.82		90744	
	PREVENTIVE MEDICINE ESTABLISHED			Blood glucose		82962		HEP B, ADOL/RISK, IM V05.3		90745	
	Physical infant – 1 yr	99391		Hemoccult		82270		HEP B, ADULT, IM V05.3		90746	
	Physical 1 yr – 4 yr	99392		Medicare Hemoccult		G0107		HEP B/HIB V06.8		90748	
	Physical 5 yr – 11 yr	99393		Hemoglobin QW		85018		INJECTIONS			
	Physical 12 yr – 17 yr	99394		Pregnancy test		81025		Allergy–1		95115	
	Physical 18 yr – 39 yr	99395		Strep test (quick) QW		86588		Allergy–2 or more		95117	
	Physical 40 yr – 64 yr	99396		Urine dip with micro		81000		Benadryl < 50 mg		J1200	
	Physical 65 yr – over	99397		Urine dip only		81002		Compazine < 10 mg		J0780	
				Urine micro only		81015		DepoMedrol 40 mg		J1030	
				Wet mount Q0111		87210		DepoMedrol 80 mg		J1040	
				Venipuncture/fingerstick		36415		Dexamethasone < 4 mg		J1100	
				Medicare venipuncture		G0001					
				SUPPLIES		99070		DIAGNOSIS			
				Medicare		A4550					
								FH heart disease		V17.3	
				FORMS				Major depression		300.00	
				Special Reports				Elevated cholesterol			

Patient: Bradfield, Maureen   **DOB:** 02/04/52   **Date of Service:** 02/12/02   **Return Visit:** 3 months

Exam case 10

Principle Family Practice Group
Harrison Brinklemeyer, MD
4555 Constitutional Boulevard
Anytown, USA 14589

Exam case 10

Patient: Maureen Bradfield   Date of service: 02/12/02   DOB: 02/04/52

This is a 50-year-old new patient, states she is feeling better than she probably ever has in her life. She has been on Zoloft now and says it really helps. Her PMH shows that she has been depressed off and on for the past 2 years. This was probably a major depression for her, though it has improved. Also looking at her labs, her total cholesterol is 247 with an LDL of 142 and HDL of 69. These are equivocal results. Her family history is very strong for heart disease, with a brother dying of a heart attack when he was 24 years old. Her mother and father both have heart disease, and it is in both families. She is S/P hysterectomy, and she is on Premarin 1.25 once per day.

EXAM: 47-year-old female in no acute distress. Eyes PERRLA (pupils equal, round and reactive to light accommodation). She is wearing knee braces. Lungs clear. Heart regular. Abdomen soft. No CVA tenderness. Extremities without clubbing, cyanosis, or edema.

ASSESSMENT:

1. Strong family history of heart disease
2. Increased cholesterol
3. Major depression

PLAN: We will start her on Zocar 20 mg 1 q day #30 with 1 refill. Check her cholesterol in 6 weeks with liver function tests and see her back in 3 months.

Harrison Brinklemeyer, MD

FIGURE 10-11
Detailed review analysis

MEDICAL RECORD REVIEW
Principle Family Practice Group
DETAILED REVIEW ANALYSIS

Physician: Harrison Brinklemeyer   Date of Review:

Patient ID	Service Date	Practice CPT® Code	History	Exam	Medical Decision Making	Documented CPT® Code

FIGURE 10-12
Summary report

PHYSICIAN MEDICAL RECORD REVIEW
Principle Family Practice Group
SUMMARY REPORT

Physician: Harrison Brinklemeyer   Date of Review:

Reviewer: _____

Number of Charts Reviewed:

One service date was reviewed for each chart reviewed for appropriate coding and supporting documentation. Each chart was reviewed in detail for completeness.

E/M documentation appeared to support service billed

E/M documentation in the record appears to support a lower level of service than billed

E/M documentation in the record appears to support a higher level of service than billed

Consultation does not meet criteria based on CMS guidelines

Other:

Other documentation coding issues:

1.

2.

3.

RECOMMENDATIONS

1.

2.

3.

TAKE THE AUDITING CHALLENGE— SURGICAL RECORDS

You have gained enough knowledge and experience to be ready to audit surgical medical records at this time. There are 10 operative notes to audit for Angela O'Graphy, MD, at the General Surgical Group. Audit all 10 cases and complete the surgery coding review analysis and summary report. Review the charge ticket for the procedure when auditing the surgical cases. It is a good idea, if you have a National Correct Coding Initiative (NCCI) book or software program, to review the edits when auditing the records. You will find a copy of the surgery audit tool along with the detailed analysis and summary reports. Make as many copies as you will need.

FIGURE 11-1

Surgery case 1 charge ticket

Surgery Case 1 Charge Ticket

Patient Name	Martha Matson
Medical Record Number/Account Number	104017
Surgeon	Angela O'Graphy
Referring Physician	Thomas Jones, MD
Assistant Surgeon	None
Anesthesiologist	Ida Numdya
Insurance Company	Medicare
Comments	Postop follow-up 1-day

Date of Surgery	Facility	Place of Service	CPT Code	Diagnosis Code(s)	Modifier	Quantity	Fee
02/14/02	Methodist Surg Cntr	OH	66984	366.9	OS	1	1200.00

Legend:

Place of Service (POS): OH, outpatient hospital; IH, inpatient hospital; ER, emergency room; O, office

Outpatient hospital surgery centers: Memorial Hospital Surgery Center
Methodist Surgery Center
University Hospital Outpatient Center
Markham Memorial Surgery Center
Acme Hospital

Hospitals: University Hospital
Methodist Hospital
Johnson County Regional Medical Center
St Vincent Hospital Center
Surgery case 1   Acme Hospital

General Surgical Group
Angela O'Graphy, MD
4555 Constitutional Boulevard
Anytown, USA 14589

OPERATIVE REPORT 1

METHODIST SURGERY CENTER

PATIENT: Martha Matson   MR# 104017

DATE OF OPERATION: 2/14/02

PREOPERATIVE DIAGNOSIS: Cataract of left eye.

POSTOPERATIVE DIAGNOSIS: Same.

OPERATION PERFORMED: Phacoemulsification of left eye cataract with posterior chamber lens implantation, Alcon Model SA6CAT, 18.5 diopters.

SURGEON: Angela O'Graphy, MD

ANESTHESIA: MAC.

ANESTHESIOLOGIST: Ida Numdya, MD

INDICATIONS FOR PROCEDURE: The patient is an 85-year-old female with advancing cataract of the left eye. Best corrected vision is 20/400. The cataract of the left eye has developed rapidly. She is experiencing extreme interference with her overall visual performance. Her left eye vision is unable to be improved with spectacles and physical examination suggests that the cataract is the primary cause of the reduced vision. The option of cataract extraction has been presented to her. The risks and benefits have been discussed. She has been provided with up-to-date printed information. The patient wishes to have the left eye cataract removed on the basis of impairment of lifestyle due to reduced vision.

DESCRIPTION OF PROCEDURE: The patient was brought to the operating room on 02/14/02. Intravenous anesthesia and retrobulbar and peribulbar block had been administered approximately 30 minutes prior to her arrival in the operating room. The left eye was prepped. A blepharostat was inserted between the lids and the surgical microscope was focused into position. A conjunctival peritomy was performed. The anterior chamber was entered at the 12 o'clock position using a keratome inserted at the end of a self-sealing limbal incision. Viscoelastic material was used as necessary throughout the case. A capsulorhexis was performed. The cataract was removed by phacoemulsification techniques without difficulty. The implant was delivered and inspected. The implant power was confirmed to be 18.5 diopters on the package. The implant was inserted into the capsular bag without difficulty. Viscoelastic material was removed from the eye. The wound was observed to be watertight. A single suture of 10-0 nylon was placed in the wound for additional security. TobraDex ointment was applied to the surface of the eye and a sterile patch taped into place. There were no complications.

She had an uneventful emergence from anesthesia and returned to the holding area in satisfactory condition. There she was monitored until stable. Postoperative instructions were reviewed and arrangements were confirmed for 1-day follow-up in my office.

Angela O'Graphy, MD

Angela O'Graphy, MD

FIGURE 11-2

Surgery case 2 charge ticket

Surgery Case 2 Charge Ticket

Patient Name	Paul Binyion
Medical Record Number/Account Number	17342
Surgeon	Angela O'Graphy
Referring Physician	None
Assistant Surgeon	None
Anesthesiologist	Local
Insurance Company	Aetna
Comments	

Date of Surgery	Facility	Place of Service	CPT Code	Diagnosis Code(s)	Modifier	Quantity	Fee
02/06/02	Office	O	25112	727.41		1	550.00

Legend:

Place of Service (POS): OH, outpatient hospital; IH, inpatient hospital; ER, emergency room; O, office

Outpatient hospital surgery centers: Memorial Hospital Surgery Center
Methodist Surgery Center
University Hospital Outpatient Center
Markham Memorial Surgery Center
Acme Hospital

Hospitals: University Hospital
Methodist Hospital
Johnson County Regional Medical Center
St Vincent Hospital Center
Acme Hospital

Surgery case 2

General Surgical Group
Angela O'Graphy, MD
4555 Constitutional Boulevard
Anytown, USA 14589

OPERATIVE REPORT 2

PATIENT: Paul Binyion   MR# 17342
DATE OF OPERATION: 02/06/02
PREOPERATIVE DIAGNOSIS: Ganglion of dorsum, right wrist.
POSTOPERATIVE DIAGNOSIS: Same (2 cm diameter).
OPERATION PERFORMED: Excision of ganglion.
SURGEON: Angela O'Graphy, MD
ANESTHESIA: Local.

DESCRIPTION OF OPERATION: The patient was taken to the operative
suite. The hand was prepped and draped in the usual manner and then
anesthetized with Xylocaine infiltration.

An incision was made overlying this large ganglion cyst, and dissection was
carried down until the cyst was encountered. There were no major
structures covering this. Small vessels were ligated. The cyst was opened,
drained of its contents, and then the cyst wall was dissected away from
surrounding structures through the areolar tissue and dissection carried
down into the joint space where a small neck was found, and it was excised.
There was good hemostasis. The subcutis was closed with PDS and the skin
closed with dermal Vicryl. A splint was then applied, and it will be worn for
about 10 days. He will be seen in the office at that time.

Angela O'Graphy, MD
Angela O'Graphy, MD

Surgery case 3 charge ticket

Surgery Case 3 Charge Ticket

Patient Name	Michael Brunson
Medical Record Number/Account Number	1045679
Surgeon	Angela O'Graphy
Referring Physician	Parker Went, MD
Assistant Surgeon	
Anesthesiologist	
Insurance Company	Medicare
Comments	Return to office 1 week

Date of Surgery	Facility	Place of Service	CPT Code	Diagnosis Code(s)	Modifier	Quantity	Fee
02/08/02	University Hospital	IH	93510	414.01 414.02 429.3		1	500.00
02/08/02	Same	IH	93539	414.01 414.02 429.3		1	550.00
02/08/02	Same	IH	93540	414.01 414.02 429.3		1	400.00
02/08/02	Same	IH	93543	414.01 414.02 429.3		1	375.00
02/08/02	Same	IH	93545	414.01 414.02 429.3		1	375.00
02/08/02	Same	IH	93555	414.01 414.02 429.3		1	375.00
02/08/02	Same	IH	93556	414.01 414.02 429.3		1	375.00

Legend:

Place of Service (POS): OH, outpatient hospital; IH, inpatient hospital; ER, emergency room; O, office

Outpatient hospital surgery centers: Memorial Hospital Surgery Center
Methodist Surgery Center
University Hospital Outpatient Center
Markham Memorial Surgery Center
Acme Hospital

Surgery case 3

General Surgical Group
Angela O'Graphy, MD
4555 Constitutional Boulevard
Anytown, USA 14589

OPERATIVE REPORT 3

PATIENT: Michael Brunson   MR # 1045679
DATE OF PROCEDURE: 02/08/02
SURGEON: Angela O'Graphy, MD

INDICATIONS: A 68-year-old man is hospitalized with unstable angina. He has been treated in the past with coronary bypass surgery. A cardiac catheterization and coronary and graft angiograms are ordered.

The surgeon performs retrograde left heart catheterization, left ventriculography, selective coronary angiography, and vein graft angiography. In addition, the cardiologist also injects the internal mammary artery to determine whether it would be a suitable arterial conduit for a second bypass operation.

IMPRESSION:
1. Arteriosclerotic heart disease of native coronary arteries (ASHD)
2. Arteriosclerotic heart disease of autologous venous grafts
3. Left ventricular hypertrophy

Angela O'Graphy, MD
Angela O'Graphy, MD

FIGURE 11-4

Surgery case 4 charge ticket

Surgery Case 4 Charge Ticket

Patient Name	Stanley Cox
Medical Record Number/Account Number	137241
Surgeon	Angela O'Graphy
Referring Physician	Stephen Lucas
Assistant Surgeon	None
Anesthesiologist	Ida Numdya
Insurance Company	Blue Cross Blue Shield
Comments	Postop follow-up 1 day

Date of Surgery	Facility	Place of Service	CPT Code	Diagnosis Code(s)	Modifier	Quantity	Fee
01/10/02	Acme Hospital	OH	66985	366.9 362.2 250.51		1	1200.00

Legend:

Place of Service (POS): OH, outpatient hospital; IH, inpatient hospital; ER, emergency room; O, office

Outpatient hospital surgery centers: Memorial Hospital Surgery Center
Methodist Surgery Center
University Hospital Outpatient Center
Markham Memorial Surgery Center
Acme Hospital

Hospitals: University Hospital
Methodist Hospital
Johnson County Regional Medical Center
St Vincent Hospital Center
Acme Hospital

Surgery case 4

General Surgical Group
Angela O'Graphy, MD
4555 Constitutional Boulevard
Anytown, USA 14589

OPERATIVE REPORT 4

PATIENT: Stanley Cox   MR# 137241
DATE OF OPERATION: 1/10/02
DIAGNOSIS: Cataract of right eye.
OPERATION PERFORMED: Phacoemulsification, right eye cataract, with
posterior chamber lens implantation, Alcon model SA6CAT 20.5 diopters
SURGEON: Angela O'Graphy, MD
ANESTHESIA: MAC.
ANESTHESIOLOGIST: Ida Numdya, MD

INDICATIONS FOR PROCEDURE: This patient is a 62-year-old male with
advancing cataract of the right eye. Best corrected vision is 20/50. He has a
posterior subcapsular type of cataract. It is bothering him tremendously
when he attempts to do close work, which is required for his occupation.
He is also experiencing significant glare. He had undergone cataract
surgery to the left eye several years ago with excellent visual recovery. He
understands the process. He is being bothered by his symptoms. The risks
and benefits of surgery have been reviewed. He has been provided with
fresh, up-to-date, pertinent information. The patient decided to have the
cataract of the right eye removed on the basis of impairment of lifestyle.

DESCRIPTION OF PROCEDURE: The patient was brought to the operating
room on 01/10/02 as an outpatient. Intravenous anesthesia and retrobulbar
block to the right eye were administered. The eye was prepped. The
blepharostat was inserted, and surgical microscope was brought into
position. Conjunctival peritomy was performed. The anterior chamber was
entered at the 12 o'clock position using a keratome inserted at the end of a
self-sealing limbal incision. Viscoelastic material was used as necessary
throughout the case. A capsulorhexis was performed. The cataract was
removed by phacoemulsification technique.

The implant was then delivered and inspected. Implant power was
confirmed to be 20.5 diopters on the package. The implant was inserted
into the capsular bag without difficulty. Viscoelastic material was removed
from the eye. The wound was observed to be fluid tight. A single 10-0
nylon suture was placed for additional security. Tobradex ointment was
applied to the surface of the eye. A sterile patch was taped into place. There
were no complications.

He had an uneventful emergence from anesthesia and returned to the
holding area in satisfactory condition. There he was monitored until stable.
Postoperative instructions were reviewed, and arrangements were made for
1-day follow-up in my office.

Angela O'Graphy, MD
Angela O'Graphy, MD

FIGURE 11-5
Surgery case 5 charge ticket

Surgery Case 5 Charge Ticket

Patient Name	Sarah Trotter
Medical Record Number/Account Number	1378512
Surgeon	Angela O'Graphy
Referring Physician	None
Assistant Surgeon	None
Anesthesiologist	Jerry Graves, MD
Insurance Company	Travelers
Comments	Return to office 1 month

Date of Surgery	Facility	Place of Service	CPT Code	Diagnosis Code(s)	Modifier	Quantity	Fee
02/10/02	Acme Hospital	IH	63042	722.10		1	1500.00

Legend:

Place of Service (POS): OH, outpatient hospital; IH, inpatient hospital; ER, emergency room; O, office

Outpatient hospital surgery centers: Memorial Hospital Surgery Center
Methodist Surgery Center
University Hospital Outpatient Center
Markham Memorial Surgery Center
Acme Hospital

Hospitals: University Hospital
Methodist Hospital
Johnson County Regional Medical Center
St Vincent Hospital Center
Acme Hospital

Surgery case 5

General Surgical Group
Angela O'Graphy, MD
4555 Constitutional Boulevard
Anytown, USA 14589

OPERATIVE REPORT 5

PATIENT: Sarah Trotter   MR# 1378512

PREOPERATIVE DIAGNOSIS: Recurrent left L4-5 lumbar disk protrusion.

POSTOPERATIVE DIAGNOSIS: Same plus left L5-S1 lumbar disk
protrusion.

PROCEDURE PERFORMED:

Redo lift L4-5 microlumbar diskectomy.

Left L5-S1 microlumbar diskectomy.

ANESTHESIA: General

ANESTHESIOLOGIST: Jerry Graves, MD

INDICATIONS FOR PROCEDURE: This 34-year-old female is one week
post left L4-5 microlumbar diskectomy. She presents with very disabling left
sciatica and is completely bedridden. She requires a morphine PCA for pain
relief. Work-up with magnetic resonance imaging scan shows a small to
moderate recurrent left L4-5 disk protrusion. She was previously known to
have a small to moderate left L5-S1 disk protrusion, which was not felt to
be symptomatic, and this still persisted on the latest study. It was felt that
her pain was most likely due to a recurrent left L4-5 disk and it was felt, as
she was bedridden, that it was reasonable to reexplore her at this point. The
nature of the procedure, the alternatives to surgery, and all the surgical risks
have been fully explained in the office.

DESCRIPTION OF PROCEDURE: The patient was brought to the operating
room in the supine position. After induction of general anesthesia she was
rolled prone on the Wilson frame with her hips flexed. She was given 1.5 g
of Zinacef intravenously. The previous Steri-Strips were carefully removed.
The patient's back was then prepped with Duraprep. After the patient had
been draped in a sterile fashion, the previous incision was reopened by
sharp dissection. By blunt dissection the plane was carried down to the
previous hemilaminectomy, which was identified with ease. Retraction was
maintained with a micro-Taylor retractor placed lateral to the facet. The
Contraves microscope was draped and the rest of the procedure was
performed under various magnifications. There was very little clot overlying
the previous hemilaminectomy and there was no scar. The left L-5 nerve
root was identified with ease. It had a normal appearance. It was not
erythematous and it did not appear to be displaced significantly, nor was it
very taut. The root was carefully mobilized with a micro-nerve root
retractor. The previous annulotomy was identified and appeared relatively
normal. I then reentered the disk space with straight and upbiting pituitary
rongeurs of varying sizes and spoon curets. A small amount of degenerative
disk material was still present within the interspace, which was carefully
removed. However, I could not identify any true extruded fragment.
After the disk space had been explored, I then explored the epidural space
superior and inferior to the disk space, out laterally in the L4 and L5
foramina and medially. However, I could not identify any extruded disk
material. In view of the paucity of the findings at L4-5, I elected to look to
L5-S1. The left L5-S1 hemilaminectomy was performed using an angled
3-mm Kerrison punch. The ligamentum flavum was sharply incised with a
15 blade knife and removed. The left S1 nerve root was identified. It had a
normal appearance. It was gently retracted medially with the nerve root

retractor. A firm annular bulge was identified corresponding to the magnetic resonance imaging appearance. The annular bulge was sharply incised with an 11 blade knife. A small amount of disk material was present, but mostly the defect seen was an osteophyte, which was not significantly displaced in the root. A small amount of disk material was removed from the L5-S1 disk space. At the completion of the diskectomy, the wound was irrigated with Bacitracin and meticulous hemostasis obtained at both levels with the bipolar and Gelfoam paste soaked in thrombin.

The wound was then closed using 0 Vicryl for the paraspinous muscles and fascia, 2-0 Vicryl for subcutaneous tissue, and 3-0 Vicryl and Steri-Strips for subcuticular skin closure. Estimated blood loss was less than 50 cc. She received no blood intraoperatively. There were no complications and she tolerated the procedure well. She was returned to the recovery room in satisfactory condition. Needle and sponge count was correct.

Angela O'Graphy, MD
Angela O'Graphy, MD

FIGURE 11-6

Surgery case 6 charge ticket

Surgery Case 6 Charge Ticket

Patient Name	Susan Dow
Medical Record Number/Account Number	1634565
Surgeon	Angela O'Graphy
Referring Physician	
Assistant Surgeon	
Anesthesiologist	None
Insurance Company	Cigna
Comments	

Date of Surgery	Facility	Place of Service	CPT Code	Diagnosis Code(s)	Modifier	Quantity	Fee
02/18/02	ACME Hospital	OH	43235	787.2		1	1000.00
02/18/02	Same	OH	43450	787.2	-51	1	850.00

Legend:

Place of Service (POS): OH, outpatient hospital; IH, inpatient hospital; ER, emergency room; O, office

Outpatient hospital surgery centers: Memorial Hospital Surgery Center
Methodist Surgery Center
University Hospital Outpatient Center
Markham Memorial Surgery Center
Acme Hospital

Hospitals: University Hospital
Methodist Hospital
Johnson County Regional Medical Center
St Vincent Hospital Center
Acme Hospital

Surgery case 6

General Surgical Group
Angela O'Graphy, MD
4555 Constitutional Boulevard
Anytown, USA 14589

OPERATIVE REPORT 6

PATIENT: Susan Dow   MR# 1634565

DATE OF OPERATION: 2/18/02

OPERATION PERFORMED: Esophagogastroduodenoscopy and Maloney dilation.

INDICATIONS FOR PROCEDURE: This is a 36-year-old female with rheumatoid arthritis who has been developing progressive dysphagia over the last week. The patient had an outpatient attempt at esophagogram in the emergency room, which suggested she had a proximal esophageal stricture; therefore, this exam is being done to evaluate this abnormality.

DESCRIPTION OF PROCEDURE: Informed consent was obtained from the patient. Demerol 60 mg, Versed 3 mg were given intravenously slowly for sedation. The patient was placed in the left lateral position.

The GIF-100 EGD scope was passed into the esophagus via the no-touch technique. The esophagus did not demonstrate a definite stricture endoscopically. Whether or not I passed it on inserting the scope, I cannot be certain. Nevertheless, there was certainly no resistance to the passage of the 9-mm scope into the proximal esophagus. The esophagogastric junction was at 40 cm. Stomach was entered and found to be within normal limits, without ulceration. The duodenal bulb and descending duodenum were both normal. The scope was then withdrawn and Maloney dilators 36, 42, 46, and 52 were passed sequentially without difficulty.

The patient tolerated both procedures well and returned to the recovery room in good condition.

IMPRESSION:

1. Possible proximal esophageal stricture.
2. Status post Maloney dilation.

Angela O'Graphy, MD
_____
Angela O'Graphy, MD

FIGURE 11-7

Surgery case 7 charge ticket

Surgery Case 7 Charge Ticket

Patient Name	Emily Stanton
Medical Record Number/Account Number	125987
Surgeon	Angela O'Graphy
Referring Physician	None
Assistant Surgeon	None
Anesthesiologist	Local
Insurance Company	M Plan
Comments	Return 3 days

Date of Surgery	Facility	Place of Service	CPT Code	Diagnosis Code(s)	Modifier	Quantity	Fee
02/15/02	Office	O	11642	173.3 140.1		2	325.00
02/15/02	Office	O	13132	173.3 140.1		1	150.00

Legend:

Place of Service (POS): OH, outpatient hospital; IH, inpatient hospital; ER, emergency room; O, office

Outpatient hospital surgery centers: Memorial Hospital Surgery Center
Methodist Surgery Center
University Hospital Outpatient Center
Markham Memorial Surgery Center
Acme Hospital

Hospitals: University Hospital
Methodist Hospital
Johnson County Regional Medical Center
St Vincent Hospital Center
Acme Hospital

Surgery case 7

General Surgical Group
Angela O'Graphy, MD
4555 Constitutional Boulevard
Anytown, USA 14589

OPERATIVE REPORT 7

PATIENT: Emily Stanton   MR#125987
DATE OF PROCEDURE: 02/15/02
PREOPERATIVE DIAGNOSIS: Nodular basal cell carcinoma, right lower lip and chin.
POSTOPERATIVE DIAGNOSIS: Same.
OPERATION PERFORMED: Excision of basal cell carcinoma and adjacent scar with complex linear repair.
SURGEON: Angela O'Graphy, MD
ANESTHESIA: Local.

DESCRIPTION OF PROCEDURE: With the patient in the supine position, the face was prepared with chlorhexidine and draped in the usual manner. The tumor measured 1.5×1.0 cm, arising in the right lateral lower lip skin and adjacent chin. Just medial and slightly superior to the tumor was an atrophic scar from a previous basal cell cancer removed 9 years earlier. Proposed lines of excision were drawn around the tumor to include the adjacent scar and the area was anesthetized with 1% Xylocaine with 1:100,000 epinephrine, buffered with sodium bicarbonate. The tumor was excised down to orbicularis oris muscle, resulting in a defect measuring 2.1 cm wide $\times$ 3.0 cm in height in the shape of an inverted teardrop. Bleeding vessels were controlled with bipolar electrocoagulation. Adjacent skin was undermined at the deep subcutaneous level medially and laterally. Consideration was given to a rotation flap repair versus a complex linear repair. It was elected to do the defect extending to the vermilion border to convert the original defect to a lazy-S ellipse. Additional undermining was accomplished and the defect was approximated with layers of 5-0 polyglactin suture deep. Final skin repair was accomplished and the defect was approximated with 6-0 nylon sutures, supported by sterile strips over surgical adhesive followed by sterile occlusive dressing.

The specimen was submitted to pathology, after staining its superior margin red, its medial and deep margin black, and its lateral margin blue for pathologic orientation. The patient tolerated the procedure well and received 1 g of acetaminophen (po) postoperatively.

PATHOLOGY REPORT: Confirms nodular basal cell carcinoma right lower lip and chin.

Angela O'Graphy, MD
Angela O'Graphy, MD

FIGURE 11-8

Surgery case 8 charge ticket

Surgery Case 8 Charge Ticket

Patient Name	John Strait
Medical Record Number/Account Number	134791
Surgeon	Angela O'Graphy
Referring Physician	Paula Pasteur, MD
Assistant Surgeon	None
Anesthesiologist	Tom Jance, MD
Insurance Company	CIGNA
Comments	

Date of Surgery	Facility	Place of Service	CPT Code	Diagnosis Code(s)	Modifier	Quantity	Fee
02/10/02	ACME Hospital	IH	31528	478.74		1	2500.00

Legend:

Place of Service (POS): OH, outpatient hospital; IH, inpatient hospital; ER, emergency room; O, office

Outpatient hospital surgery centers: Memorial Hospital Surgery Center
Methodist Surgery Center
University Hospital Outpatient Center
Markham Memorial Surgery Center
Acme Hospital

Hospitals: University Hospital
Methodist Hospital
Johnson County Regional Medical Center
St Vincent Hospital Center
Acme Hospital

Surgery case 8

General Surgical Group
Angela O'Graphy, MD
4555 Constitutional Boulevard
Anytown, USA 14589

OPERATIVE REPORT 8

PATIENT: John Strait   MR# 134791
DATE OF PROCEDURE: 02/10/02
SURGEON: Angela O'Graphy, MD
PREOPERATIVE DIAGNOSIS: Laryngeal stenosis.
POSTOPERATIVE DIAGNOSIS: Same.
ANESTHESIOLOGIST: Tom Jance, MD

INDICATIONS: This 1-year-old male infant was born prematurely at a gestational age of approximately 29 weeks. The patient developed respiratory distress and was intubated for 3 weeks. At this time, the patient subsequently failed extubation and a tracheostomy tube was placed. The patient's respiratory failure was felt to be secondary to subglottic stenosis. Previous endoscopic evaluation with laryngeal dilation was performed. The patient presents for possible ablation of subglottic tissue. The patient was prepped and draped in the usual fashion. A laryngoscope was inserted orally and examination of the larynx and pharynx revealed no abnormalities. The glottis closed as a reflex to the laryngoscope coming in contact. The telescope was withdrawn. There appeared to be subglottic narrowing. The larynx was initially dilated. A fibrous mass was visualized just above the previously inserted tracheostomy tube, somewhat obscuring visualization. The telescope was passed through the cords and stenotic area for better visualization. On close inspection it appeared to be a thick, firm mass attached to the anterior tracheal wall, just above the level of the tracheal stoma. This represented a reactive tissue fibroma.

The telescope was advanced along the left lateral tracheal wall past the level of this fibrous lesion and past the tracheostomy tube to the level of the carina. After inspection, the laryngoscope was withdrawn and the patient sent to recovery in stable condition.

Angela O'Graphy, MD
Angela O'Graphy, MD

Surgery case 9 charge ticket

Surgery Case 9 Charge Ticket

Patient Name	Tray Smith
Medical Record Number/Account Number	144121
Surgeon	Angela O'Graphy
Referring Physician	Gary Creedon, MD
Assistant Surgeon	
Anesthesiologist	Jerry Graves, MD
Insurance Company	Consolidated Insurance
Comments	Return 2 weeks for follow-up visit in office

Date of Surgery	Facility	Place of Service	CPT Code	Diagnosis Code(s)	Modifier	Quantity	Fee
02/06/02	Markham Surgery Center	OH	29881	836.0		1	2200.00

Legend:

Place of Service (POS): OH, outpatient hospital; IH, inpatient hospital; ER, emergency room; O, office

Outpatient hospital surgery centers:
Memorial Hospital Surgery Center
Methodist Surgery Center
University Hospital Outpatient Center
Markham Memorial Surgery Center
Acme Hospital

Hospitals:
University Hospital
Methodist Hospital
Johnson County Regional Medical Center
St Vincent Hospital Center
Acme Hospital

Surgery case 9

General Surgical Group
Angela O'Graphy, MD
4555 Constitutional Boulevard
Anytown, USA 14589

OPERATIVE REPORT 9

PATIENT: Tray Smith   MR# 144121
DATE OF OPERATION: 02/06/02
PREOPERATIVE DIAGNOSIS: Left knee medial meniscal tear, displacing.
POSTOPERATIVE DIAGNOSIS: Left knee locked bucket-handle medial meniscal tear.
OPERATION PERFORMED: Left knee
Exam under anesthesia.
Video arthroscopy.
Partial medial meniscectomy.
SURGEON: Angela O'Graphy, MD
ANESTHESIA: General.
ANESTHESIOLOGIST: Jerry Graves, MD

INDICATIONS FOR PROCEDURE: The patient is a 19-year-old male who presents for treatment of his left knee with which he has been having problems. It is hindering him while he plays basketball. He has had intermittent locking of the knee and intermittent catching of the knee. Recently he has twisted his knee and locked it. He has developed swelling and medial side pain. Secondary to this he is brought to the operating room at this time for treatment.

INTERPRETIVE FINDINGS: Examination under anesthesia reveals a stable knee. The video arthroscopy examination reveals smooth articular surfaces throughout the entire knee. He has a lateral meniscus that is normal. His medial meniscus shows a locked bucket-handle medial meniscal tear, which underwent excision. The cruciate ligament is intact.

DESCRIPTION OF PROCEDURE: On 02/06/98, the patient was taken to the operating room. After adequate general anesthesia, the left lower extremity was prepped with alcohol, painted with Betadine, and draped in a sterile fashion. The tourniquet was inflated to 300 mm Hg of pressure.

The arthroscope was introduced through the anteromedial portal with visualization of the patellofemoral joint, negative. The medial compartment was entered where the medial meniscus was visualized and probed. It was a locked bucket-handle medial meniscal tear noted with a rim remaining with some tearing. It underwent reduction followed by excision. It was removed through a combination of anteromedial and anterolateral portals through a combination of biter, shaver, and punch. Once the fragment had been removed, the remaining rim was trimmed of its remaining fragments with the shaver. The medial femoral condyle was smooth, as was the medial tibial plateau. Intercondylar notch area revealed intact cruciate ligament. The lateral compartment revealed a normal-appearing lateral meniscus and chondral surfaces.

At this time, a final inspection of the knee revealed no additional pathology. Therefore, attention was turned toward the closure. The knee was well irrigated with overhead solution followed by the removal of arthroscopic instrumentation with tips intact. The portal sites were closed with a simple Prolene stitch followed by injection of Marcaine 0.25% with epinephrine. The patient was transferred to the recovery room cart and taken to the recovery room in satisfactory condition, having tolerated the procedure well.

Angela O'Graphy, MD
Angela O'Graphy, MD

FIGURE 11-10

Surgery case 10 charge ticket

Surgery Case 10 Charge Ticket

Patient Name	Howard Burns
Medical Record Number/Account Number	1354654
Surgeon	Angela O'Graphy
Referring Physician	Kim Shirt, MD
Assistant Surgeon	
Anesthesiologist	Jerry Graves, MD
Insurance Company	Medicaid
Comments	

Date of Surgery	Facility	Place of Service	CPT Code	Diagnosis Code(s)	Modifier	Quantity	Fee
02/06/02	Markham Surgery Center	OH	30140	478.1	-51	1	1800.00

Legend:

Place of Service (POS): OH, outpatient hospital; IH, inpatient hospital; ER, emergency room; O, office

Outpatient hospital surgery centers: Memorial Hospital Surgery Center
Methodist Surgery Center
University Hospital Outpatient Center
Markham Memorial Surgery Center
Acme Hospital

Hospitals: University Hospital
Methodist Hospital
Johnson County Regional Medical Center
St Vincent Hospital Center
Acme Hospital

Surgery case 10

General Surgical Group
Angela O'Graphy, MD
4555 Constitutional Boulevard
Anytown, USA 14589

OPERATIVE REPORT 10

PATIENT: Howard Burns   MR# 1354654

DATE OF OPERATION: 02/06/02

PREOPERATIVE DIAGNOSIS: Inferior turbinate hypertrophy, nasal obstruction.

POSTOPERATIVE DIAGNOSIS: Same.

OPERATION PERFORMED: Bilateral submucous resection of inferior turbinates.

SURGEON: Angela O'Graphy, MD

ANESTHESIA: General endotracheal.

ANESTHESIOLOGIST: Jerry Graves, MD

ESTIMATED BLOOD LOSS: Minimal.

FLUIDS: Crystalloid.

COMPLICATIONS: None.

INDICATIONS FOR PROCEDURE: The patient is a 47-year-old gentleman with a long history of nasal obstruction secondary to inferior turbinate hypertrophy. The patient previously underwent very conservative submucous resection of inferior turbinates and continues to have some nasal obstruction. Treatment with nasal steroids was ineffective. Treatment options including risks, benefits, and potential complications were thoroughly discussed with the patient. He indicated he understood and agreed to consent to the above procedure.

DESCRIPTION OF PROCEDURE: On 02/06/98, the patient was taken to the operating room and placed in supine position. General anesthesia was administered via endotracheal tube without complications.

The patient was prepared and draped in the usual manner. Four percent cocaine-saturated neurosurgical cottonoids was placed in either side of the nose. After a sufficient length of time had elapsed, the cottonoids were removed.

Incision was made along the inferior border of the turbinates and the flaps were elevated. Anterior and inferior redundant mucosa was then removed. The turbinates were lateralized. The patient had improved airway. The patient tolerated the procedure well. The patient was awakened and extubated in the operating room and taken to the recovery room in stable condition.

Angela O'Graphy, MD
Angela O'Graphy, MD

F I G U R E 11-11
Surgery audit tool

SURGERY AUDIT TOOL

Patient Name _____ MR# _____

Date of Birth _____ Date of Visit _____ Insurance Carrier _____

Surgical Service (s) Billed _____

Diagnosis Code (s) Billed _____

Comments _____

Documented	Y	N	N/A	Comments
Preoperative information	☐	☐	☐	
Patient demographics	☐	☐	☐	
Surgery date	☐	☐	☐	
Preoperative anesthesia	☐	☐	☐	
Indication for procedure	☐	☐	☐	
Diagnostic reports	☐	☐	☐	
Intraoperative information	☐	☐	☐	
Preoperative diagnosis	☐	☐	☐	
Postoperative diagnosis	☐	☐	☐	
Surgeon/assistant/cosurgeons	☐	☐	☐	
Procedure title	☐	☐	☐	
Findings	☐	☐	☐	
Procedure details	☐	☐	☐	
Tissue/organ removed	☐	☐	☐	
Materials removed/inserted	☐	☐	☐	
Closure information	☐	☐	☐	
Blood loss/replacement	☐	☐	☐	
Wound status	☐	☐	☐	
Drainage	☐	☐	☐	
Complications noted	☐	☐	☐	
Postoperative condition of patient	☐	☐	☐	
IV infusion record	☐	☐	☐	
Signatures	☐	☐	☐	
Legibility	☐	☐	☐	
Supports procedure (CPT/HCPCS)	☐	☐	☐	
Supports medical necessity (ICD-9-CM)	☐	☐	☐	

FIGURE 11-12
Summary report

SUMMARY REPORT

Physician: Angela O'Graphy, MD   Date of Review:

Reviewer:

Number of Operative Notes Reviewed:

Operative notes were reviewed for completeness and appropriateness of care along with coding documentation and medical necessity.

Documentation in the operative note appears to provide preoperative information

Surgery date appears to be documented in the note

Preoperative anesthesia appears to be documented in the note

Indication for procedure appears to be documented in the operative report

Preoperative diagnosis appears to be documented in the operative report

Postoperative diagnosis appears to be documented in the note and supported by findings

Surgeon/assistant/cosurgeons are listed in the operative note

Findings appear to be indicated in the operative report

Procedure details appear to be documented appropriately in the operative report

Postoperative condition of patient appears to be indicated in the operative report

The operative report appears to support procedure (CPT/HCPCS)

The operative report appears to support medical necessity (ICD-9-CM)

Other Documentation and Coding Issues:

1.

2.

3.

4.

5.

RECOMMENDATIONS

1.

2.

3.

4.

5.

FIGURE 11-13
General surgical group summary report

GENERAL SURGICAL GROUP
SUMMARY REPORT

Physician: Angela O'Graphy, MD   Date of Review:

Reviewer:

Number of Operative Notes Reviewed:

Billed   Documented

Patient	CPT® Code	ICD-9-CM Code	MOD	CPT® Code	ICD-9-CM Code	MOD

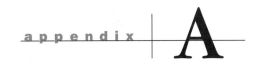
*CMS EXAM TABLES FOR 1997 GUIDELINES

GENERAL MULTI-SYSTEM EXAMINATION

System/Body Area	Elements of Examination
Constitutional	■ Measurement of **any three of the following seven** vital signs: 1) sitting or standing blood pressure, 2) supine blood pressure, 3) pulse rate and regularity, 4) respiration, 5) temperature, 6) height, 7) weight (May be measured and recorded by ancillary staff) ■ General appearance of patient (eg, development, nutrition, body habitus, deformities, attention to grooming)
Eyes	■ Inspection of conjunctivae and lids ■ Examination of pupils and irises (eg, reaction to light and accommodation, size and symmetry) ■ Ophthalmoscopic examination of optic discs (eg, size, C/D ratio, appearance) and posterior segments (eg, vessel changes, exudates, hemorrhages)
Ears, Nose, Mouth and Throat	■ External inspection of ears and nose (eg, overall appearance, scars, lesions, masses) ■ Otoscopic examination of external auditory canals and tympanic membranes ■ Assessment of hearing (eg, whispered voice, finger rub, tuning fork) ■ Inspection of nasal mucosa, septum and turbinates ■ Inspection of lips, teeth and gums ■ Examination of oropharynx: oral mucosa, salivary glands, hard and soft palates, tongue, tonsils and posterior pharynx
Neck	■ Examination of neck (eg, masses, overall appearance, symmetry, tracheal position, crepitus) ■ Examination of thyroid (eg, enlargement, tenderness, mass)

System/Body Area	Elements of Examination
Respiratory	■ Assessment of respiratory effort (eg, intercostal retractions, use of accessory muscles, diaphragmatic movement) ■ Percussion of chest (eg, dullness, flatness, hyperresonance) ■ Palpation of chest (eg, tactile fremitus) ■ Auscultation of lungs (eg, breath sounds, adventitious sounds, rubs)

Cardiovascular	■ Palpation of heart (eg, location, size, thrills)
	■ Auscultation of heart with notation of abnormal sounds and murmurs
	Examination of:
	  • carotid arteries (eg, pulse amplitude, bruits)
	  • abdominal aorta (eg, size, bruits)
	  • femoral arteries (eg, pulse amplitude, bruits)
	  • pedal pulses (eg, pulse amplitude)
	  • extremities for edema and/or varicosities

Chest (Breasts)	■ Inspection of breasts (eg, symmetry, nipple discharge) ■ Palpation of breasts and axillae (eg, masses or lumps, tenderness)
Gastrointestinal (Abdomen)	■ Examination of abdomen with notation of presence of masses or tenderness ■ Examination of liver and spleen ■ Examination for presence or absence of hernia ■ Examination (when indicated) of anus, perineum and rectum, including sphincter tone, presence of hemorrhoids, rectal masses ■ Obtain stool sample for occult blood test when indicated

Genitourinary	**MALE:**
	■ Examination of the scrotal contents (eg, hydrocele, spermatocele, tenderness of cord, testicular mass)
	■ Examination of the penis
	■ Digital rectal examination of prostate gland (eg, size, symmetry, nodularity, tenderness)
	FEMALE:
	■ Pelvic examination (with or without specimen collection for smears and cultures), including
	  • Examination of external genitalia (eg, general appearance, hair distribution, lesions) and vagina (eg, general appearance, estrogen effect, discharge, lesions, pelvic support, cystocele, rectocele)
	  • Examination of urethra (eg, masses, tenderness, scarring)
	  • Examination of bladder (eg, fullness, masses, tenderness)
	  • Cervix (eg, general appearance, lesions, discharge)

System/Body Area	Elements of Examination
Genitourinary (cont.)	■ Uterus (eg, size, contour, position, mobility, tenderness, consistency, descent or support) ■ Adnexa/parametria (eg, masses, tenderness, organomegaly, nodularity)
Lymphatic	Palpation of lymph nodes in **two or more** areas: ■ Neck ■ Axillae ■ Groin ■ Other
Musculoskeletal	■ Examination of gait and station ■ Inspection and/or palpation of digits and nails (eg, clubbing, cyanosis, inflammatory conditions, petechiae, ischemia, infections, nodes) Examination of joints, bones and muscles of **one or more of the following six** areas: 1) head and neck; 2) spine, ribs and pelvis; 3) right upper extremity; 4) left upper extremity; 5) right lower extremity; and 6) left lower extremity. The examination of a given area includes: • Inspection and/or palpation with notation of presence of any misalignment, asymmetry, crepitation, defects, tenderness, masses, effusions • Assessment of range of motion with notation of any pain, crepitation or contracture • Assessment of stability with notation of any dislocation (luxation), subluxation or laxity • Assessment of muscle strength and tone (eg, flaccid, cogwheel, spastic) with notation of any atrophy or abnormal movement
Skin	■ Inspection of skin and subcutaneous tissue (eg, rashes, lesions, ulcers) ■ Palpation of skin and subcutaneous tissue (eg, induration, subcutaneous nodules, tightening)
Neurologic	■ Test cranial nerves with notation of any deficits ■ Examination of deep tendon reflexes with notation of pathological reflexes (eg, Babinski) ■ Examination of sensation (eg, by touch, pin, vibration, proprioception)
Psychiatric	■ Description of patient's judgment and insight Brief assessment of mental status including: • orientation to time, place and person • recent and remote memory • mood and affect (eg, depression, anxiety, agitation)

Content and Documentation Requirements

Level of Exam	Perform and Document:
Problem Focused	**One to five** elements identified by a bullet.
Expanded Problem Focused	**At least six** elements identified by a bullet.
Detailed	**At least two** elements identified by a bullet from each of six areas/systems OR **at least twelve elements** identified by a bullet in two or more areas/systems.
Comprehensive	Perform **all** elements identified by a bullet in at least nine organ systems or body areas and document at least two elements identified by a bullet from each of nine areas/systems.

CARDIOVASCULAR EXAMINATION

System/Body Area	Elements of Examination
Constitutional	▪ Measurement of **any three of the following seven** vital signs: 1) sitting or standing blood pressure, 2) supine blood pressure, 3) pulse rate and regularity, 4) respiration, 5) temperature, 6) height, 7) weight (May be measured and recorded by ancillary staff) ▪ General appearance of patient (eg, development, nutrition, body habitus, deformities, attention to grooming)
Head and Face	
Eyes	▪ Inspection of conjunctivae and lids (eg, xanthelasma)
Ears, Nose, Mouth and Throat	▪ Inspection of teeth, gums and palate ▪ Inspection of oral mucosa with notation of presence of pallor or cyanosis
Neck	▪ Examination of jugular veins (eg, distention; a, v or cannon a waves) ▪ Examination of thyroid (eg, enlargement, tenderness, mass)
Respiratory	▪ Assessment of respiratory effort (eg, intercostal retractions, use of accessory muscles, diaphragmatic movement) ▪ Auscultation of lungs (eg, breath sounds, adventitious sounds, rubs)
Cardiovascular	▪ Palpation of heart (eg, location, size and forcefulness of the point of maximal impact; thrills; lifts; palpable S3 or S4) ▪ Auscultation of heart including sounds, abnormal sounds and murmurs ▪ Measurement of blood pressure in two or more extremities when indicated (eg, aortic dissection, coarctation) Examination of: • Carotid arteries (eg, waveform, pulse amplitude, bruits, apical-carotid delay)

System/Body Area	Elements of Examination
	• Abdominal aorta (eg, size, bruits) • Femoral arteries (eg, pulse amplitude, bruits) • Pedal pulses (eg, pulse amplitude) • Extremities for peripheral edema and/or varicosities
Chest (Breasts)	
Gastrointestinal (Abdomen)	■ Examination of abdomen with notation of presence of masses or tenderness ■ Examination of liver and spleen ■ Obtain stool sample for occult blood from patients who are being considered for thrombolytic or anticoagulant therapy
Genitourinary (Abdomen)	
Lymphatic	
Musculoskeletal	■ Examination of the back with notation of kyphosis or scoliosis ■ Examination of gait with notation of ability to undergo exercise testing and/or participation in exercise programs ■ Assessment of muscle strength and tone (eg, flaccid, cogwheel, spastic) with notation of any atrophy and abnormal movements
Extremities	■ Inspection and palpation of digits and nails (eg, clubbing, cyanosis, inflammation, petechiae, ischemia, infections, Osler's nodes)
Skin	■ Inspection and/or palpation of skin and subcutaneous tissue (eg, stasis dermatitis, ulcers, scars, xanthomas)
Neurological/ Psychiatric	Brief assessment of mental status including • Orientation to time, place and person, • Mood and affect (eg, depression, anxiety, agitation)

Content and Documentation Requirements

Level of Exam	Perform and Document:
Problem Focused	**One to five** elements identified by a bullet.
Expanded Problem Focused	**At least six** elements identified by a bullet.
Detailed	**At least twelve** elements identified by a bullet.
Comprehensive	Perform **all** elements identified by a bullet; document every element in each box with a shaded border and at least one element in each box with an unshaded border.

EAR, NOSE AND THROAT EXAMINATION

System/Body Area	Elements of Examination
Constitutional	■ Measurement of **any three of the following seven** vital signs: 1) sitting or standing blood pressure, 2) supine blood pressure, 3) pulse rate and regularity, 4) respiration, 5) temperature, 6) height, 7) weight (May be measured and recorded by ancillary staff) ■ General appearance of patient (eg, development, nutrition, body habitus, deformities, attention to grooming) ■ Assessment of ability to communicate (eg, use of sign language or other communication aids) and quality of voice
Head and Face	■ Inspection of head and face (eg, overall appearance, scars, lesions and masses) ■ Palpation and/or percussion of face with notation of presence or absence of sinus tenderness ■ Examination of salivary glands ■ Assessment of facial strength
Eyes	■ Test ocular motility including primary gaze alignment
Ears, Nose, Mouth and Throat	■ Otoscopic examination of external auditory canals and tympanic membranes including pneumo-otoscopy with notation of mobility of membranes ■ Assessment of hearing with tuning forks and clinical speech reception thresholds (eg, whispered voice, finger rub) ■ External inspection of ears and nose (eg, overall appearance, scars, lesions and masses) ■ Inspection of nasal mucosa, septum and turbinates ■ Inspection of lips, teeth and gums ■ Examination of oropharynx: oral mucosa, hard and soft palates, tongue, tonsils and posterior pharynx (eg, asymmetry, lesions, hydration of mucosal surfaces) ■ Inspection of pharyngeal walls and pyriform sinuses (eg, pooling of saliva, asymmetry, lesions) ■ Examination by mirror of larynx including the condition of the epiglottis, false vocal cords, true vocal cords and mobility of larynx (Use of mirror not required in children) ■ Examination by mirror of nasopharynx including appearance of the mucosa, adenoids, posterior choanae and eustachian tubes (Use of mirror not required in children)
Neck	■ Examination of neck (eg, masses, overall appearance, symmetry, tracheal position, crepitus)

System/Body Area	Elements of Examination
Neck (cont.)	■ Examination of thyroid (eg, enlargement, tenderness, mass)
Respiratory	■ Inspection of chest including symmetry, expansion and/or assessment of respiratory effort (eg, intercostal retractions, use of accessory muscles, diaphragmatic movement) ■ Auscultation of lungs (eg, breath sounds, adventitious sounds, rubs)
Cardiovascular	■ Auscultation of heart with notation of abnormal sounds and murmurs ■ Examination of peripheral vascular system by observation (eg, swelling, varicosities) and palpation (eg, pulses, temperature, edema, tenderness)
Chest (Breasts)	
Gastrointestinal (Abdomen)	
Genitourinary	
Lymphatic	■ Palpation of lymph nodes in neck, axillae, groin and/or other location
Musculoskeletal	
Extremities	
Skin	
Neurological/ Psychiatric	■ Test cranial nerves with notation of any deficits Brief assessment of mental status including • Orientation to time, place and person • Mood and affect (eg, depression, anxiety, agitation)

Content and Documentation Requirements

Level of Exam	Perform and Document:
Problem Focused	**One to five** elements identified by a bullet.
Expanded Problem Focused	**At least six** elements identified by a bullet.
Detailed	**At least twelve** elements identified by a bullet.
Comprehensive	Perform **all** elements identified by a bullet; document every element in each box with a shaded border and at least one element in each box with an unshaded border.

EYE EXAMINATION

System/Body Area	Elements of Examination
Constitutional	
Head and Face	

Eyes	■ Test visual acuity (Does not include determination of refractive error)
	■ Gross visual field testing by confrontation
	■ Test ocular motility including primary gaze alignment
	■ Inspection of bulbar and palpebral conjunctivae
	■ Examination of ocular adnexae including lids (eg, ptosis or lagophthalmos), lacrimal glands, lacrimal drainage, orbits and preauricular lymph nodes
	■ Examination of pupils and irises including shape, direct and consensual reaction (afferent pupil), size (eg, anisocoria) and morphology
	■ Slit lamp examination of the corneas including epithelium, stroma, endothelium and tear film
	■ Slit lamp examination of the anterior chambers including depth, cells and flare
	■ Slit lamp examination of the lenses including clarity, anterior and posterior capsule, cortex and nucleus
	■ Measurement of intraocular pressures (except in children and patients with trauma or infectious disease)
	Ophthalmoscopic examination through dilated pupils (unless contraindicated) of
	  • Optic discs including size, C/D ratio, appearance (eg, atrophy, cupping, tumor elevation) and nerve fiber layer
	  • Posterior segments including retina and vessels (eg, exudates and hemorrhages)

Ears, Nose, Mouth and Throat	
Neck	
Respiratory	
Cardiovascular	
Chest (Breasts)	
Gastrointestinal (Abdomen)	
Genitourinary	
Lymphatic	
Musculoskeletal	
Extremities	

System/Body Area	Elements of Examination
Skin	
Neurological/ Psychiatric	Brief assessment of mental status including • Orientation to time, place and person • Mood and affect (eg, depression, anxiety, agitation)

Content and Documentation Requirements

Level of Exam	Perform and Document:
Problem Focused	**One to five** elements identified by a bullet.
Expanded Problem Focused	**At least six** elements identified by a bullet.
Detailed	**At least nine** elements identified by a bullet.
Comprehensive	Perform **all** elements identified by a bullet; document every element in each box with a shaded border and at least one element in each box with an unshaded border.

GENITOURINARY EXAMINATION

System/Body Area	Elements of Examination
Constitutional	▪ Measurement of **any three of the following seven** vital signs: 1) sitting or standing blood pressure, 2) supine blood pressure, 3) pulse rate and regularity, 4) respiration, 5) temperature, 6) height, 7) weight (May be measured and recorded by ancillary staff) ▪ General appearance of patient (eg, development, nutrition, body habitus, deformities, attention to grooming)
Head and Face	
Eyes	
Ears, Nose, Mouth and Throat	
Neck	▪ Examination of neck (eg, masses, overall appearance, symmetry, tracheal position, crepitus) ▪ Examination of thyroid (eg, enlargement, tenderness, mass)
Respiratory	▪ Assessment of respiratory effort (eg, intercostal retractions, use of accessory muscles, diaphragmatic movement) ▪ Auscultation of lungs (eg, breath sounds, adventitious sounds, rubs)

System/Body Area	Elements of Examination
Cardiovascular	■ Auscultation of heart with notation of abnormal sounds and murmurs ■ Examination of peripheral vascular system by observation (eg, swelling, varicosities) and palpation (eg, pulses, temperature, edema, tenderness)
Chest (Breasts)	[See genitourinary (female)]
Gastrointestinal (Abdomen)	■ Examination of abdomen with notation of presence of masses or tenderness ■ Examination for presence or absence of hernia ■ Examination of liver and spleen ■ Obtain stool sample for occult blood test when indicated

Genitourinary	**MALE:**
	■ Inspection of anus and perineum
	Examination (with or without specimen collection for smears and cultures) of genitalia including:
	  • Scrotum (eg, lesions, cysts, rashes)
	  • Epididymides (eg, size, symmetry, masses)
	■ Testes (eg, size, symmetry, masses)
	  • Urethral meatus (eg, size, location, lesions, discharge)
	  • Penis (eg, lesions, presence or absence of foreskin, foreskin retractability, plaque, masses, scarring, deformities)
	Digital rectal examination including:
	■ Prostate gland (eg, size, symmetry, nodularity, tenderness)
	  • Seminal vesicles (eg, symmetry, tenderness, masses, enlargement)
	■ Sphincter tone, presence of hemorrhoids, rectal masses

Genitourinary	**FEMALE:**
	Includes **at least seven of the following eleven** elements identified by bullets:
	■ Inspection and palpation of breasts (eg, masses or lumps, tenderness, symmetry, nipple discharge)
	■ Digital rectal examination including sphincter tone, presence of hemorrhoids, rectal masses
	Pelvic examination (with or without specimen collection for smears and cultures) including:
	  • External genitalia (eg, general appearance, hair distribution, lesions)
	  • Urethral meatus (eg, size, location, lesions, prolapse)
	  • Urethra (eg, masses, tenderness, scarring)
	  • Bladder (eg, fullness, masses, tenderness)
	  • Vagina (eg, general appearance, estrogen effect, discharge, lesions, pelvic support, cystocele, rectocele)

System/Body Area	Elements of Examination
Genitourinary (cont.)	• Cervix (eg, general appearance, lesions, discharge) • Uterus (eg, size, contour, position, mobility, tenderness, consistency, descent or support) • Adnexa/parametria (eg, masses, tenderness, organomegaly, nodularity) • Anus and perineum
Lymphatic	• Palpation of lymph nodes in neck, axillae, groin and/or other location
Musculoskeletal	
Extremities	
Skin	■ Inspection and/or palpation of skin and subcutaneous tissue (eg, rashes, lesions, ulcers)
Neurological/ Psychiatric	Brief assessment of mental status including • Orientation (eg, time, place and person) and • Mood and affect (eg, depression, anxiety, agitation)

Content and Documentation Requirements

Level of Exam	Perform and Document:
Problem Focused	**One to five** elements identified by a bullet.
Expanded Problem Focused	**At least six** elements identified by a bullet.
Detailed	**At least twelve** elements identified by a bullet.
Comprehensive	Perform **all** elements identified by a bullet; document every element in each box with a shaded border and at least one element in each box with an unshaded border.

HEMATOLOGIC/LYMPHATIC/ IMMUNOLOGIC EXAMINATION

System/Body Area	Elements of Examination
Constitutional	■ Measurement of **any three of the following seven** vital signs: 1) sitting or standing blood pressure, 2) supine blood pressure, 3) pulse rate and regularity, 4) respiration, 5) temperature, 6) height, 7) weight (May be measured and recorded by ancillary staff) ■ General appearance of patient (eg, development, nutrition, body habitus, deformities, attention to grooming)

System/Body Area	Elements of Examination
Head and Face	◼ Palpation and/or percussion of face with notation of presence or absence of sinus tenderness
Eyes	◼ Inspection of conjunctivae and lids
Ears, Nose, Mouth and Throat	◼ Otoscopic examination of external auditory canals and tympanic membranes ◼ Inspection of nasal mucosa, septum and turbinates ◼ Inspection of teeth and gums ◼ Examination of oropharynx (eg, oral mucosa, hard and soft palates, tongue, tonsils, posterior pharynx)
Neck	• Examination of neck (eg, masses, overall appearance, symmetry, tracheal position, crepitus) • Examination of thyroid (eg, enlargement, tenderness, mass)
Respiratory	◼ Assessment of respiratory effort (eg, intercostal retractions, use of accessory muscles, diaphragmatic movement) ◼ Auscultation of lungs (eg, breath sounds, adventitious sounds, rubs)
Cardiovascular	◼ Auscultation of heart with notation of abnormal sounds and murmurs ◼ Examination of peripheral vascular system by observation (eg, swelling, varicosities) and palpation (eg, pulses, temperature, edema, tenderness)
Chest (Breasts)	
Gastrointestinal (Abdomen)	◼ Examination of abdomen with notation of presence of masses or tenderness ◼ Examination of liver and spleen
Genitourinary	
Lymphatic	◼ Palpation of lymph nodes in neck, axillae, groin, and/or other location
Musculoskeletal	
Extremities	◼ Inspection and palpation of digits and nails (eg, clubbing, cyanosis, inflammation, petechiae, ischemia, infections, nodes)
Skin	◼ Inspection and/or palpation of skin and subcutaneous tissue (eg, rashes, lesions, ulcers, ecchymoses, bruises)
Neurological/ Psychiatric	Brief assessment of mental status including • Orientation to time, place and person • Mood and affect (eg, depression, anxiety, agitation)

Content and Documentation Requirements

Level of Exam	Perform and Document:
Problem Focused	**One to five** elements identified by a bullet.
Expanded Problem Focused	**At least six** elements identified by a bullet.
Detailed	**At least twelve** elements identified by a bullet.
Comprehensive	Perform **all** elements identified by a bullet; document every element in each box with a shaded border and at least one element in each box with an unshaded border.

MUSCULOSKELETAL EXAMINATION

System/Body Area	Elements of Examination
Constitutional	■ Measurement of **any three of the following seven** vital signs: 1) sitting or standing blood pressure, 2) supine blood pressure, 3) pulse rate and regularity, 4) respiration, 5) temperature, 6) height, 7) weight (May be measured and recorded by ancillary staff) ■ General appearance of patient (eg, development, nutrition, body habitus, deformities, attention to grooming)
Head and Face	
Eyes	
Ears, Nose, Mouth and Throat	
Neck	
Respiratory	
Cardiovascular	■ Examination of peripheral vascular system by observation (eg, swelling, varicosities) and palpation (eg, pulses, temperature, edema, tenderness)
Chest (Breasts)	
Gastrointestinal	
(Abdomen)	
Genitourinary	
Lymphatic	■ Palpation of lymph nodes in neck, axillae, groin and/or other location
Musculoskeletal	■ Examination of gait and station Examination of joint(s), bone(s) and muscle(s)/tendon(s) of **four of the following six** areas: 1) head and neck; 2) spine, ribs and pelvis; 3) right upper extremity; 4) left upper extremity; 5) right lower extremity; and 6) left lower extremity. The examination of a given area includes:

System/Body Area	Elements of Examination
	• Inspection, percussion and/or palpation with notation of any misalignment, asymmetry, crepitation, defects, tenderness, masses or effusions • Assessment of range of motion with notation of any pain (eg, straight leg raising), crepitation or contracture • Assessment of stability with notation of any dislocation (luxation), subluxation or laxity • Assessment of muscle strength and tone (eg, flaccid, cogwheel, spastic) with notation of any atrophy or abnormal movements NOTE: For the comprehensive level of examination, all four of the elements identified by a bullet must be performed and documented for each of four anatomic areas. For the three lower levels of examination, each element is counted separately for each body area. For example, assessing range of motion in two extremities constitutes two elements.
Extremities	[See musculoskeletal and skin]
Skin	■ Inspection and/or palpation of skin and subcutaneous tissue (eg, scars, rashes, lesions, cafe-au-lait spots, ulcers) in **four of the following six** areas: 1) head and neck; 2) trunk; 3) right upper extremity; 4) left upper extremity; 5) right lower extremity; and 6) left lower extremity. NOTE: For the comprehensive level, the examination of all four anatomic areas must be performed and documented. For the three lower levels of examination, each body area is counted separately. For example, inspection and/or palpation of the skin and subcutaneous tissue of two extremities constitutes two elements.
Neurological/ Psychiatric	■ Test coordination (eg, finger/nose, heel/ knee/shin, rapid alternating movements in the upper and lower extremities, evaluation of fine motor coordination in young children) ■ Examination of deep tendon reflexes and/or nerve stretch test with notation of pathological reflexes (eg, Babinski) ■ Examination of sensation (eg, by touch, pin, vibration, proprioception) Brief assessment of mental status including • Orientation to time, place and person • Mood and affect (eg, depression, anxiety, agitation)

Content and Documentation Requirements

Level of Exam	Perform and Document:
Problem Focused	**One to five** elements identified by a bullet.
Expanded Problem Focused	**At least six** elements identified by a bullet.
Detailed	**At least twelve** elements identified by a bullet.
Comprehensive	Perform **all** elements identified by a bullet; document every element in each box with a shaded border and at least one element in each box with an unshaded border.

NEUROLOGICAL EXAMINATION

System/Body Area	Elements of Examination
Constitutional	▪ Measurement of **any three of the following seven** vital signs: 1) sitting or standing blood pressure, 2) supine blood pressure, 3) pulse rate and regularity, 4) respiration, 5) temperature, 6) height, 7) weight (May be measured and recorded by ancillary staff) ▪ General appearance of patient (eg, development, nutrition, body habitus, deformities, attention to grooming)
Head and Face	
Eyes	• Ophthalmoscopic examination of optic discs (eg, size, C/D ratio, appearance) and posterior segments (eg, vessel changes, exudates, hemorrhages)
Ears, Nose, Mouth and Throat	
Neck	
Respiratory	
Cardiovascular	• Examination of carotid arteries (eg, pulse amplitude, bruits) ▪ Auscultation of heart with notation of abnormal sounds and murmurs ▪ Examination of peripheral vascular system by observation (eg, swelling, varicosities) and palpation (eg, pulses, temperature, edema, tenderness)
Chest (Breasts)	
Gastrointestinal	
(Abdomen)	
Genitourinary	
Lymphatic	

System/Body Area	Elements of Examination
Musculoskeletal	■ Examination of gait and station Assessment of motor function including: • Muscle strength in upper and lower extremities • Muscle tone in upper and lower extremities (eg, flaccid, cogwheel, spastic) with notation of any atrophy or abnormal movements (eg, fasciculation, tardive dyskinesia)
Extremities	[See Musculoskeletal]
Skin	
Neurological	Evaluation of higher integrative functions including: • Orientation to time, place and person • Recent and remote memory • Attention span and concentration • Language (eg, naming objects, repeating phrases, spontaneous speech) • Fund of knowledge (eg, awareness of current events, past history, vocabulary) Test the following cranial nerves: • 2nd cranial nerve (eg, visual acuity, visual fields, fundi) • 3rd, 4th and 6th cranial nerves (eg, pupils, eye movements) • 5th cranial nerve (eg, facial sensation, corneal reflexes) • 7th cranial nerve (eg, facial symmetry, strength) • 8th cranial nerve (eg, hearing with tuning fork, whispered voice and/or finger rub) • 9th cranial nerve (eg, spontaneous or reflex palate movement) • 11th cranial nerve (eg, shoulder shrug strength) • 12th cranial nerve (eg, tongue protrusion) ■ Examination of sensation (eg, by touch, pin, vibration, proprioception) ■ Examination of deep tendon reflexes in upper and lower extremities with notation of pathological reflexes (eg, Babinski) ■ Test coordination (eg, finger/nose, heel/knee/shin, rapid alternating movements in the upper and lower extremities, evaluation of fine motor coordination in young children)
Psychiatric	

Content and Documentation Requirements

Level of Exam	Perform and Document:
Problem Focused	One to five elements identified by a bullet.
Expanded Problem Focused	At least six elements identified by a bullet.
Detailed	At least twelve elements identified by a bullet.
Comprehensive	Perform all elements identified by a bullet; document every element in each box with a shaded border and at least one element in each box with an unshaded border.

PSYCHIATRIC EXAMINATION

System/Body Area	Elements of Examination
Constitutional	■ Measurement of **any three of the following seven** vital signs: 1) sitting or standing blood pressure, 2) supine blood pressure, 3) pulse rate and regularity, 4) respiration, 5) temperature, 6) height, 7) weight (May be measured and recorded by ancillary staff) ■ General appearance of patient (eg, development, nutrition, body habitus, deformities, attention to grooming)
Head and Face	
Eyes	
Ears, Nose, Mouth and Throat	
Neck	
Respiratory	
Cardiovascular	
Chest (Breasts)	
Gastrointestinal	
(Abdomen)	
Genitourinary	
Lymphatic	
Musculoskeletal	■ Assessment of muscle strength and tone (eg, flaccid, cogwheel, spastic) with notation of any atrophy and abnormal movements ■ Examination of gait and station
Extremities	
Skin	
Neurological	

System/Body Area	Elements of Examination
Psychiatric	◼ Description of speech including: rate; volume; articulation; coherence; and spontaneity with notation of abnormalities (eg, perseveration, paucity of language)
	◼ Description of thought processes including: rate of thoughts; content of thoughts (eg, logical vs illogical, tangential); abstract reasoning; and computation
	◼ Description of associations (eg, loose, tangential, circumstantial, intact)
	◼ Description of abnormal or psychotic thoughts including: hallucinations; delusions; preoccupation with violence; homicidal or suicidal ideation; and obsessions
	◼ Description of the patient's judgment (eg, concerning everyday activities and social situations) and insight (eg, concerning psychiatric condition)
	Complete mental status examination including
	• Orientation to time, place and person
	• Recent and remote memory
	• Attention span and concentration
	• Language (eg, naming objects, repeating phrases)
	• Fund of knowledge (eg, awareness of current events, past history, vocabulary)
	• Mood and affect (eg, depression, anxiety, agitation, hypomania, lability)

Content and Documentation Requirements

Level of Exam	Perform and Document:
Problem Focused	**One to five** elements identified by a bullet.
Expanded Problem Focused	**At least six** elements identified by a bullet.
Detailed	**At least nine** elements identified by a bullet.
Comprehensive	Perform **all** elements identified by a bullet; document every element in each box with a shaded border and at least one element in each box with an unshaded border.

RESPIRATORY EXAMINATION

System/Body Area	Elements of Examination
Constitutional	■ Measurement of **any three of the following seven** vital signs: 1) sitting or standing blood pressure, 2) supine blood pressure, 3) pulse rate and regularity, 4) respiration, 5) temperature, 6) height, 7) weight (May be measured and recorded by ancillary staff) ■ General appearance of patient (eg, development, nutrition, body habitus, deformities, attention to grooming)
Head and Face	
Eyes	
Ears, Nose, Mouth and Throat	■ Inspection of nasal mucosa, septum and turbinates ■ Inspection of teeth and gums ■ Examination of oropharynx (eg, oral mucosa, hard and soft palates, tongue, tonsils and posterior pharynx)
Neck	■ Examination of neck (eg, masses, overall appearance, symmetry, tracheal position, crepitus) ■ Examination of thyroid (eg, enlargement, tenderness, mass) ■ Examination of jugular veins (eg, distention; a, v or cannon a waves)
Respiratory	■ Inspection of chest with notation of symmetry and expansion ■ Assessment of respiratory effort (eg, intercostal retractions, use of accessory muscles, diaphragmatic movement) ■ Percussion of chest (eg, dullness, flatness, hyperresonance) ■ Palpation of chest (eg, tactile fremitus) ■ Auscultation of lungs (eg, breath sounds, adventitious sounds, rubs)
Cardiovascular	■ Auscultation of heart including sounds, abnormal sounds and murmurs ■ Examination of peripheral vascular system by observation (eg, swelling, varicosities) and palpation (eg, pulses, temperature, edema, tenderness)
Chest (Breasts)	
Gastrointestinal (Abdomen)	■ Examination of abdomen with notation of presence of masses or tenderness ■ Examination of liver and spleen
Genitourinary	
Lymphatic	■ Palpation of lymph nodes in neck, axillae, groin and/or other location

System/Body Area	Elements of Examination
Musculoskeletal	■ Assessment of muscle strength and tone (eg, flaccid, cogwheel, spastic) with notation of any atrophy and abnormal movements ■ Examination of gait and station
Extremities	■ Inspection and palpation of digits and nails (eg, clubbing, cyanosis, inflammation, petechiae, ischemia, infections, nodes)
Skin	■ Inspection and/or palpation of skin and subcutaneous tissue (eg, rashes, lesions, ulcers)
Neurological/ Psychiatric	Brief assessment of mental status including • Orientation to time, place and person • Mood and affect (eg, depression, anxiety, agitation)

Content and Documentation Requirements

Level of Exam	Perform and Document:
Problem Focused	**One to five** elements identified by a bullet.
Expanded Problem Focused	**At least six** elements identified by a bullet.
Detailed	**At least twelve** elements identified by a bullet.
Comprehensive	Perform **all** elements identified by a bullet; document every element in each box with a shaded border and at least one element in each box with an unshaded border.

SKIN EXAMINATION

System/Body Area	Elements of Examination
Constitutional	■ Measurement of any **three of the following seven** vital signs: 1) sitting or standing blood pressure, 2) supine blood pressure, 3) pulse rate and regularity, 4) respiration, 5) temperature, 6) height, 7) weight (May be measured and recorded by ancillary staff) ■ General appearance of patient (eg, development, nutrition, body habitus, deformities, attention to grooming)
Head and Face	
Eyes	■ Inspection of conjunctivae and lids
Ears, Nose, Mouth and Throat	■ Inspection of lips, teeth and gums ■ Examination of oropharynx (eg, oral mucosa, hard and soft palates, tongue, tonsils, posterior pharynx)

System/Body Area	Elements of Examination
Neck	■ Examination of thyroid (eg, enlargement, tenderness, mass)
Respiratory	
Cardiovascular	■ Examination of peripheral vascular system by observation (eg, swelling, varicosities) and palpation (eg, pulses, temperature, edema, tenderness)
Chest (Breasts)	
Gastrointestinal (Abdomen)	■ Examination of liver and spleen ■ Examination of anus for condyloma and other lesion
Genitourinary	
Lymphatic	■ Palpation of lymph nodes in neck, axillae, groin and/or other location
Musculoskeletal	
Extremities	■ Inspection and palpation of digits and nails (eg, clubbing, cyanosis, inflammation, petechiae, ischemia, infections, nodes)
Skin	■ Palpation of scalp and inspection of hair of scalp, eyebrows, face, chest, pubic area (when indicated) and extremities ■ Inspection and/or palpation of skin and subcutaneous tissue (eg, rashes, lesions, ulcers, susceptibility to and presence of photo damage) in **eight of the following ten** areas: ■ Head, including the face and ■ Neck ■ Chest, including breasts and axillae ■ Abdomen ■ Genitalia, groin, buttocks ■ Back ■ Right upper extremity ■ Left upper extremity ■ Right lower extremity ■ Left lower extremity NOTE: For the comprehensive level, the examination of at least eight anatomic areas must be performed and documented. For the three lower levels of examination, each body area is counted separately. For example, inspection and/or palpation of the skin and subcutaneous tissue of the right upper extremity and the left upper extremity constitutes two elements. ■ Inspection of eccrine and apocrine glands of skin and subcutaneous tissue with identification and location of any hyperhidrosis, chromhidroses or bromhidrosis
Neurological/ Psychiatric	Brief assessment of mental status including • Orientation to time, place and person • Mood and affect (eg, depression, anxiety, agitation)

Content and Documentation Requirements

Level of Exam	Perform and Document:
Problem Focused	**One to five** elements identified by a bullet.
Expanded Problem Focused	**At least six** elements identified by a bullet.
Detailed	**At least twelve** elements identified by a bullet.
Comprehensive	Perform **all** elements identified by a bullet; document every element in each box with a shaded border and at least one element in each box with an unshaded border.

*CMS DOCUMENTATION GUIDELINES FOR 1995 AND 1997

1995 DOCUMENTATION GUIDELINES FOR EVALUATION & MANAGEMENT SERVICES

I.   INTRODUCTION

WHAT IS DOCUMENTATION AND WHY IS IT IMPORTANT?

Medical record documentation is required to record pertinent facts, findings, and observations about an individual's health history including past and present illnesses, examinations, tests, treatments, and outcomes. The medical record chronologically documents the care of the patient and is an important element contributing to high quality care. The medical record facilitates:

- the ability of the physician and other health care professionals to evaluate and plan the patient's immediate treatment, and to monitor his/her health care over time;
- communication and continuity of care among physicians and other health care professionals involved in the patient's care;
- accurate and timely claims review and payment;
- appropriate utilization review and quality of care evaluations; and
- collection of data that may be useful for research and education.

An appropriately documented medical record can reduce many of the "hassles" associated with claims processing and may serve as a legal document to verify the care provided, if necessary.

WHAT DO PAYERS WANT AND WHY?

Because payers have a contractual obligation to enrollees, they may require reasonable documentation that services are consistent with the insurance coverage provided. They may request information to validate:

- the site of service;
- the medical necessity and appropriateness of the diagnostic and/or therapeutic services provided; and/or
- that services provided have been accurately reported.

*Centers for Medicare and Medicaid Services (CMS)

II. GENERAL PRINCIPLES OF MEDICAL RECORD DOCUMENTATION

The principles of documentation listed below are applicable to all types of medical and surgical services in all settings. For Evaluation and Management (E/M) services, the nature and amount of physician work and documentation varies by type of service, place of service and the patient's status. The general principles listed below may be modified to account for these variable circumstances in providing E/M services.

1. The medical record should be complete and legible.

2. The documentation of each patient encounter should include:

   ■ reason for the encounter and relevant history, physical examination findings and prior diagnostic test results;

   ■ assessment, clinical impression or diagnosis;

   ■ plan for care; and

   ■ date and legible identity of the observer.

3. If not documented, the rationale for ordering diagnostic and other ancillary services should be easily inferred.

4. Past and present diagnoses should be accessible to the treating and/or consulting physician.

5. Appropriate health risk factors should be identified.

6. The patient's progress, response to and changes in treatment, and revision of diagnosis should be documented.

7. The CPT and ICD-9-CM codes reported on the health insurance claim form or billing statement should be supported by the documentation in the medical record.

III. DOCUMENTATION OF E/M SERVICES

This publication provides definitions and documentation guidelines for the three *key* components of E/M services and for visits which consist predominately of counseling or coordination of care. The three key components—history, examination, and medical decision making—appear in the descriptors for office and other outpatient services, hospital observation services, hospital inpatient services, consultations, emergency department services, nursing facility services, domiciliary care services, and home services. While some of the text of CPT has been repeated in this publication, the reader should refer to CPT for the complete descriptors for E/M services and instructions for selecting a level of service. Documentation guidelines are identified by the symbol •*DG.*

The descriptors for the levels of E/M services recognize seven components which are used in defining the levels of E/M services. These components are:

■ history;

■ examination;

■ medical decision making;

■ counseling;

■ coordination of care;

■ nature of presenting problem; and

■ time.

The first three of these components (ie, history, examination and medical decision making) are the *key* components in selecting the level of E/M services. An exception to this rule is the case of visits which consist predominantly of counseling or coordination of care; for these services time is the key or controlling factor to qualify for a particular level of E/M service.

For certain groups of patients, the recorded information may vary slightly from that described here. Specifically, the medical records of infants, children, adolescents and pregnant women may have additional or modified information recorded in each history and examination area.

As an example, newborn records may include under history of the present illness (HPI) the details of mother's pregnancy and the infant's status at birth; social history will focus on family structure; family history will focus on congenital anomalies and hereditary disorders in the family. In addition, information on growth and development and/or nutrition will be recorded. Although not specifically defined in these documentation guidelines, these patient group variations on history and examination are appropriate.

A. DOCUMENTATION OF HISTORY

The levels of E/M services are based on four types of history (Problem Focused, Expanded Problem Focused, Detailed, and Comprehensive). Each type of history includes some or all of the following elements:

■ Chief complaint (CC);

■ History of present illness (HPI);

■ Review of systems (ROS); and

■ Past, family and/or social history (PFSH).

The extent of history of present illness, review of systems and past, family and/or social history that is obtained and documented is dependent upon clinical judgment and the nature of the presenting problem(s).

The chart below shows the progression of the elements required for each type of history. To qualify for a given type of history, all three elements in the table must be met. (A chief complaint is indicated at all levels.)

History of Present Illness (HPI)	Review of Systems (ROS)	Past, Family, and/or Social History (PFSH)	Type of History
Brief	N/A	N/A	Problem Focused
Brief	Problem Pertinent	N/A	Expanded Problem Focused
Extended	Extended	Pertinent	Detailed
Extended	Complete	Complete	Comprehensive

•DG: *The CC, ROS and PFSH may be listed as separate elements of history, or they may be included in the description of the history of the present illness.*

•DG: *A ROS and/or a PFSH obtained during an earlier encounter does not need to be re-recorded if there is evidence that the physician reviewed and updated the previous information. This may occur when a physician updates his or her own record or in an institutional setting or group practice where many physicians use a common record. The review and update may be documented by:*

   ■ *describing any new ROS and/or PFSH information or noting there has been no change in the information; and*

   ■ *noting the date and location of the earlier ROS and/or PFSH.*

•DG: *The ROS and/or PFSH may be recorded by ancillary staff or on a form completed by the patient. To document that the physician reviewed the information, there must be a notation supplementing or confirming the information recorded by others.*

•DG: *If the physician is unable to obtain a history from the patient or other source, the record should describe the patient's condition or other circumstance which precludes obtaining a history.*

Definitions and specific documentation guidelines for each of the elements of history are listed below.

CHIEF COMPLAINT (CC)

The CC is a concise statement describing the symptom, problem, condition, diagnosis, physician recommended return, or other factor that is the reason for the encounter.

•*DG: The medical record should clearly reflect the chief complaint.*

HISTORY OF PRESENT ILLNESS (HPI)

The HPI is a chronological description of the development of the patient's present illness from the first sign and/or symptom or from the previous encounter to the present. It includes the following elements:

- location,
- quality,
- severity,
- duration,
- timing,
- context,
- modifying factors, and
- associated signs and symptoms.

Brief and *extended* HPIs are distinguished by the amount of detail needed to accurately characterize the clinical problem(s).

A *brief* HPI consists of one to three elements of the HPI.

•*DG: The medical record should describe one to three elements of the present illness (HPI).*

An *extended* HPI consists of four or more elements of the HPI.

•*DG: The medical record should describe four or more elements of the present illness (HPI) or associated comorbidities.*

REVIEW OF SYSTEMS (ROS)

A ROS is an inventory of body systems obtained through a series of questions seeking to identify signs and/or symptoms which the patient may be experiencing or has experienced.

For purposes of ROS, the following systems are recognized:

- Constitutional symptoms (eg, fever, weight loss)
- Eyes
- Ears, Nose, Mouth, Throat
- Cardiovascular
- Respiratory
- Gastrointestinal
- Genitourinary
- Musculoskeletal
- Integumentary (skin and/or breast)
- Neurological
- Psychiatric
- Endocrine
- Hematologic/Lymphatic
- Allergic/Immunologic

A *problem pertinent* ROS inquires about the system directly related to the problem(s) identified in the HPI.

•DG: *The patient's positive responses and pertinent negatives for the system related to the problem should be documented.*

An *extended* ROS inquires about the system directly related to the problem(s) identified in the HPI and a limited number of additional systems.

•DG: *The patient's positive responses and pertinent negatives for two to nine systems should be documented.*

A *complete* ROS inquires about the system(s) directly related to the problem(s) identified in the HPI <u>plus</u> all additional body systems.

•DG: *At least ten organ systems must be reviewed. Those systems with positive or pertinent negative responses must be individually documented. For the remaining systems, a notation indicating all other systems are negative is permissible. In the absence of such a notation, at least ten systems must be individually documented.*

PAST, FAMILY AND/OR SOCIAL HISTORY (PFSH)

The PFSH consists of a review of three areas:

- past history (the patient's past experiences with illnesses, operations, injuries and treatments);
- family history (a review of medical events in the patient's family, including diseases which may be hereditary or place the patient at risk); and
- social history (an age-appropriate review of past and current activities).

For the categories of subsequent hospital care, follow-up inpatient consultations and subsequent nursing facility care, CPT requires only an "interval" history. It is not necessary to record information about the PFSH.

A *pertinent* PFSH is a review of the history area(s) directly related to the problem(s) identified in the HPI.

•DG: *At least one specific item from <u>any</u> of the three history areas must be documented for a pertinent PFSH .*

A *complete* PFSH is of a review of two or all three of the PFSH history areas, depending on the category of the E/M service. A review of all three history areas is required for services that by their nature include a comprehensive assessment or reassessment of the patient. A review of two of the three history areas is sufficient for other services.

•DG: *At least one specific item from <u>two</u> of the three history areas must be documented for a complete PFSH for the following categories of E/M services: office or other outpatient services, established patient; emergency department; subsequent nursing facility care; domiciliary care, established patient; and home care, established patient.*

•DG: *At least one specific item from <u>each</u> of the three history areas must be documented for a complete PFSH for the following categories of E/M services: office or other outpatient services, new patient; hospital observation services; hospital inpatient services, initial care; consultations; comprehensive nursing facility assessments; domiciliary care, new patient; and home care, new patient.*

B.   DOCUMENTATION OF EXAMINATION

The levels of E/M services are based on four types of examination that are defined as follows:

- *Problem Focused*—a limited examination of the affected body area or organ system.
- *Expanded Problem Focused*—a limited examination of the affected body area or organ system and other symptomatic or related organ system(s).
- *Detailed*—an extended examination of the affected body area(s) and other symptomatic or related organ system(s).
- *Comprehensive*—a general multisystem examination or complete examination of a single organ system.

For purposes of examination, the following *body areas* are recognized:

- Head, including the face
- Neck
- Chest, including breasts and axillae
- Abdomen
- Genitalia, groin, buttocks
- Back, including spine
- Each extremity

For purposes of examination, the following *organ systems* are recognized:

- Constitutional (eg, vital signs, general appearance)
- Eyes
- Ears, nose, mouth and throat
- Cardiovascular
- Respiratory
- Gastrointestinal
- Genitourinary
- Musculoskeletal
- Skin
- Neurologic
- Psychiatric
- Hematologic/lymphatic/immunologic

The extent of examinations performed and documented is dependent upon clinical judgment and the nature of the presenting problem(s). They range from limited examinations of single body areas to general multisystem or complete single organ system examinations.

- •DG: *Specific abnormal and relevant negative findings of the examination of the affected or symptomatic body area(s) or organ system(s) should be documented. A notation of "abnormal" without elaboration is insufficient.*
- •DG: *Abnormal or unexpected findings of the examination of the unaffected or asymptomatic body area(s) or organ system(s) should be described.*
- •DG: *A brief statement or notation indicating "negative" or "normal" is sufficient to document normal findings related to unaffected area(s) or asymptomatic organ system(s).*
- •DG: *The medical record for a general multisystem examination should include findings about 8 or more of the 12 organ systems.*

C. DOCUMENTATION OF THE COMPLEXITY OF MEDICAL DECISION MAKING

The levels of E/M services recognize four types of medical decision making (straightforward, low complexity, moderate complexity and high complexity). Medical decision making refers to the complexity of establishing a diagnosis and/or selecting a management option as measured by:

- the number of possible diagnoses and/or the number of management options that must be considered;
- the amount and/or complexity of medical records, diagnostic tests, and/or other information that must be obtained, reviewed and analyzed; and
- the risk of significant complications, morbidity and/or mortality, as well as comorbidities, associated with the patient's presenting problem(s), the diagnostic procedure(s) and/or the possible management options.

The chart below shows the progression of the elements required for each level of medical decision making. To qualify for a given type of decision making, two of the three elements in the table must be either met or exceeded. Each of the elements of medical decision making is described below.

Number of diagnoses or management options	Amount and/or complexity of data to be reviewed	Risk of complications and/or morbidity or mortality	Type of decision making
Minimal	Minimal or None	Minimal	Straightforward
Limited	Limited	Low	Low Complexity
Multiple	Moderate	Moderate	Moderate Complexity
Extensive	Extensive	High	High Complexity

NUMBER OF DIAGNOSES OR MANAGEMENT OPTIONS

The number of possible diagnoses and/or the number of management options that must be considered is based on the number and types of problems addressed during the encounter, the complexity of establishing a diagnosis and the management decisions that are made by the physician.

Generally, decision making with respect to a diagnosed problem is easier than that for an identified but undiagnosed problem. The number and type of diagnostic tests employed may be an indicator of the number of possible diagnoses. Problems which are improving or resolving are less complex than those which are worsening or failing to change as expected. The need to seek advice from others is another indicator of complexity of diagnostic or management problems.

- •DG: *For each encounter, an assessment, clinical impression, or diagnosis should be documented. It may be explicitly stated or implied in documented decisions regarding management plans and/or further evaluation.*

   For a presenting problem with an established diagnosis the record should reflect whether the problem is: a) improved, well controlled, resolving or resolved; or, b) inadequately controlled, worsening, or failing to change as expected.

   For a presenting problem without an established diagnosis, the assessment or clinical impression may be stated in the form of a differential diagnoses or as "possible," "probable," or "rule out" (R/O) diagnoses.

- •DG: *The initiation of, or changes in, treatment should be documented. Treatment includes a wide range of management options including patient instructions, nursing instructions, therapies, and medications.*

- •DG: *If referrals are made, consultations requested or advice sought, the record should indicate to whom or where the referral or consultation is made or from whom the advice is requested.*

AMOUNT AND/OR COMPLEXITY OF DATA TO BE REVIEWED

The amount and complexity of data to be reviewed is based on the types of diagnostic testing ordered or reviewed. A decision to obtain and review old medical records and/or obtain history from sources other than the patient increases the amount and complexity of data to be reviewed.

Discussion of contradictory or unexpected test results with the physician who performed or interpreted the test is an indication of the complexity of data being reviewed. On occasion the physician who ordered a test may personally review the image, tracing or specimen to supplement information from the physician who prepared the test report or interpretation; this is another indication of the complexity of data being reviewed.

- *DG:* *If a diagnostic service (test or procedure) is ordered, planned, scheduled, or performed at the time of the E/M encounter, the type of service, eg, lab or x-ray, should be documented.*

- *DG:* *The review of lab, radiology and/or other diagnostic tests should be documented. An entry in a progress note such as "WBC elevated" or "chest x-ray unremarkable" is acceptable. Alternatively, the review may be documented by initialing and dating the report containing the test results.*

- *DG:* *A decision to obtain old records or decision to obtain additional history from the family, caretaker or other source to supplement that obtained from the patient should be documented.*

- *DG:* *Relevant finding from the review of old records, and/or the receipt of additional history from the family, caretaker or other source should be documented. If there is no relevant information beyond that already obtained, that fact should be documented. A notation of "old records reviewed" or "additional history obtained from family" without elaboration is insufficient.*

- *DG:* *The results of discussion of laboratory, radiology or other diagnostic tests with the physician who performed or interpreted the study should be documented.*

- *DG:* *The direct visualization and independent interpretation of an image, tracing or specimen previously or subsequently interpreted by another physician should be documented.*

RISK OF SIGNIFICANT COMPLICATIONS, MORBIDITY, AND/OR MORTALITY

The risk of significant complications, morbidity, and/or mortality is based on the risks associated with the presenting problem(s), the diagnostic procedure(s), and the possible management options.

- *DG:* *Comorbidities/underlying diseases or other factors that increase the complexity of medical decision making by increasing the risk of complications, morbidity, and/or mortality should be documented.*

- *DG:* *If a surgical or invasive diagnostic procedure is ordered, planned or scheduled at the time of the E/M encounter, the type of procedure, eg, laparoscopy, should be documented.*

- *DG:* *If a surgical or invasive diagnostic procedure is performed at the time of the E/M encounter, the specific procedure should be documented.*

- *DG:* *The referral for or decision to perform a surgical or invasive diagnostic procedure on an urgent basis should be documented or implied.*

The following table may be used to help determine whether the risk of significant complications, morbidity, and/or mortality is *minimal, low, moderate,* or *high.* Because the determination of risk is complex and not readily quantifiable, the table includes common clinical examples rather than absolute measures of risk. The assessment of risk of the presenting problem(s) is based on the risk related to the disease process anticipated between the present encounter and the next one. The assessment of risk of selecting diagnostic procedures and management options is based on the risk during and immediately following any procedures or treatment. The highest level of risk in any one category (presenting problem[s], diagnostic procedure[s], or management options) determines the overall risk.

TABLE OF RISK

Level of Risk	Presenting Problem(s)	Diagnostic Procedure(s) Ordered	Management Options Selected
Minimal	• One self-limited or minor problem, eg cold, insect bite, tinea corporis	• Laboratory tests requiring venipuncture • Chest x-rays • EKG/EEG • Urinalysis • Ultrasound, eg, echocardiography • KOH prep	• Rest • Gargles • Elastic bandages • Superficial dressings
Low	• Two or more self-limited or minor problems • One stable chronic illness, eg, well-controlled hypertension or non–insulin-dependent diabetes, cataract, BPH • Acute uncomplicated illness or injury, eg, cystitis, allergic rhinitis, simple sprain	• Physiologic tests not under stress, eg, pulmonary function tests • Noncardiovascular imaging studies with contrast, eg, barium enema • Superficial needle biopsies • Clinical laboratory tests requiring arterial puncture • Skin biopsies	• Over-the-counter drugs • Minor surgery with no identified risk factors • Physical therapy • Occupational therapy • IV fluids without additives
Moderate	• One or more chronic illnesses with mild exacerbation, progression, or side effects of treatment • Two or more stable chronic illnesses • Undiagnosed new problem with uncertain prognosis, eg, lump in breast • Acute illness with systemic symptoms, eg, pyelonephritis, pneumonitis, colitis • Acute complicated injury, eg, head injury with brief loss of consciousness	• Physiologic tests under stress, eg, cardiac stress test, fetal contraction stress test • Diagnostic endoscopies with no identified risk factors • Deep needle or incisional biopsy • Cardiovascular imaging studies with contrast and no identified risk factors, eg, arteriogram, cardiac catheterization • Obtain fluid from body cavity, eg, lumbar puncture, thoracentesis, culdocentesis	• Minor surgery with identified risk factors • Elective major surgery (open, percutaneous or endoscopic) with no identified risk factors • Prescription drug management • Therapeutic nuclear medicine • IV fluids with additives • Closed treatment of fracture or dislocation without manipulation
High	• One or more chronic illnesses with severe exacerbation, progression, or side effects of treatment • Acute or chronic illnesses or injuries that pose a threat to life or bodily function, eg, multiple trauma, acute MI, pulmonary embolus, severe respiratory distress, progressive severe rheumatoid arthritis, psychiatric illness with potential threat to self or others, peritonitis, acute renal failure • An abrupt change in neurologic status, eg, seizure, TIA, weakness, or sensory loss	• Cardiovascular imaging studies with contrast with identified risk factors • Cardiac electrophysiological tests • Diagnostic endoscopies with identified risk factors • Discography	• Elective major surgery (open, percutaneous or endoscopic) with identified risk factors • Emergency major surgery (open, percutaneous or endoscopic) • Parenteral controlled substances • Drug therapy requiring intensive monitoring for toxicity • Decision not to resuscitate or to deescalate care because of poor prognosis

C. DOCUMENTATION OF AN ENCOUNTER DOMINATED BY
     COUNSELING OR COORDINATION OF CARE

In the case where counseling and/or coordination of care dominates (more
than 50%) of the physician/patient and/or family encounter (face-to-face time
in the office or other outpatient setting or floor/unit time in the hospital or
nursing facility), time is considered the key or controlling factor to qualify for a
particular level of E/M services.

•*DG: If the physician elects to report the level of service based on counseling and/or
       coordination of care, the total length of time of the encounter (face-to-face or
       floor time, as appropriate) should be documented and the record should
       describe the counseling and/or activities to coordinate care.*

1997 DOCUMENTATION GUIDELINES FOR EVALUATION AND MANAGEMENT SERVICES

I. INTRODUCTION

WHAT IS DOCUMENTATION AND WHY IS IT IMPORTANT?
Medical record documentation is required to record pertinent facts, findings, and observations about an individual's health history including past and present illnesses, examinations, tests, treatments, and outcomes. The medical record chronologically documents the care of the patient and is an important element contributing to high quality care. The medical record facilitates:

- the ability of the physician and other health care professionals to evaluate and plan the patient's immediate treatment, and to monitor his/her health care over time;
- communication and continuity of care among physicians and other health care professionals involved in the patient's care;
- accurate and timely claims review and payment;
- appropriate utilization review and quality of care evaluations; and
- collection of data that may be useful for research and education.

An appropriately documented medical record can reduce many of the "hassles" associated with claims processing and may serve as a legal document to verify the care provided, if necessary.

WHAT DO PAYERS WANT AND WHY?
Because payers have a contractual obligation to enrollees, they may require reasonable documentation that services are consistent with the insurance coverage provided. They may request information to validate:

- the site of service;
- the medical necessity and appropriateness of the diagnostic and/or therapeutic services provided; and/or
- that services provided have been accurately reported.

II. GENERAL PRINCIPLES OF MEDICAL RECORD DOCUMENTATION
The principles of documentation listed below are applicable to all types of medical and surgical services in all settings. For Evaluation and Management (E/M) services, the nature and amount of physician work and documentation varies by type of service, place of service and the patient's status. The general principles listed below may be modified to account for these variable circumstances in providing E/M services.

1. The medical record should be complete and legible.
2. The documentation of each patient encounter should include:
    - reason for the encounter and relevant history, physical examination findings and prior diagnostic test results;
    - assessment, clinical impression or diagnosis;
    - plan for care; and
    - date and legible identity of the observer.
3. If not documented, the rationale for ordering diagnostic and other ancillary services should be easily inferred.
4. Past and present diagnoses should be accessible to the treating and/or consulting physician.
5. Appropriate health risk factors should be identified.
6. The patient's progress, response to and changes in treatment, and revision of diagnosis should be documented.

7. The CPT and ICD-9-CM codes reported on the health insurance claim form or billing statement should be supported by the documentation in the medical record.

III. DOCUMENTATION OF E/M SERVICES

This publication provides definitions and documentation guidelines for the three key components of E/M services and for visits which consist predominately of counseling or coordination of care. The three *key* components—history, examination, and medical decision making—appear in the descriptors for office and other outpatient services, hospital observation services, hospital inpatient services, consultations, emergency department services, nursing facility services, domiciliary care services, and home services. While some of the text of CPT has been repeated in this publication, the reader should refer to CPT for the complete descriptors for E/M services and instructions for selecting a level of service. Documentation guidelines are identified by the symbol •*DG*.

The descriptors for the levels of E/M services recognize seven components which are used in defining the levels of E/M services. These components are:

- history;
- examination;
- medical decision making;
- counseling;
- coordination of care;
- nature of presenting problem; and
- time.

The first three of these components (ie, history, examination and medical decision making) are the key components in selecting the level of E/M services. In the case of visits which consist <u>predominantly</u> of counseling or coordination of care, time is the key or controlling factor to qualify for a particular level of E/M service.

Because the level of E/M service is dependent on two or three key components, performance and documentation of one component (eg, examination) at the highest level does not necessarily mean that the encounter in its entirety qualifies for the highest level of E/M service.

These Documentation Guidelines for E/M services reflect the needs of the typical adult population. For certain groups of patients, the recorded information may vary slightly from that described here. Specifically, the medical records of infants, children, adolescents and pregnant women may have additional or modified information recorded in each history and examination area.

As an example, newborn records may include under history of the present illness (HPI) the details of mother's pregnancy and the infant's status at birth; social history will focus on family structure; family history will focus on congenital anomalies and hereditary disorders in the family. In addition, the content of a pediatric examination will vary with the age and development of the child. Although not specifically defined in these documentation guidelines, these patient group variations on history and examination are appropriate.

A. DOCUMENTATION OF HISTORY

The levels of E/M services are based on four types of history (Problem Focused, Expanded Problem Focused, Detailed, and Comprehensive). Each type of history includes some or all of the following elements:

- Chief complaint (CC);
- History of present illness (HPI);

- Review of systems (ROS); and
- Past, family and/or social history (PFSH).

The extent of history of present illness, review of systems and past, family and/or social history that is obtained and documented is dependent upon clinical judgment and the nature of the presenting problem(s).

The chart below shows the progression of the elements required for each type of history. To qualify for a given type of history all three elements in the table must be met. (A chief complaint is indicated at all levels.)

History of Present Illness (HPI)	Review of Systems (ROS)	Past, Family, and/or Social History (PFSH)	Type of History
Brief	N/A	N/A	*Problem Focused*
Brief	Problem Pertinent	N/A	*Expanded Problem Focused*
Extended	Extended	Pertinent	*Detailed*
Extended	Complete	Complete	*Comprehensive*

- *DG: The CC, ROS and PFSH may be listed as separate elements of history, or they may be included in the description of the history of the present illness.*
- *DG: A ROS and/or a PFSH obtained during an earlier encounter does not need to be re-recorded if there is evidence that the physician reviewed and updated the previous information. This may occur when a physician updates his or her own record or in an institutional setting or group practice where many physicians use a common record. The review and update may be documented by:*
  - *describing any new ROS and/or PFSH information or noting there has been no change in the information; and*
  - *noting the date and location of the earlier ROS and/or PFSH.*
- *DG: The ROS and/or PFSH may be recorded by ancillary staff or on a form completed by the patient. To document that the physician reviewed the information, there must be a notation supplementing or confirming the information recorded by others.*
- *DG: If the physician is unable to obtain a history from the patient or other source, the record should describe the patient's condition or other circumstance which precludes obtaining a history.*

Definitions and specific documentation guidelines for each of the elements of history are listed below.

CHIEF COMPLAINT (CC)

The CC is a concise statement describing the symptom, problem, condition, diagnosis, physician recommended return, or other factor that is the reason for the encounter, usually stated in the patient's words.

- *DG: The medical record should clearly reflect the chief complaint.*

HISTORY OF PRESENT ILLNESS (HPI)

The HPI is a chronological description of the development of the patient's present illness from the first sign and/or symptom or from the previous encounter to the present. It includes the following elements:

- location,
- quality,

- severity,
- duration,
- timing,
- context,
- modifying factors, and
- associated signs and symptoms.

Brief and *extended* HPIs are distinguished by the amount of detail needed to accurately characterize the clinical problem(s).

A *brief* HPI consists of one to three elements of the HPI.

•*DG: The medical record should describe one to three elements of the present illness (HPI).*

An *extended* HPI consists of at least four elements of the HPI or the status of at least three chronic or inactive conditions.

•*DG: The medical record should describe at least four elements of the present illness (HPI), or the status of at least three chronic or inactive conditions.*

REVIEW OF SYSTEMS (ROS)

A ROS is an inventory of body systems obtained through a series of questions seeking to identify signs and/or symptoms which the patient may be experiencing or has experienced.

For purposes of ROS, the following systems are recognized:

- Constitutional symptoms (eg, fever, weight loss)
- Eyes
- Ears, Nose, Mouth, Throat
- Cardiovascular
- Respiratory
- Gastrointestinal
- Genitourinary
- Musculoskeletal
- Integumentary (skin and/or breast)
- Neurological
- Psychiatric
- Endocrine
- Hematologic/Lymphatic
- Allergic/Immunologic

A *problem pertinent* ROS inquires about the system directly related to the problem(s) identified in the HPI.

•*DG: The patient's positive responses and pertinent negatives for the system related to the problem should be documented.*

An *extended* ROS inquires about the system directly related to the problem(s) identified in the HPI and a limited number of additional systems.

•*DG: The patient's positive responses and pertinent negatives for two to nine systems should be documented.*

A *complete* ROS inquires about the system(s) directly related to the problem(s) identified in the HPI *plus* all additional body systems.

•*DG: At least ten organ systems must be reviewed. Those systems with positive or pertinent negative responses must be individually documented. For the*

*remaining systems, a notation indicating all other systems are negative is
permissible. In the absence of such a notation, at least ten systems must be
individually documented.*

PAST, FAMILY AND/OR SOCIAL HISTORY (PFSH)

The PFSH consists of a review of three areas:

- past history (the patient's past experiences with illnesses, operations, injuries and treatments);
- family history (a review of medical events in the patient's family, including diseases which may be hereditary or place the patient at risk); and
- social history (an age appropriate review of past and current activities).

For certain categories of E/M services that include only an interval history, it is
not necessary to record information about the PFSH. Those categories are
subsequent hospital care, follow-up inpatient consultations and subsequent
nursing facility care.

A *pertinent* PFSH is a review of the history area(s) directly related to the
problem(s) identified in the HPI.

•*DG: At least one specific item from any of the three history areas must be
documented for a pertinent PFSH .*

A *complete* PFSH is of a review of two or all three of the PFSH history areas,
depending on the category of the E/M service. A review of all three history
areas is required for services that by their nature include a comprehensive
assessment or reassessment of the patient. A review of two of the three history
areas is sufficient for other services.

•*DG: At least one specific item from two of the three history areas must be
documented for a complete PFSH for the following categories of E/M services:
office or other outpatient services, established patient; emergency department;
domiciliary care, established patient; and home care, established patient.*

•*DG: At least one specific item from each of the three history areas must be
documented for a complete PFSH for the following categories of E/M services:
office or other outpatient services, new patient; hospital observation services;
hospital inpatient services, initial care; consultations; comprehensive nursing
facility assessments; domiciliary care, new patient; and home care, new
patient.*

B.   DOCUMENTATION OF EXAMINATION

The levels of E/M services are based on four types of examination:

- *Problem Focused*—a limited examination of the affected body area or organ system.
- *Expanded Problem Focused*—a limited examination of the affected body area or organ system and any symptomatic or related body area(s) or organ system(s).
- *Detailed*—an extended examination of the affected body area(s) or organ system(s) and any other symptomatic or related body area(s) or organ system(s).
- *Comprehensive*—a general multi-system examination, or complete examination of a single organ system and other symptomatic or related body area(s) or organ system(s).

These types of examinations have been defined for general multisystem and
the following single organ systems:

- Cardiovascular
- Ears, Nose, Mouth and Throat
- Eyes
- Genitourinary (Female)
- Genitourinary (Male)
- Hematologic/Lymphatic/Immunologic
- Musculoskeletal
- Neurological
- Psychiatric
- Respiratory
- Skin

A general multisystem examination or a single organ system examination may be performed by any physician regardless of specialty. The type (general multisystem or single organ system) and content of examination are selected by the examining physician and are based upon clinical judgment, the patient's history, and the nature of the presenting problem(s).

The content and documentation requirements for each type and level of examination are summarized below and described in detail in tables beginning on page 306. In the tables, organ systems and body areas recognized by CPT for purposes of describing examinations are shown in the left column. The content, or individual elements, of the examination pertaining to that body area or organ system are identified by bullets (■) in the right column.

Parenthetical examples, "(eg, . . .)," have been used for clarification and to provide guidance regarding documentation. Documentation for each element must satisfy any numeric requirements (such as "Measurement of *any three of the following seven* . . .") included in the description of the element. Elements with multiple components but with no specific numeric requirement (such as "Examination of *liver* and *spleen*") require documentation of at least one component. It is possible for a given examination to be expanded beyond what is defined here. When that occurs, findings related to the additional systems and/or areas should be documented.

- •*DG: Specific abnormal and relevant negative findings of the examination of the affected or symptomatic body area(s) or organ system(s) should be documented. A notation of "abnormal" without elaboration is insufficient.*
- •*DG: Abnormal or unexpected findings of the examination of any asymptomatic body area(s) or organ system(s) should be described.*
- •*DG: A brief statement or notation indicating "negative" or "normal" is sufficient to document normal findings related to unaffected area(s) or asymptomatic organ system(s).*

GENERAL MULTISYSTEM EXAMINATIONS

General multisystem examinations are described in detail later. To qualify for a given level of multisystem examination, the following content and documentation requirements should be met:

- *Problem Focused Examination*—should include performance and documentation of one to five elements identified by a bullet (■) in one or more organ system(s) or body area(s).
- *Expanded Problem Focused Examination*—should include performance and documentation of at least six elements identified by a bullet (■) in one or more organ system(s) or body area(s).
- *Detailed Examination*—should include at least six organ systems or body areas. For each system/area selected, performance and documentation of at

least two elements identified by a bullet (■) is expected. Alternatively, a detailed examination may include performance and documentation of at least twelve elements identified by a bullet (■) in two or more organ systems or body areas.

■ *Comprehensive Examination*—should include at least nine organ systems or body areas. For each system/area selected, all elements of the examination identified by a bullet (■) should be performed, unless specific directions limit the content of the examination. For each area/system, documentation of at least two elements identified by a bullet is expected.

SINGLE ORGAN SYSTEM EXAMINATIONS

The single organ system examinations are recognized by CPT. Variations among these examinations in the organ systems and body areas identified in the left columns and in the elements of the examinations described in the right columns reflect differing emphases among specialties. To qualify for a given level of single organ system examination, the following content and documentation requirements should be met:

■ *Problem Focused Examination*—should include performance and documentation of one to five elements identified by a bullet (■), whether in a box with a shaded or unshaded border.

■ *Expanded Problem Focused Examination*—should include performance and documentation of at least six elements identified by a bullet (■), whether in a box with a shaded or unshaded border.

■ *Detailed Examination*—examinations other than the eye and psychiatric examinations should include performance and documentation of at least twelve elements identified by a bullet (■), whether in box with a shaded or unshaded border.

> Eye and psychiatric examinations should include the performance and documentation of at least nine elements identified by a bullet (■), whether in a box with a shaded or unshaded border.

■ *Comprehensive Examination*—should include performance of all elements identified by a bullet (■), whether in a shaded or unshaded box. Documentation of every element in each box with a shaded border and at least one element in each box with an unshaded border is expected.

Exam tables are located in Appendix A.

DOCUMENTATION OF THE COMPLEXITY OF MEDICAL DECISION MAKING

The levels of E/M services recognize four types of medical decision making (straightforward, low complexity, moderate complexity and high complexity). Medical decision making refers to the complexity of establishing a diagnosis and/or selecting a management option as measured by:

■ the number of possible diagnoses and/or the number of management options that must be considered;

■ the amount and/or complexity of medical records, diagnostic tests, and/or other information that must be obtained, reviewed and analyzed; and

■ the risk of significant complications, morbidity and/or mortality, as well as comorbidities, associated with the patient's presenting problem(s), the diagnostic procedure(s) and/or the possible management options.

The chart on the next page shows the progression of the elements required for each level of medical decision making. To qualify for a given type of decision making, **two of the three elements in the table must be either met or exceeded.**

Number of diagnoses or management options	Amount and/or complexity of data to be reviewed	Risk of complications and/or morbidity or mortality	Type of decision making
Minimal	Minimal or None	Minimal	*Straightforward*
Limited	Limited	Low	*Low Complexity*
Multiple	Moderate	Moderate	*Moderate Complexity*
Extensive	Extensive	High	*High Complexity*

Each of the elements of medical decision making is described below.

NUMBER OF DIAGNOSES OR MANAGEMENT OPTIONS

The number of possible diagnoses and/or the number of management options that must be considered is based on the number and types of problems addressed during the encounter, the complexity of establishing a diagnosis and the management decisions that are made by the physician.

Generally, decision making with respect to a diagnosed problem is easier than that for an identified but undiagnosed problem. The number and type of diagnostic tests employed may be an indicator of the number of possible diagnoses. Problems which are improving or resolving are less complex than those which are worsening or failing to change as expected. The need to seek advice from others is another indicator of complexity of diagnostic or management problems.

- •DG: *For each encounter, an assessment, clinical impression, or diagnosis should be documented. It may be explicitly stated or implied in documented decisions regarding management plans and/or further evaluation.*

  For a presenting problem with an established diagnosis the record should reflect whether the problem is: a) improved, well controlled, resolving or resolved; or, b) inadequately controlled, worsening, or failing to change as expected.

  For a presenting problem without an established diagnosis, the assessment or clinical impression may be stated in the form of differential diagnoses or as a "possible," "probable," or "rule out" (R/O) diagnosis.

- •DG: *The initiation of, or changes in, treatment should be documented. Treatment includes a wide range of management options including patient instructions, nursing instructions, therapies, and medications.*

- •DG: *If referrals are made, consultations requested or advice sought, the record should indicate to whom or where the referral or consultation is made or from whom the advice is requested.*

AMOUNT AND/OR COMPLEXITY OF DATA TO BE REVIEWED

The amount and complexity of data to be reviewed is based on the types of diagnostic testing ordered or reviewed. A decision to obtain and review old medical records and/or obtain history from sources other than the patient increases the amount and complexity of data to be reviewed.

Discussion of contradictory or unexpected test results with the physician who performed or interpreted the test is an indication of the complexity of data being reviewed. On occasion the physician who ordered a test may personally review the image, tracing or specimen to supplement information from the physician who prepared the test report or interpretation; this is another indication of the complexity of data being reviewed.

- •*DG: If a diagnostic service (test or procedure) is ordered, planned, scheduled, or performed at the time of the E/M encounter, the type of service, eg, lab or x-ray, should be documented.*

- •*DG: The review of lab, radiology and/or other diagnostic tests should be documented. A simple notation such as "WBC elevated" or "chest x-ray unremarkable" is acceptable. Alternatively, the review may be documented by initialing and dating the report containing the test results.*

- •*DG: A decision to obtain old records or decision to obtain additional history from the family, caretaker or other source to supplement that obtained from the patient should be documented.*

- •*DG: Relevant findings from the review of old records, and/or the receipt of additional history from the family, caretaker or other source to supplement that obtained from the patient should be documented. If there is no relevant information beyond that already obtained, that fact should be documented. A notation of "old records reviewed" or "additional history obtained from family" without elaboration is insufficient.*

- •*DG: The results of discussion of laboratory, radiology or other diagnostic tests with the physician who performed or interpreted the study should be documented.*

- •*DG: The direct visualization and independent interpretation of an image, tracing or specimen previously or subsequently interpreted by another physician should be documented.*

RISK OF SIGNIFICANT COMPLICATIONS, MORBIDITY, AND/OR MORTALITY

The risk of significant complications, morbidity, and/or mortality is based on the risks associated with the presenting problem(s), the diagnostic procedure(s), and the possible management options.

- •*DG: Comorbidities/underlying diseases or other factors that increase the complexity of medical decision making by increasing the risk of complications, morbidity, and/or mortality should be documented.*

- •*DG: If a surgical or invasive diagnostic procedure is ordered, planned or scheduled at the time of the E/M encounter, the type of procedure, eg, laparoscopy, should be documented.*

- •*DG: If a surgical or invasive diagnostic procedure is performed at the time of the E/M encounter, the specific procedure should be documented.*

- •*DG: The referral for or decision to perform a surgical or invasive diagnostic procedure on an urgent basis should be documented or implied.*

The following table may be used to help determine whether the risk of significant complications, morbidity, and/or mortality is *minimal, low, moderate,* or *high.* Because the determination of risk is complex and not readily quantifiable, the table includes common clinical examples rather than absolute measures of risk. The assessment of risk of the presenting problem(s) is based on the risk related to the disease process anticipated between the present encounter and the next one. The assessment of risk of selecting diagnostic procedures and management options is based on the risk during and immediately following any procedures or treatment. **The highest level of risk in any one category (presenting problem[s], diagnostic procedure[s], or management options) determines the overall risk.**

TABLE OF RISK

Level of Risk	Presenting Problem(s)	Diagnostic Procedure(s) Ordered	Management Options Selected
Minimal	• One self-limited or minor problem, eg cold, insect bite, tinea corporis	• Laboratory tests requiring venipuncture • Chest x-rays • EKG/EEG • Urinalysis • Ultrasound, eg, echocardiography • KOH prep	• Rest • Gargles • Elastic bandages • Superficial dressings
Low	• Two or more self-limited or minor problems • One stable chronic illness, eg, well-controlled hypertension or non–insulin-dependent diabetes, cataract, BPH • Acute uncomplicated illness or injury, eg, cystitis, allergic rhinitis, simple sprain	• Physiologic tests not under stress, eg, pulmonary function tests • Noncardiovascular imaging studies with contrast, eg, barium enema • Superficial needle biopsies • Clinical laboratory tests requiring arterial puncture • Skin biopsies	• Over-the-counter drugs • Minor surgery with no identified risk factors • Physical therapy • Occupational therapy • IV fluids without additives
Moderate	• One or more chronic illnesses with mild exacerbation, progression, or side effects of treatment • Two or more stable chronic illnesses • Undiagnosed new problem with uncertain prognosis, eg, lump in breast • Acute illness with systemic symptoms, eg, pyelonephritis, pneumonitis, colitis • Acute complicated injury, eg, head injury with brief loss of consciousness	• Physiologic tests under stress, eg, cardiac stress test, fetal contraction stress test • Diagnostic endoscopies with no identified risk factors • Deep needle or incisional biopsy • Cardiovascular imaging studies with contrast and no identified risk factors, eg, arteriogram, cardiac catheterization • Obtain fluid from body cavity, eg, lumbar puncture, thoracentesis, culdocentesis	• Minor surgery with identified risk factors • Elective major surgery (open, percutaneous or endoscopic) with no identified risk factors • Prescription drug management • Therapeutic nuclear medicine • IV fluids with additives • Closed treatment of fracture or dislocation without manipulation
High	• One or more chronic illnesses with severe exacerbation, progression, or side effects of treatment • Acute or chronic illnesses or injuries that pose a threat to life or bodily function, eg, multiple trauma, acute MI, pulmonary embolus, severe respiratory distress, progressive severe rheumatoid arthritis, psychiatric illness with potential threat to self or others, peritonitis, acute renal failure • An abrupt change in neurologic status, eg, seizure, TIA, weakness, or sensory loss	• Cardiovascular imaging studies with contrast with identified risk factors • Cardiac electrophysiological tests • Diagnostic endoscopies with identified risk factors • Discography	• Elective major surgery (open, percutaneous or endoscopic) with identified risk factors • Emergency major surgery (open, percutaneous or endoscopic) • Parenteral controlled substances • Drug therapy requiring intensive monitoring for toxicity • Decision not to resuscitate or to deescalate care because of poor prognosis

D. DOCUMENTATION OF AN ENCOUNTER DOMINATED BY COUNSELING OR COORDINATION OF CARE

In the case where counseling and/or coordination of care dominates (more than 50%) of the physician/patient and/or family encounter (face-to-face time in the office or other or outpatient setting, floor/unit time in the hospital or nursing facility), time is considered the key or controlling factor to qualify for a particular level of E/M services.

•*DG:* *If the physician elects to report the level of service based on counseling and/or coordination of care, the total length of time of the encounter (face-to-face or floor time, as appropriate) should be documented and the record should describe the counseling and/or activities to coordinate care.*

AUDIT FORMS

Form 1: Detailed review analysis

MEDICAL RECORD REVIEW
DETAILED REVIEW ANALYSIS

Physician: Date of Review:

Reviewer:

Number of Charts Reviewed:

Patient ID	Service Date	Practice CPT® Code	History	Exam	Medical Decision Making	Documented CPT® Code

Form 2: Summary report

PHYSICIAN MEDICAL RECORD REVIEW
SUMMARY REPORT

Physician: Date of Review:

Reviewer:

Number of Charts Reviewed:

One service date was reviewed for each chart reviewed for appropriate coding and supporting documentation. Each chart was reviewed in detail for completeness.

E/M office visit documentation appears to support service billed.

E/M documentation in the record appears to support a lower level of service than billed.

E/M documentation in the record appears to support a higher level of service than billed.

E/M consultation documentation in the record appears to support a lower level of service than billed.

E/M documentation appears to be missing dictation and/or a handwritten note.

E/M documentation appears to bill the wrong category of service.

E/M documentation in the record appears to be missing a key component: history, examination, and/or medical decision making.

Other Documentation and Coding Issues:

1.

2.

3.

4.

RECOMMENDATIONS

1.

2.

3.

4.

CONFIDENTIAL

Form 3: E/M audit tool #1

E/M Audit Tool #1
Patient Information

Patient: Visit Date: History Level

Examined By: Exam Level

Patient Status: DOB: Decision Making

Service Type: Sex: Insurance Carrier

CPT® Code(s) Billed   DOCUMENTED   DIAGNOSIS CODE(S) BILLED   DOCUMENTED

History

History of Present Illness
- ☐ location
- ☐ quality
- ☐ severity
- ☐ duration
- ☐ timing
- ☐ context
- ☐ modifying factors
- ☐ associated signs and symptoms
- ☐ No. of chronic diseases

History _____

Review of Systems
- ☐ Constitutional symptoms
- ☐ Eyes
- ☐ Ears, nose, mouth, throat
- ☐ Cardiovascular
- ☐ Respiratory
- ☐ Gastrointestinal
- ☐ Genitourinary
- ☐ Integumentary
- ☐ Musculoskeletal

- ☐ Neurologic
- ☐ Psychiatric
- ☐ Endocrine

- ☐ Hematologic/lymphatic
- ☐ Allergic/immunologic

Past, Family & Social History

PAST
- ☐ current medication
- ☐ prior illnesses and injuries
- ☐ operations and hospitalizations
- ☐ age-appropriate immunizations
- ☐ allergies   ☐ dietary status

FAMILY
- ☐ health status or cause of death of parents, siblings, and children
- ☐ hereditary or high-risk diseases
- ☐ diseases related to CC, HPI, ROS

SOCIAL
- ☐ living arrangements
- ☐ marital status   ☐ sexual history
- ☐ occupational history
- ☐ use of drugs, alcohol, or tobacco
- ☐ extent of education
- ☐ current employment   ☐ other

☐ PFSH Form reviewed, no change   ☐ PFSH form reviewed, updated   ☐ PFSH form new

General Multi-System Examination

Constitutional
- ☐ 3 of 7 (2 BP, pulse, respir, tmp, hgt, wgt)
- ☐ General Appearance

Eyes
- ☐ Conjunctivae, Lids
- ☐ Eyes: Pupils, Irises
- ☐ Ophthal exam—Optic discs, Pos Seg

ENT
- ☐ Ears, Nose
- ☐ Oto exam—Aud canals,Tymp membr
- ☐ Hearing
- ☐ Nasal mucosa, Septum, Turbinates
- ☐ ENTM: Lips, Teeth, Gums
- ☐ Oropharynx—oral mucosa, palates

Neck
- ☐ Neck
- ☐ Thyroid

Respiratory
- ☐ Respiratory effort
- ☐ Percussion of chest
- ☐ Palpation of chest
- ☐ Auscultation of lungs

Cardiovascular
- ☐ Palpation of heart
- ☐ Auscultation of heart (& sounds)
- ☐ Carotid arteriesAbdominal aorta
- ☐ Femoral arteries
- ☐ Pedal pulses
- ☐ Extrem for periph edema/varicosities

Chest
- ☐ Inspect Breasts
- ☐ Palpation of Breasts & Axillae

Gastrointestinal
- ☐ Abd (+/- masses or tenderness)
- ☐ Liver, Spleen
- ☐ Hernia (+/-)
- ☐ Anus, Perineum, Rectum
- ☐ Stool for occult blood

GU/Female
- ☐ Female: Genitalia, Vagina
- ☐ Female Urethra
- ☐ Bladder
- ☐ Cervix
- ☐ Uterus
- ☐ Adnexa/parametria

GU/Male
- ☐ Scrotal Contents
- ☐ Penis
- ☐ Digital Rectal of Prostate

Lymphatic
- ☐ Lymph: Neck
- ☐ Lymph: Axillae
- ☐ Lymph: Groin
- ☐ Lymph: Other

Musculoskeletal
- ☐ Gait (...ability to exercise)
- ☐ Palpation Digits, Nails
- ☐ Head/Neck: Inspect, Percuss, Palp
- ☐ Head/Neck: Motion (+/-pain, crepit)
- ☐ Head/Neck: Stability (+/- lux, sublux)
- ☐ Head/Neck: Muscle strength & tone
- ☐ Spine/Rib/Pelv: Inspect, Percuss, Palp
- ☐ Spine/Rib/Pelv: Motion
- ☐ Spine/Rib/Pelv: Stability
- ☐ Spine/Rib/Pelv: Strength and tone

- ☐ R. Up Extrem: Inspect, Percuss, Palp
- ☐ R. Up Extrem: Motion (+/- pain, crepit)
- ☐ R. Up Extrem: Stability (+/- lux, sublux)
- ☐ R. Up Extrem: Muscle strength & tone
- ☐ L. Up Extrem: Inspect, Percuss, Palp
- ☐ L. Up Extrem: Motion (+/- pain, crepit)
- ☐ L. Up Extrem: Muscle strength & tone
- ☐ R. Low Extrem: Inspect, Percuss, Palp
- ☐ R. Low Extrem: Motion (+/-pain, crepit)
- ☐ R. Low Extrem: Stability (+/- lux, laxity)
- ☐ R. Low Extrem: Muscle strength & tone
- ☐ L. Low Extrem: Inspect, Percuss, Palp
- ☐ L. Low Extrem: Motion (+/-pain, crepit)
- ☐ L. Low Extrem: Stability (+/- lux, sublux)
- ☐ L. Low Extrem: Muscle strength & tone

Skin
- ☐ Skin: Inspect Skin & Subcut tissues
- ☐ Skin: Palpation Skin & Subcut tissues

Neuro
- ☐ Neuro: Cranial nerves (+/- deficits)
- ☐ Neuro: DTRs (+/- pathological reflexes)
- ☐ Neuro: Sensations

Psychiatry
- ☐ Psych: Judgment, Insight
- ☐ Psych: Mood, Affect (depression, anxiety)

Exam Documented _____

Form 3: E/M audit tool #1 (continued)

Number of Diagnoses/Management Options	Points
Self-limited or minor (Stable, improved, or worsened) ➡ Maximum 2 points in this category.	1
Established problem (to examining MD); stable or improved	1
Established problem (to examining MD); worsening	2
New problem (to examining MD); no additional workup planned ➡ Maximum 1 point in this category.	3
New problem (to examining MD); additional workup (eg, admit/transfer)	4
Total	

Amount and/or Complexity of Data Reviewed	Points
Lab ordered and/or reviewed (regardless of # ordered)	1
X-ray ordered and/or reviewed (regardless of # ordered)	1
Medicine section (90701-99199) ordered and/or reviewed	1
Discussion of test results with performing physician	1
Decision to obtain old record and/or obtain hx from someone other than patient	1
Review and summary of old records and/or obtaining hx from someone other than patient and/or discussion with other health provider	2
Independent visualization of image, tracing, or specimen (not simply review of report)	2
Total	

TABLE OF RISK

Level of Risk	Presenting Problem(s)	Diagnostic Procedure(s) Ordered	Management Options Selected
Minimal	•One self-limited or minor problem, eg, cold, insect bite, tinea corporis	• Laboratory tests requiring venipuncture • Chest x-rays • EKG/EEG • Urinalysis • Ultrasound, eg, echocardiography • KOH prep	• Rest • Gargles • Elastic bandages • Superficial dressings
Low	• Two or more self-limited or minor problems • One stable chronic illness, eg, well-controlled hypertension, non-insulin-dependent diabetes, cataract, BPH • Acute uncomplicated illness or injury, eg, cystitis, allergic rhinitis, simple sprain	• Physiologic tests not under stress, eg, pulmonary function tests • Noncardiovascular imaging studies with contrast, eg, barium enema • Superficial needle biopsies • Clinical laboratory tests requiring arterial puncture • Skin biopsies	• Over-the-counter drugs • Minor surgery with no identified risk factors • Physical therapy • Occupational therapy • IV fluids without additives
Moderate	• One or more chronic illnesses with mild exacerbation, progression, or side effects of treatment • Two or more stable chronic illnesses • Undiagnosed new problem with uncertain prognosis, eg, lump in breast • Acute illness with systemic symptoms, eg, pyelonephritis, pneumonitis, colitis • Acute complicated injury, eg, head injury with brief loss of consciousness	• Physiologic tests under stress, eg, cardiac stress test, fetal contraction stress test • Diagnostic endoscopies with no identified risk factors • Deep needle or incisional biopsy • Cardiovascular imaging studies with contrast and no identified risk factors, eg, arteriogram, cardiac catheterization • Obtain fluid from body cavity, eg, lumbar puncture, thoracentesis, culdocentesis	• Minor surgery with identified risk factors • Elective major surgery (open, percutaneous, or endoscopic) with no identified risk factors • Prescription drug management • Therapeutic nuclear medicine • IV fluids with additives • Closed treatment of fracture or dislocation without manipulation
High	• One or more chronic illnesses with severe exacerbation, progression, or side effects of treatment • Acute or chronic illnesses or injuries that pose a threat to life or bodily function, eg, multiple trauma, acute MI, pulmonary embolus, severe respiratory distress, progressive severe rheumatoid arthritis, psychiatric illness with imminent threat to self or others, peritonitis, acute renal failure • An abrupt change in neurologic status, eg, seizure, TIA, weakness, sensory loss	• Cardiovascular imaging studies with contrast with identified risk factors • Cardiac electrophysiological tests • Diagnostic endoscopies with identified risk factors • Discography	• Elective major surgery (open, percutaneous, or endoscopic) with identified risk factors • Emergency major surgery (open, percutaneous, or endoscopic) • Parenteral controlled substances • Drug therapy requiring intensive monitoring for toxicity • Decision not to resuscitate or to deescalate care because of poor prognosis

Medical Decision Making	SF	LOW	MOD	HIGH
Number of Diagnoses or Treatment Options	1	2	3	4
Amount and/or Complexity of Data to be Reviewed	1	2	3	4
Risk of Complications, Morbidity, Mortality	Minimal	Low	Moderate	High
E/M Level=2 out of 3				

MDM _____

Chart Note
☐ Dictated ☐ Handwritten
☐ Form ☐ Illegible
☐ Note signed
☐ Signature missing

Other Services or Modalities:

Auditor:

Form 4: Alternate audit tool #2

Alternate Audit Tool #2

Physician _____   Date of Audit: _____

Patient Name _____DOB _____

Date of Service_____ Date of Birth_____ Insurance _____

Practice CPT Code(s) Selected _____

Documented Diagnose(s) _____

❑ New Patient   ❑ Established Patient   ❑ Office Visit   ❑ Consultation   ❑ Hospital

❑ Hospital Subsequent   ❑ Critical Care   ❑ Preventive   ❑ Other Procedures _____

HISTORY (Elements: Chief Complaint, History of Present Illness (HPI), Review of Systems (ROS), Past Medical, Family, Social History (PFSH)

History of Present Illness (HPI) Elements	Review of Systems	History
HPI ELEMENTS	**ROS Elements**	❑ Past Medical
		❑ Family History
❑ Location	❑ Constitutional	❑ Social History
❑ Quality	❑ Eyes	
❑ Severity	❑ ENT/mouth	
❑ Duration	❑ CV	
❑ Timing	❑ Resp	
❑ Context	❑ GI	
❑ Modifying Factors	❑ GU	Problem Focused N/A
❑ Associated Signs and Symptoms	❑ Musculoskeletal	
❑ Status of 3 or More Chronic	❑ Integ/Skin/Breast	
❑ Conditions	❑ Neurological	
	❑ Psych	
	❑ Endo	
	❑ Hem/lymph	
	❑ Allerg/Immuno	
Problem Focused (Min-1)	Problem Focused N/A	Expanded Problem Focused N/A
Expanded Problem Focused (Min-1)	Expanded Problem Focused (2-9 systems)	Detailed 1
Detailed		Comprehensive
AT LEAST 4 or at least 3 Chronic DX	Detailed (2-9 systems)	2-Established 3-New
Comprehensive	Comprehensive (Min-10 required)	
AT LEAST 4 or at least 3 Chronic DX		

History: ☐ Problem Focused   ☐ Expanded Problem Focused   ☐ Detailed   ☐ Comprehensive

Form 4: Alternate audit tool #2 (continued)

GENERAL MULTISYSTEM EXAMINATION

Exam	At least 1 element identified by a bullet from any system	6 items identified by a bullet from any system	2 items identified by a bullet from a minimum of 6 systems (12)	2 items identified by a bullet from a minimum of 9 systems (18)
Constitutional	❑ Any One of Three Vitals ❑ General Appearance of Patient			
Eyes	❑ Conjunctiva and Lids ❑ Pupils & Irises ❑ Optic Discs			
ENT	❑ External Ears & Nose ❑ Hearing ❑ EACs & TM ❑ Nasal Mucosa Septum & Turbinates ❑ Exam of Oropharynx; oral mucosa, salivary glands, hard and soft palates, tongue, tonsils, and posterior pharynx			
Neck	❑ Neck ❑ Thyroid			
Respiratory	❑ Respiratory Effort ❑ Percussion ❑ Palpation ❑ Auscultation			
Cardiovascular	❑ Palpation of Heart ❑ Auscultation ❑ Carotids ❑ Abdominal Aorta ❑ Femoral ❑ Pedal Pulses ❑ Extremities for Edema and Varicosities			
Chest	❑ Inspection of Breasts ❑ Palpation of Breast and Axillae			
GI (Abdomen)	❑ Masses/Tenderness ❑ Liver and Spleen ❑ Hernia ❑ Anus, Perineum, & Rectum ❑ Occult Test			
GU	Male: ❑ Scrotal Contents ❑ Penis ❑ Prostate Glands Female: ❑ External Genitalia ❑ Urethra ❑ Bladder ❑ Cervix ❑ Uterus ❑ Adnexa/Parametria			
Lymph	❑ Lymph Nodes in 2 or More Areas ❑ Neck ❑ Axillae ❑ Groin ❑ Other			
Musculoskeletal	❑ Gait & Station ❑ Digits & Nails Muscles of at Least One Area 1) Head, Neck 2). Spine, Ribs, Pelvis 3) Right Upper Extremity 4) Left Upper Extremity 5) Right Lower Extremity 6) Left LowerExtremity; With Exam Including ❑ Inspection and/or Palpation ❑ ROM ❑ Stability ❑ Strength & Tone			
Skin	❑ Inspection of Skin and Subcutaneous Tissues ❑ Palpation of Skin and Subcutaneous Tissues			
Neuro	❑Cranial Nerves ❑Reflexes ❑Sensation ❑ Judgment & Insight ❑Orientation to Time and Place/Person			
Psychiatric	❑ Memory ❑ Mood ❑ Mental Status Exam Complete ❑ Orientation to Time and Place/Person ❑ Recent and Remote Memory ❑ Attention Span and Concentration ❑ Language (naming objects, repeating phrases etc) ❑ Judgment & Insight			

☐ Problem Focused   ☐ Expanded Problem Focused   ☐ Detailed   ☐ Comprehensive

Level of Exam 1995 _____   Level of Exam 1997 _____

Form 4: **Alternate audit tool #2** (continued)

Medical Decision Making   Audit of Evaluation and Management Service

Number of Diagnoses and Management Options	Points Assigned	Points Per Category	Amount and Complexity of Data	Points Assigned	Points Per Category
Self-Limiting or Minor Problems (Stable, Improved, or Worsening) Maximum of 2 points can be given	1		Ordered and/or reviewed clinical lab	1	
Established Problem – Stable or Improved	1		Ordered and/or reviewed radiology	1	
Established Problem – Worsening	2		Discussed tests with performing or interpreting physician	1	
New Problem – No Additional Workup Planned Maximum of 1 problem given credit	3		Ordered and/or reviewed test in the CPT Medicine section	1	
New Problem – Additional workup Planned	4		Independent visualization and direct view of image, tracing, specimen	2	
Total Points:			Decision to obtain old records or additional history from someone other than patient, eg, family, caretaker, previous physician	1	
			Reviewed and summarized old records and/or obtained history from someone other than patient	2	
			Total Points		

Table of Risk—The Highest Level in ONE Area Determines the Overall Risk

Level of Risk	Presenting Problem(s) or	Diagnostic Procedure or	Management Options
Minimal	❏ One self-limited or minor problem, ie, cold, insect bite, tinea corporis	❏ Laboratory tests requiring venipuncture ❏ Chest x-ray ❏ EKG/EEG ❏ Urinalysis ❏ Ultrasound, eg, echocardiography ❏ KOH prep	❏ Rest ❏ Gargles ❏ Elastic bandages ❏ Superficial dressing
Low	❏ Two or more self-limited or minor problems ❏ One stable chronic illness, eg, well-controlled hypertension, non–insulin-dependent diabetes, cataract, BPH ❏ Acute uncomplicated illness or injury, eg, cystitis, allergic rhinitis, simple sprain	❏ Physiological tests not under stress, eg, pulmonary function test ❏ Noncardiovascular imaging studies with contrast, eg, barium enema ❏ Superficial needle biopsies ❏ Clinical laboratory tests requiring arterial puncture ❏ Skin biopsies	❏ Over-the-counter drugs ❏ Minor surgery with no identified ❏ risk factors ❏ Physical therapy ❏ Occupational therapy ❏ IV fluids without additives
Moderate	❏ One or more chronic illnesses with mild exacerbation, progression, or side effects of treatment ❏ Two or more stable chronic illnesses ❏ Undiagnosed new problem with uncertain prognosis, eg, lump in breast ❏ Acute illness with systemic symptoms, eg, pyelonephritis, pneumonitis, colitis	❏ Physiological tests under stress, eg, cardiac stress test, fetal contraction stress test ❏ Diagnostic endoscopies with no identified risk factors ❏ Deep needle or incisional biopsy ❏ Cardiovascular imaging studies with contrast and no identified risk factors, eg, arteriogram, cardiac catheterization ❏ Obtain fluid from body cavity, eg, lumbar puncture, thoracentesis, culdocentesis	❏ Minor surgery with identified risk factors ❏ Elective major surgery (open, percutaneous, or endoscopic) with no identified risk factors ❏ Prescription drug management ❏ Therapeutic nuclear medicine ❏ IV fluids with additives ❏ Closed treatment of fracture or dislocation w/o manipulation
High	❏ One or more chronic illnesses w/severe exacerbation, progression, or side effects of treatment ❏ Acute or chronic illness or injuries that pose a threat to life or bodily function eg, multiple trauma, acute MI, pulmonary embolus, severe respiratory distress, progressive severe rheumatoid arthritis, psychiatric illness w/potential threat to self or others, peritonitis, acute renal failure ❏ An abrupt change in neurologic status, eg, seizure, TIA, weakness, or sensory loss	❏ Cardiovascular imaging studies with contrast with identified risk factors ❏ Cardiac electrophysiological tests ❏ Diagnostic endoscopies with identified risk factors ❏ Discography	❏ Elective major surgery (open, percutaneous, or endoscopic) with identified risk factors ❏ Emergency major surgery (open, percutaneous, or endoscopic) ❏ Parenteral control substances ❏ Drug therapy requiring intensive monitoring for toxicity ❏ Decision not to resuscitate or to deescalate care because of poor prognosis

Form 4: Alternate audit tool #2 (continued)

Decision Making Total: 2 of 3 Must Meet

Points Assigned	1	2	3	4
Number of Diagnoses	❐ Minimal	❐ Limited	❐ Multiple	❐ Extensive
Amount of Data	❐ Minimal	❐ Limited	❐ Moderate	❐ Extensive
Risk of Complications	❐ Minimal	❐ Low	❐ Moderate	❐ High
Levels	❐ Straightforward	❐ Low Complexity	❐ Moderate Complexity	❐ High Complexity

Level of Service: History _____ Exam _____ Medical Decision Making

Chart Note

☐ Dictated ☐ Handwritten _____ ☐ Form ☐ Illegible ☐ Note signed

☐ Signature missing ☐ Diagnosis code(s) supported

Diagnosis Code(s) Billed_____

Other Services Billed _____

Comments:

Auditor's Signature _____

Form 5: Alternate audit tool #3

PT: _____ Provider: _____

DOS: _____ Billed: _____ Supported: _____

History

Audit of Evaluation and Management Service

Chief Complaint/Reason for Encounter: _____

❏ Brief HPI 1 to 3 Elements

❏ Extended HPI 4+ Elements or 3 Chronic Illnesses

❏ Pertinent ROS (One System)

❏ Extended ROS (2 to 9 Systems)

❏ Complete ROS (10+ Systems)

History of Present Illness			Review of Systems		
Location	✓	Documentation	Systems	✓	Documentation
Location			Constitut. (fever, wt. loss)		
Quality			Eyes		
Severity			Ears/Nose/Mouth/Throat		
Timing			Cardiovascular		
Assoc.Signs/Symptoms			Respiratory		
Duration			Gastrointest. (abdominal)		
Modifying Factors			Genitourinary		
Context			Musculoskeletal		
			Integumentary		
OR			Neurological		
Status of 3 Chronic Illnesses or Inactive Problems=extended			Psychiatric		
1.			Endocrine		
2.			Hematologic/Lymphatic		
3.			Allergic/Immunologic		

❏ Documented, "All Other Systems Negative"

Past Medical History		Family History		Social History	
Past Illness		Family Illness		Smoking	
Past Surgeries		Hereditary Diseases		Drug Use	
Allergies				Living Arrangements	
Current Medications				Employment	
Past Hospitalizations				Other:	

HISTORY TOTAL:

❏ Problem Focused	❏ Expanded Problem Focused	❏ Detailed	❏ Complete
CC, Brief HPI, No ROS No PFSH	CC, Brief HPI, 1 ROS No PFSH	CC, Extended HPI, 2-9 ROS Pertinent PFSH	CC, Extended HPI, 10+ ROS Complete PFSH

* Preventive Medicine requires no CC or HPI, but does require a complete ROS and PFSH.

EXAM TOTAL:

❏ Problem Focused	❏ Expanded Problem Focused	❏ Detailed	❏ Complete
1 – 5 _____Elements	6 – 11 _____Elements	12 (9) _____Elements	_____Elements

Form 5: Alternate audit tool #3 (continued)

Medical Decision Making   **Audit of Evaluation and Management Service**

Number of Diagnoses and Management Options	Points Assigned	Points Per Category	Amount and Complexity of Data	Points Assigned	Points Per Category
Self-Limiting or Minor Problems (Stable, Improved, or Worsening) Maximum of 2 points can be given	1		Ordered and/or reviewed clinical lab	1	
Established Problem – Stable, Improved	1		Ordered and/or reviewed radiology	1	
Established Problem – Worsening	2		Discussed tests with performing or interpreting physician	1	
New Problem – No Additional Workup Planned Maximum of 1 problem given credit	3		Ordered and/or reviewed test in the CPT Medicine section	1	
New Problem – Additional workup Planned	4		Independent visualization and direct view of image, tracing, specimen	2	
Total Points:			Decision to obtain old records or additional history from someone other than patient, eg, family, caretaker, previous physician	1	
			Reviewed and summarized old records and/or obtained history from someone other than patient	2	
			Total Points		

Table of Risk—The Highest Level in ONE Area Determines the Overall Risk

Level of Risk	Presenting Problem(s) or	Diagnostic Procedure or	Management Options
Minimal	❏ One self-limited or minor problem, ie, cold, insect bite, tinea corporis	❏ Laboratory tests requiring venipuncture ❏ Chest x-ray ❏ EKG/EEG ❏ Urinalysis ❏ Ultrasound, eg, echocardiography ❏ KOH prep	❏ Rest ❏ Gargles ❏ Elastic bandages ❏ Superficial dressing
Low	❏ Two or more self-limited or minor problems ❏ One stable chronic illness, eg, well-controlled hypertension, non–insulin-dependent diabetes, cataract, BPH ❏ Acute uncomplicated illness or injury, eg, cystitis, allergic rhinitis, simple sprain	❏ Physiological tests not under stress, eg, pulmonary function test ❏ Noncardiovascular imaging studies with contrast, eg, barium enema ❏ Superficial needle biopsies ❏ Clinical laboratory tests requiring arterial puncture ❏ Skin biopsies	❏ Over-the-counter drugs ❏ Minor surgery with no identified risk factors ❏ Physical therapy ❏ Occupational therapy ❏ IV fluids without additives
Moderate	❏ One or more chronic illnesses with mild exacerbation, progression, or side effects of treatment ❏ Two or more stable chronic illnesses ❏ Undiagnosed new problem with uncertain prognosis, eg, lump in breast ❏ Acute illness with systemic symptoms, eg, pyelonephritis, pneumonitis, colitis	❏ Physiological tests under stress, eg, cardiac stress test, fetal contraction stress test ❏ Diagnostic endoscopies with no identified risk factors ❏ Deep needle or incisional biopsy ❏ Cardiovascular imaging studies with contrast and no identified risk factors, eg, arteriogram, cardiac catheterization ❏ Obtain fluid from body cavity, eg, lumbar puncture, thoracentesis, culdocentesis	❏ Minor surgery with identified risk factors. ❏ Elective major surgery (open, percutaneous, or endoscopic) with no identified risk factors ❏ Prescription drug management ❏ Therapeutic nuclear medicine ❏ IV fluids with additives ❏ Closed treatment of fracture or dislocation w/o manipulation
High	❏ One or more chronic illnesses w/severe exacerbation, progression, or side effects of treatment ❏ Acute or chronic illness or injuries that pose a threat to life or bodily function, eg, multiple trauma, acute MI, pulmonary embolus, severe respiratory distress, progressive severe rheumatoid arthritis, psychiatric illness w/potential threat to self or others, peritonitis, acute renal failure ❏ An abrupt change in neurologic status, eg, seizure, TIA, weakness, or sensory loss	❏ Cardiovascular imaging studies with contrast with identified risk factors ❏ Cardiac electrophysiological tests ❏ Diagnostic endoscopies with identified risk factors ❏ Discography	❏ Elective major surgery (open, percutaneous, or endoscopic) with identified risk factors ❏ Emergency major surgery (open percutaneous or endoscopic) ❏ Parenteral control substances ❏ Drug therapy requiring intensive monitoring for toxicity ❏ Decision not to resuscitate or to deescalate care because of poor prognosis

Decision Making Total: 2 of 3 Must Meet

Points Assigned	1	2	3	4
Number of Diagnoses	❏ Minimal	❏ Limited	❏ Multiple	❏ Extensive
Amount of Data	❏ Minimal	❏ Limited	❏ Moderate	❏ Extensive
Risk of Complications	❏ Minimal	❏ Low	❏ Moderate	❏ High
Levels	❏ Straightforward	❏ Low Complexity	❏ Moderate Complexity	❏ High Complexity

Auditor's Signature: _____

Form 6: OB/GYN audit tool

OB/GYN Audit Tool
Patient Information

Patient:	**Visit Date:**	**History Level**
Examined By:		**Exam Level**
Patient Status:	**DOB:**	**Decision Making**
Service Type:	**Sex:**	**Insurance Carrier**

CPT® Code(s) Billed   DOCUMENTED   DIAGNOSIS CODE(S) BILLED   DOCUMENTED

History

History of Present Illness
- ☐ location
- ☐ quality
- ☐ severity
- ☐ duration
- ☐ timing
- ☐ context
- ☐ modifying factors
- ☐ associated signs and symptoms
- ☐ No. of chronic diseases

History _____

Review of Systems
- ☐ Constitutional symptoms
- ☐ Eyes
- ☐ Ears, nose, mouth, throat
- ☐ Cardiovascular
- ☐ Respiratory
- ☐ Gastrointestinal
- ☐ Genitourinary
- ☐ Integumentary
- ☐ Musculoskeletal
- ☐ Neurologic
- ☐ Psychiatric
- ☐ Endocrine
- ☐ Hematologic/lymphatic
- ☐ Allergic/immunologic

Past, Family, & Social History
PAST
- ☐ current medication
- ☐ prior illnesses and injuries
- ☐ operations and hospitalizations
- ☐ age-appropriate immunizations
- ☐ allergies   ☐ dietary status

FAMILY
- ☐ health status or cause of death of parents, siblings, and children
- ☐ hereditary or high-risk diseases
- ☐ diseases related to CC, HPI, ROS

SOCIAL
- ☐ living arrangements
- ☐ marital status   ☐ sexual history
- ☐ occupational history
- ☐ use of drugs, alcohol, or tobacco
- ☐ extent of education
- ☐ current employment   ☐ other

☐ PFSH Form reviewed, no change ☐ PFSH form reviewed, updated ☐ PFSH form new

---

General Multisystem Examination

Constitutional
- ☐ 3 of 7 (2 BP, pulse, respir, tmp, hgt, wgt)
- ☐ General appearance

Neck
- ☐ Neck
- ☐ Thyroid

Respiratory
- ☐ Respiratory effort
- ☐ Percussion of chest
- ☐ Palpation of chest
- ☐ Auscultation of lungs

Cardiovascular
- ☐ Auscultation of heart (& sounds)
- ☐ Carotid arteries
- ☐ Abdominal aorta
- ☐ Femoral arteries
- ☐ Pedal pulses
- ☐ Extrem for periph edema/varicosities

Gastrointestinal
- ☐ Abd   (+/- masses or tenderness)
- ☐ Liver, Spleen
- ☐ Hernia (+/-)
- ☐ Anus, Perineum, Rectum
- ☐ Stool for Occult Blood

GU/Female
- ☐ Inspect Breasts
- ☐ Palpation of Breasts & Axillae
- ☐ Female: Genitalia, Vagina
- ☐ Female Urethra
- ☐ Urethral meatus
- ☐ Bladder
- ☐ Vagina
- ☐ Cervix
- ☐ Uterus
- ☐ Adnexa/parametria
- ☐ Anus and perineum

Lymphatic
- ☐ Lymph: Neck
- ☐ Lymph: Axillae
- ☐ Lymph: Groin
- ☐ Lymph: Other

Skin
- ☐ Skin: Inspect Skin & Subcut Tissues
- ☐ Skin: Palpation Skin & Subcut Tissues

Neuro
- ☐ Assessment of Mental Status
- ☐ Neuro: Cranial Nerves (+/- deficits)
- ☐ Neuro: DTRs (+/- pathological reflexes)
- ☐ Neuro: Sensations

Psychiatry
- ☐ Psych: Orientation, Time, Place, etc
- ☐ Psych: Mood, Affect (depression, anxiety)

Exam Documented _____

Form 6: OB/GYN audit tool (continued)

Number of Diagnoses/Management Options	Points
Self-limited or minor (stable, improved or worsened) ➡ Maximum 2 points in this category	1
Established problem (to examining MD); stable or improved	1
Established problem (to examining MD); worsening	2
New problem (to examining MD); no additional workup planned ➡ Maximum 1 point in this category	3
New problem (to examining MD); additional workup (eg, admit/transfer)	4
Total	

Amount and/or Complexity of Data Reviewed	Points
Lab ordered and/or reviewed (regardless of # ordered)	1
X-ray ordered and/or reviewed (regardless of # ordered)	1
Medicine section (90701-99199) ordered and/or reviewed	1
Discussion of test results with performing physician	1
Decision to obtain old record and/or obtain hx from someone other than patient	1
Review and summary of old records and/or obtaining hx from someone other than patient and/or discussion with other health provider	2
Independent visualization of image, tracing, or specimen (not simply review of report)	2
Total	

TABLE OF RISK

Level of Risk	Presenting Problem(s)	Diagnostic Procedure(s) Ordered	Management Options Selected
Minimal	• One self-limited or minor problem, eg, cold, insect bite, tinea corporis	• Laboratory tests requiring venipuncture • Chest x-rays • EKG/EEG • Urinalysis • Ultrasound, eg, echocardiography • KOH prep	• Rest • Gargles • Elastic bandages • Superficial dressings
Low	• Two or more self-limited or minor problems • One stable chronic illness, eg, well-controlled hypertension, non–insulin-dependent diabetes, cataract, BPH • Acute uncomplicated illness or injury, eg, cystitis, allergic rhinitis, simple sprain	• Physiologic tests not under stress, eg, pulmonary function tests • Noncardiovascular imaging studies with contrast, eg, barium enema • Superficial needle biopsies • Clinical laboratory tests requiring arterial puncture • Skin biopsies	• Over-the-counter drugs • Minor surgery with no identified risk factors • Physical therapy • Occupational therapy • IV fluids without additives
Moderate	• One or more chronic illnesses with mild exacerbation, progression, or side effects of treatment • Two or more stable chronic illnesses • Undiagnosed new problem with uncertain prognosis, eg, lump in breast • Acute illness with systemic symptoms, eg, pyelonephritis, pneumonitis, colitis • Acute complicated injury, eg, head injury with brief loss of consciousness	• Physiologic tests under stress, eg, cardiac stress test, fetal contraction stress test • Diagnostic endoscopies with no identified risk factors • Deep needle or incisional biopsy • Cardiovascular imaging studies with contrast and no identified risk factors, eg, arteriogram, cardiac catheterization • Obtain fluid from body cavity, eg, lumbar puncture, thoracentesis, culdocentesis	• Minor surgery with identified risk factors • Elective major surgery (open, percutaneous, or endoscopic) with no identified risk factors • Prescription drug management • Therapeutic nuclear medicine • IV fluids with additives • Closed treatment of fracture or dislocation without manipulation
High	• One or more chronic illnesses with severe exacerbation, progression, or side effects of treatment • Acute or chronic illnesses or injuries that pose a threat to life or bodily function, eg, multiple trauma, acute MI, pulmonary embolus, severe respiratory distress, progressive severe rheumatoid arthritis, psychiatric illness with potential threat to self or others, peritonitis, acute renal failure • An abrupt change in neurologic status, eg, seizure, TIA, weakness, sensory loss	• Cardiovascular imaging studies with contrast with identified risk factors • Cardiac electrophysiological tests • Diagnostic endoscopies with identified risk factors • Discography	• Elective major surgery (open, percutaneous, or endoscopic) with identified risk factors • Emergency major surgery (open, percutaneous, or endoscopic) • Parenteral controlled substances • Drug therapy requiring intensive monitoring for toxicity • Decision not to resuscitate or to deescalate care because of poor prognosis

Medical Decision Making	SF	LOW	MOD	HIGH
Number of Diagnoses or Treatment Options	1	2	3	4
Amount and/or Complexity of Data to be Reviewed	1	2	3	4
Risk of Complications, Morbidity, Mortality	Minimal	Low	Moderate	High
E/M Level=2 out of 3				

MDM _____

Chart Note

☐ Dictated   ☐ Handwritten
☐ Form   ☐ Illegible
☐ Note signed
☐ Signature missing

Other Services Billed:

Auditor: _____

Form 7: Surgery audit tool

Surgery Audit Tool

Patient Name _____MR# _____

Date of Birth _____Date of Visit _____Insurance Carrier:_____

Surgical Service (s) billed _____

Diagnosis Code (s) billed _____

Comments _____

Documented	Y	N	N/A	Comments
Preoperative information	☐	☐	☐	
Patient demographics	☐	☐	☐	
Surgery date	☐	☐	☐	
Preoperative anesthesia	☐	☐	☐	
Indication for procedure	☐	☐	☐	
Diagnostic reports	☐	☐	☐	
Intraoperative information	☐	☐	☐	
Preoperative diagnosis	☐	☐	☐	
Postoperative diagnosis	☐	☐	☐	
Surgeon/assistant/cosurgeons	☐	☐	☐	
Procedure title	☐	☐	☐	
Findings	☐	☐	☐	
Procedure details	☐	☐	☐	
Tissue/organ removed	☐	☐	☐	
Materials removed/inserted	☐	☐	☐	
Closure information	☐	☐	☐	
Blood loss/replacement	☐	☐	☐	
Wound status	☐	☐	☐	
Drainage	☐	☐	☐	
Complications noted	☐	☐	☐	
Postoperative condition of patient	☐	☐	☐	
IV infusion record	☐	☐	☐	
Signatures	☐	☐	☐	
Legibility	☐	☐	☐	
Supports procedure (CPT/HCPCS)	☐	☐	☐	
Supports medical necessity (ICD-9-CM)	☐	☐	☐	

Form 8: Surgery summary report

SURGERY SUMMARY REPORT

Physician: Date of Review:

Reviewer:

Number of Operative Notes Reviewed:

Operative notes were reviewed for completeness and appropriateness of care along with coding documentation and medical necessity.

Documentation in the operative note appears to provide preoperative information.

Surgery date appears to be documented in the note.

Preoperative anesthesia appears to be documented in the note.

Indication for procedure appears to be documented in the operative report.

Preoperative diagnosis appears to be documented in the operative report.

Postoperative diagnosis appears to be documented in the note and supported by findings.

Surgeon/assistant/cosurgeons are listed in the operative note.

Findings appear to be indicated in the operative report.

Procedure details appear to be documented appropriately in the operative report.

Postoperative condition of patient appears to be indicated in the operative report.

The operative report appears to support procedure (CPT®/HCPCS).

The operative report appears to support medical necessity (ICD-9-CM).

Other Documentation and Coding Issues:

1.

2.

3.

4.

Form 8: **Surgery summary report** (continued)

SURGERY SUMMARY REPORT

RECOMMENDATIONS

1.

2.

3.

4.

5.

Form 9: Surgery detailed analysis

GENERAL SURGICAL GROUP
SURGERY DETAILED ANALYSIS

Physician: Date of Review:

Reviewer:

Number of Operative Notes Reviewed:

Billed   Documented

Patient	CPT® Code	ICD-9-CM Code	MOD	CPT® Code	ICD-9-CM Code	MOD

Valuable Websites

GENERAL MEDICAL PAGES

http://www.ncbi.nlm.nih.gov/PubMed/

http://www.medscape.com/Home/network/MedStudent/MedStudent.html

http://www.coloradohealthnet.org/

http://www.AcronymFinder.com/

http://www.vh.org/

http://www.vh.org/Patients/IHB/OrgSys.html

http://www.msms.doe.k12.ms.us/biology/anatomy/apmain.html

http://www.medsite.com/

http://www.adam.com/upgradedefault.htm

http://cgl.microsoft.com/clipgallerylive/cg130/eula.asp?nInterface=0

http://cgl.microsoft.com/clipgallerylive/default.asp?nEULA=1&nInterface=0

http://www.mtdesk.com/mt.shtml

GOVERNMENT

http://www.ahcpr.gov	Agency for Healthcare Policy and Research
http://www.access.gpo.gov/nara/cfr	Code of Federal Regulations
http://www.dhhs.gov	Department of Health & Human Services
http://www.fda.gov/medbull	FDA Medical Bulletin Information for Health Professionals from the U.S. FDA
http://www.access.gpo.gov/nara/cfr	Federal Register
http://www.fedworld.gov	Fedworld Information Network
http://www.access.gpo.gov	Government Printing Office
http://www.hcfa.gov	Centers for Medicare and Medicaid (CMS)
http://www.hcfa.gov/pubforms/06%5Fcim/ci35.htm	Coverage Issues Manual for Medical Procedures
http://www.healthfinder.gov	Healthfinder (trademark)
http://aspe.os.dhhs.gov	Health Insurance Portability and Accountability Act
http://www.umdnj.edu/homeweb/index.htm	Information for State Health Policy
http://www.jcaho.org	Joint Commission on Accreditation of Healthcare Organizations
http://www.cdc.gov	National Center for Health Statistics

http://www.ncqa.org	National Center for Quality Assurance
http://www.nih.gov	National Institutes of Health
http://www.hhs.gov/progorg/oig/	Office of Inspector General (OIG)
http://rarediseases.info.nih.gov/ord/	Office of Rare Diseases
http://www.ssa.gov	Social Security Online
http://thomas.loc.gov	Thomas provides legislative information
http://www.dhhs.gov/progorg/oig	U.S. Department of Health and Human Services' Office of the Inspector General
http://www.xact.org/	Xact med Clinical Laboratory Billing Guide

HEALTH MANAGEMENT, CODING, AND TRAINING RESOURCES

http://www.integsoft.com/appeals/tal/index.htm	The Appeal Letter published quarterly by Appeal Solutions to assist medical providers in appealing denied insurance claims
http://www.aapcnatl.org	American Academy of Professional Coders
http://www.mxcity.com/cgi- bin/resource?4&MxCity.com/category=29843	(Hot topics: heading–Coding Compliance)
http://www.justcoding.com	JustCoding.com
http://www.medicaretraining.com/cbt.htm	Online Medicare Coding/Billing Training from First Coast Service Options
http://www.nlm.nih.gov/databases/freemedl.html	Medline (U.S. National Library of Medicine)
http://206.132.0.133/medline/basic.cfm	Medsite's clinical information search tool
http://www.ache.org	American College of Healthcare Executives
http://www.aclm.org	American College of Legal Medicine
http://www.ahima.org	American Health Management Information Association
http://www.hcca-info.org	Health Care Compliance Association
http://www.hfma.org	Healthcare Financial Management Association
http://www.physicianswebsites.com	Medical Association of Billers
http://www.mgma.com/index.html	Medical Group Management Association
http://www.who.ch	World Health Organization
http://www.ama-assn.org	American Medical Association
http://www.medprofs.com	MPI (Medical Professionals, Inc.)

MEDICOLEGAL

http://www.nhcaa.org	National Healthcare Antifraud Association
http://www.healthlawyers.org	American Health Lawyers Association
http://www.internets.com/mednets/smedgovt.htm	MedNets Government Searchable Databases
http://www.mediregs.com/index.html	MediRegs a Gov. search engine
http://aspe.os.dhhs.gov	Health Insurance Portability and Accountability Act

TERMINOLOGY

Abuse   A practice that results in unnecessary costs to a government program, in which it is not possible to determine if the error was committed knowingly or willingly. These incidents or practices are not considered fraudulent, but inconsistent with accepted medical business or fiscal practice.

Add on Codes   Any CPT® code that states "in addition to" is an adjunct code and does not require the use of modifier -51.

Advance Beneficiary Notice (ABN)   A written notification that must be signed prior to rendering services to a Medicare beneficiary that could potentially be denied or deemed "not medically necessary". A modifier must be used on the HCFA 1500 claim form to indicate to Medicare that the Advanced Beneficiary Notice is on file. The notice is sometimes referred to as a "Medicare Waiver of Liability". Once an ABN is on file, the patient is lawfully liable for the charges if Medicare denies payment for the services.

Ambulatory Surgery Center   An independent surgical facility licensed by the state health department for the purpose of performing outpatient surgeries on patients expected to be discharged the same day.

Audit   An examination of the systems used to make sure a practitioner is billing and coding correctly. These systems are sometimes called "monitors." For instance, an audit checks the thermometer on a regular basis to make sure it is working properly.

Audit Tool   A form, sometimes referred to as a tally sheet, that is used to perform a medical record review (chart audit) and documents the findings of each individual medical record audited.

Balanced Budget Act of 1997 (BBA)   Similar to HIPAA, the Balanced Budget Act of 1997 passed by Congress allocated a great deal of money to prevent fraud and abuse in the health care industry.

Baseline Audit   The first audit performed for an individual practitioner or group to determine the problematic areas in coding, billing, documentation and/or compliance.

Beneficiary   A term for a patient enrolled in the Medicare program.

Bilateral Procedures   When the surgical procedure is unilateral, and performed bilaterally, report the CPT® code once and use a modifier -50 to the code. Modifier -50 identifies a procedure performed identically on the opposite side of the body. If the surgical code is inherently bilateral, the CPT® code is reported once without modifier -50, even if the procedure is performed on both sides.

Care Plan Oversight   These are codes used to report the services of a physician who is providing ongoing review and revision of a patient's care plan involving complex or multi-disciplinary care.

Category of Service   This phrase refers to location of service (ie, home, office, hospital, consultation, etc) and determination if the patient is new or established.

Charge ticket   Routing slip personalized for the medical group or practice, which encompasses patient demographics, charges, Current Procedural Terminology Codes (CPT®) and may also include diagnostic codes (ICD-9-CM). A copy is normally given to a patient when he/she leaves the office.

Chart Entries   Dated entries made by a physician, practitioner, nurse, or office staff in the patient medical record.

Chief Complaint   Concise statement describing the symptoms, problems, condition, diagnosis, or other factor that is the reason for the encounter.

Compliance   An effort to reduce fraud in a medical organization by reducing coding, billing, and reimbursement errors and improving quality and standards in the medical facility.

Compliance Officer   A person designated by an organization to oversee compliance, address problematic areas, develop policies and standards, and oversee compliance activities.

Compliance Plan   A key plan for ensuring compliance with laws and regulations, which includes policies and procedures for the medical organization. It includes seven key elements.

Complications following surgery   Any additional services requiring the intervention of the surgeon during the postoperative period of the surgery when additional trips to the operating room or abnormal medical intervention is necessary.

Comprehensive Exam   Includes a complete single-organ system examination or a general multi-system examination including systems and body areas.

Consent for Treatment   An agreement that the patient signs allowing the provider to treat the patient.

Consultation   A type of service provided by a physician whose advice or opinion regarding evaluation and/or management of a specific problem is requested by another physician or other appropriate source.

Corporate Compliance   A program that ensures that a company is following both its own policies and the government's laws and regulations. A compliance program is a way for a company to monitor itself through a system of checks and balances

Correct Coding Initiative   In 1996, the Centers for Medicare and Medicaid (CMS) implemented a national policy aimed at controlling improper or incorrect practices in the filing of Medicare Part B claims.

Corrective Action   The action steps of identifying problem areas and implementing a plan to change patterns and promote correct coding, documentation and billing.

Counseling   A discussion with the patient and/or family members regarding diagnostic results, instructions for management, prognosis, and other items related to the patient's condition.

CPT® Coding   Current Procedural Terminology Coding–The American Medical Association publishes the updated CPT® (Current Procedural Terminology) book annually. The CPT® nomenclature is an alphanumeric coding system with two (2) digit add-on descriptors (modifiers) which describes medical services. It is a widely accepted method of communicating to payers the descriptions of procedures and services provided to patients.

Critical Care Services   Defined by CPT® as "the direct delivery by a physician(s) of medical care for a critically ill or critically injured patient. A critical illness or injury acutely impairs one or more vital organ systems such that the patient's survival is jeopardized."

Detailed Analysis Report   A report that summarizes the charts reviewed, the codes selected by the practitioner versus the correct codes documented in a table format.

Detailed Exam   Includes an extended examination of the affected body area(s) and other symptomatic or related organ system(s).

Detailed History   Includes a chief complaint; extended history of present illness; extended review of systems including a limited number of additional systems; pertinent past, family, and/or social history directly related to the patient's problems.

Diagnosis/Impression   The impression or condition of the patient after the history and examination is performed.

DOJ   Department of Justice–A federal agency that handles the investigation and enforcement of federal criminal laws, including proven cases of fraudulent health care claims.

Domiciliary care These codes are used to report care given to patients residing in a long term care facility that provides room and board, as well as other personal assistance services. The facility's services do not include a medical component.

Documentation A method for recording facts chronologically including detailed observations about the patient's health status as seen in medical reports and chart notes.

Downcoding An action that occurs when the coding system used on a claim submitted to an insurance carrier does not match the coding system used by the company receiving the claim. If they do not match, the claims examiner has an opportunity to substitute a code with a lower value, which of course means lower reimbursement.

E/M Evaluation and Management–Refers to codes that physicians use to describe their evaluations of patients. Codes usually range from 1 (lowest complexity) to 5 (highest complexity). Elements that go into determining an appropriate E/M code level include 1) taking a history from patient, 2) examination of the patient and 3) creating a diagnosis or care plan (called Medical Decision Making).

Excision/Destruction Includes procedures that remove or cut out a particular body area or part. All ectomy (e.g., excision or surgically cutting into) are found under this subheading.

Emergency Department Services In this context, types of codes used by hospital-based and non-hospital based physicians that clearly define an emergency department as an organized hospital-based facility for the provision of unscheduled episodic services to patients who present for immediate medical attention. The facility must be available 24 hours a day. No distinction is made between a new or established patient in the emergency department.

Encounter Form A form used to record all services and diagnoses applicable to an individual patient encounter.

Established Patient A patient who has received any professional services within the past three (3) years from a physician, or another physician of the same specialty belonging to the same group practice within the past three (3) years.

Expanded Problem Focused Examination A limited exam of the affected body area or organ system and other symptomatic or related organ system(s).

False Claim A practitioner knowingly makes, uses, or causes to be made or uses a false record or statement to get a claim paid by a government payor.

False Claims Act A federal law that was enacted in 1863 when Lincoln was president. The False Claims Act allows the government to sue those who submit incorrect claims for reimbursement from the government. Often these claims are honest billing errors, but the government still considers them false claims. An intent to defraud is not required. There are steep fines for submitting a false claim to the government—between $5,000 and $10,000 for each claim falsely submitted plus triple damages. Having an effective corporate compliance program in place can reduce these fines.

Family History   A review and written summary of the historical medical data in the patient's family that includes such information as cause of death, known specific diseases, and hereditary conditions/diseases.

Federal Sentencing Guidelines   Set of criteria used by the government for sentencing individuals and organizations for any federal crime, including health care fraud. Organizations that have effective compliance programs in place can reduce fines and penalties under the Federal Sentencing Guidelines.

Fragmented or Unbundled Billing   An important issue in today's health care reimbursement arena. Medicare, Medicaid and other insurers carefully review charges and code applications due to this common and problematic practice. Often unbundling occurs because the office is submitting obsolete codes from outdated CPT® books. Very few offices intentionally fragment bills with the intent to commit fraud.

Fraud   Deliberately misrepresenting facts to deceive or mislead another party, or intentionally providing false information to the government with the purpose of defrauding the government.

HCPCS Coding   The HCFA Common Procedural Coding System used for reporting outpatient health care services provided to government insurance carriers. This system contains alphanumeric codes for reporting physician and non-physician services not included in the CPT® nomenclature.

Global days   The time period that the carrier includes for follow up care following the surgical service. Each individual insurance carrier defines the number of global days for each procedure.

Health Care Insurance Portability and Accountability Act (HIPAA)
Legislation passed by Congress in 1996 that contains provisions for insured persons enrolled in employer-sponsored insurance programs to retain the right to new health care insurance when they change jobs. This is without regard to their current health status. Also referred to as the Kennedy-Kassebaum bill.

High Severity   A type of presenting problem in which the risk of morbidity without treatment is high to extreme; there is moderate to high risk of mortality without treatment; or high probability of severe; prolonged functional impairment.

HIPAA   The Health Insurance Portability and Accountability Act was passed by Congress in 1996. The portability part of this Act made headlines when it was first released, because it allows employees to take their health

insurance with them when they change jobs. The accountability aspect of
HIPAA gives the government its power to investigate health care providers
they believe are committing fraud. One of the most significant parts of this
Act is that a fund was created that will continue to finance fraud
investigations and additional staff members.

History of Present Illness   A description of the chronological
development of the patient's present illness from first onset of symptoms.
This includes a description of location, quality, severity, timing, duration,
modifying factors, and associated signs and symptoms significantly related
to the present problem(s).

Home Services   CPT® codes are used to report any health care services
provided at the patient's home or other private residence.

Hospital Inpatient   In this context, CPT® codes that are used to
report E/M hospital inpatient services and admission to a hospital
setting.

Hospital Observation   CPT® codes used to report E/M services provided
to patients designated or admitted as "observation status" in a hospital,
though it is not necessary that the patient be located in an observation area
designated by the hospital.

ICD-9-CM   The International Classification of Diseases, Ninth Revision,
Clinical Modification is a numeric coding system for diagnoses and
procedures.

Incision   Provide descriptions of those surgical services that involve cutting
into the body. All otomy (eg, cutting, making an incision into) procedures
are located under the subheading of "Incision." Incision codes include
various drainage, exploration, piercing, puncture, and centesis procedures.

Insurance Carrier   An insurance company that underwrites polices that
cover health care services.

Introduction or Removal   Includes procedures that scope, irrigate, inject,
insert, remove, or replace into various body areas.

Intraoperative services   Those services that are normally a usual and
necessary part of a surgical procedure (eg, local, metacarpal, digital block,
topical anesthesia, the operation itself)

Intermediary (or Fiscal Intermediary)   An insurance company that
contracts with Medicare and other government health care programs to pay
the claims of health care providers with government funds.

Key Components   The three elements (history, examination, and medical
decision making) that make up the evaluation and management services
provided by physicians and other healthcare providers to bill a specific level
of service.

Level of E/M service   The level of visit or service dependent on three key components, history, examination, and medical decision making. Counseling, coordination of care, and time are also contributory elements in the selection of the level of service.

LMRP or Local Medical Review Policy   A Local Medical Review Policy may designate that certain ICD-9-CM codes be present on a medical order to be considered medically necessary and reimbursed. If not, then an ABN (see above) may be required.

Low Severity   A type of presenting problem in which the risk of morbidity without treatment is low, there is little to no risk of mortality without treatment; and full recovery is expected.

Medical Coding   The act of assigning a code to a medical service to submit to an insurance carrier for reimbursement.

Medical Decision Making   The decision making process based on the nature of the presenting problem, that takes into account differential diagnosis, treatment options, complexity, and potential for complications.

Medical History   History of the patient's past illnesses, surgical procedures, allergies, medications, and other pertinent facts related to the patient's past illnesses and problems.

Medically Necessary (or Medical Necessity)   Medically necessary procedures are those that need to be done based on the patient's current condition. This condition must be documented in the patient's chart. Medicare considers medically unnecessary procedures (when the reason for performing the procedure is not properly documented) to be an example of fraudulent billing.

Medical Record   Written or graphic information documenting facts and pertinent data during rendering of patient care.

Medicaid   A federally aided, state-operated program that assists low-income persons in need of medical care.

Medicare   A federal health care program for the elderly and disabled that pays a portion of a beneficiary's medical costs. There are two parts of Medicare coverage: Part A and Part B, which refer to differing levels of coverage for physicians and hospitals. Medicare is administered by the Centers for Medicare and Medicaid (CMS).

Medicare Secondary Payor (MSP)   The government requires that providers ask Medicare beneficiaries a series of questions to determine if another insurance program should be billed first, before Medicare is billed. This other insurance program is considered primary and should pay the majority of the bill. Once the primary insurance has paid, then Medicare should pay appropriate remaining costs.

Medication Sheet   A data sheet which is an up-to-date listing of the patient's medications and/or failures. This information is located in the patient's medical record.

Minimal Severity   A type of presenting problem that may not require the presence of a physician, but in which services are rendered under a physician's supervision.

Moderate Severity   A type of presenting problem in which the risk of morbidity without treatment is moderate; there is a moderate risk of mortality without treatment, uncertain prognosis or increased probability of prolonged functional impairment.

Multiple Procedures   Use Modifier -51 to identify multiple procedures when rendered on the same date of service, at the same operative session. When a procedure is performed with another separately identifiable procedure, the highest valued code is listed as the primary procedure and additional procedures are listed with -51.

New Patient   A patient who has not received any professional service from the physician, or another physician of the same specialty belonging to the same group practice within the past three (3) years.

Office of Inspector General (OIG)   An Agency within the Department of Health and Human Services (HHS) charged with the responsibility for enforcement of federal law.

Record Retention   A recommended time period that records in a medical organization should be kept.

Operation Restore Trust   This is an effort by the government to concentrate on specific abuses within the health care industry.

Operative Note   A formal or informal (depending on setting) form of documentation indicating the procedure performed and all-pertinent details of the surgery.

Other/Miscellaneous procedures   Inclusive of those medical procedures that are unique and do not associate with other groupings. Some of these procedures include endoscopy, arthrodesis, manipulation, amputation, suture, fracture, dislocation, splints, strapping, casts, and unlisted procedures.

Outpatient Services   Services provided in the physician's office or other outpatient setting or ambulatory facility.

Patient Encounter Form   A form used to record the patient visit.

Patient Registration Form   A detailed form to record the patient demographic information and insurance information.

Past Medical History   A review of the patient's previous experiences with trauma, illness, and treatments that includes previous surgery and hospitalizations, current medications, allergies, and other pertinent prior medical encounters.

Postoperative visits   Follow-up visits after surgery during the postoperative period of the surgery (0-90 days normally) related to the recovery from the surgery. Each carrier defines global days individually.

Preventive Medicine   In this context, codes for reporting services provided to patients to promote health and prevent illness or injury, including routine examinations performed in the absence of patient complaints or symptoms and counseling, or risk factor reduction intervention.

Problem Focused Exam   A limited exam of the affected body area or organ system.

Prolonged Services   In this context, codes for reporting prolonged service that is beyond the usual service. This includes both codes for direct face-to-face contact and codes for prolonged services without direct face-to-face contact with the patient in an inpatient or outpatient setting.

Problem List   A list of the patient's chronic medical problems and/or conditions. This information is located in the patient's medical record.

Record Retention   Time limit that each individual state and/or insurance carrier requires records to be kept.

Repair/Reconstruction   Describes those procedures that surgically improve and repair improperly functioning, deformed, or painful parts of the body. All "orrhaphy" (suturing) or "plasty" (surgical repair) procedures are found under this subheading.

Review of Systems   An inventory of body systems which is part of the history which indicates negative or positive responses to medical problems.

Risk Table   The table published by the Centers for Medicare and Medicaid that identifies the presenting problem and/or diagnoses, amount of data ordered or reviewed, and management options.

Separate Procedures   A separate procedure is a component of a more complex service and is usually not identified separately. When performed alone, or if unrelated or distinct from other service(s) performed, it may be reported separately. A procedure that is carried out as an integral part of the total service does not warrant a separate identification. Separate procedures codes are often misread and coded with related cases. Related cases refer to procedures with the same diagnosis, same operative area, and same indication. Linking these procedures is referred to as fragmented billing.

SOAP   Acronym for method of documentation; subjective, objective, assessment and plan.

Social History   An age-appropriate review of events and activities that include information regarding marital status, use of alcohol, tobacco or drugs, education, employment, and sexual history.

Special E/M Services   In this context, codes used to report evaluation and /or examinations for the purpose of establishing baseline information for insurance certification, work related information, or medical disability evaluation. No active management or treatment is performed during the encounter.

Subsequent Audits   Audits performed on a routine basis to monitor coding and documentation practices.

Summary Report   A report of audit findings in a simple, easy to read format that indicates incorrect coding, documentation and/or billing errors with recommendations for improvement.

System Review   A body system inventory acquired from a series of questions asked of the patient. The purpose is to ascertain signs or symptoms that the patient may be experiencing, to clarify the differential diagnoses and to identify the need for further testing.

Tally Sheet   Most commonly referred to as the audit tool. (See definition of audit tool.)

Third Party Payer   Insurance carrier which intervenes to pay hospital or medical bills.

Treatment Plan   Plan of care involving the complexity of the physician's medical decision making.

Unbundling/Bundling   Medicare pays for many tests and procedures as a group. For instance, the medical practice will receive payment for a particular diagnosis, and all services related to that diagnosis will be "bundled" into one payment. Unbundling refers to the practice of charging for a service individually when it should have already been covered as part of a group payment. For lab services, the government now says that "panel" tests—lab tests that are grouped or bundled together—must be unbundled if any of the tests are not medically necessary.

Upcoding   In addition to codes for diagnoses, every procedure performed by a health care provider also has a code that corresponds to it. If a procedure requires complex tasks or a large amount of time, it has a higher code number assigned to it. Upcoding refers to the inappropriate practice of assigning a higher procedure code than what was actually performed. Medicare requires that all procedures performed on a patient be written in the patient's chart. What is written in the chart must match the procedure code level given.

Answer Key

CHAPTER 1

Test Your Knowledge

1.	False	5.	False	9.	b	13.	b
2.	False	6.	False	10.	d	14.	d
3.	True	7.	True	11.	c	15.	c
4.	True	8.	c	12.	c		

CHAPTER 2

Checkpoint Exercises 2-1

1.	O	5.	O	9.	S
2.	P	6.	P	10.	O
3.	O	7.	S		
4.	A	8.	P		

Test Your Knowledge

1. United Kingdom, St. Bartholomew's Hospital; Dated 1123 AD
2. *The Doctor, His Patient, and the Illness*
3. Problem-oriented medical record
4. Problem list, history, examination, laboratory findings, plan of care, daily SOAP
5. Data collection, formulation of problems, devising a management plan, reviewing the medical problems, and revising the plan when necessary
6. Heading, body
7. Draw a line through the error, note "error," and initial it
8. Subjective, Objective, Assessment, Plan
9. Site of service, documented level or type of service or procedure, medical necessity
10. Aid to memory, support for continuity of care, provision of witness to an event for legal, financial, and regulatory purposes

11. Any three of the following: outpatient office visit, consultation, medications and prescriptions, immunization records, laboratory tests and results, x-rays—imaging and diagnostic studies, surgical services and operative reports, pathology services

12. Any three of the following: claim form negligence, supporting level of service billed, document medical histories, provide a method in which health statistics are tracked, act as a legal document, justify to insurance companies the charges billed based on the medical care provided, assess quality of care

CHAPTER 3

Test Your Knowledge

1.	False	6.	False	11.	99212	16.	99202
2.	False	7.	False	12.	99201	17.	99201
3.	True	8.	False	13.	99212		
4.	True	9.	True	14.	99214		
5.	False	10.	True	15.	99385		

CHAPTER 4

Test Your Knowledge

1.	E/M	5.	E/M	9.	C	13.	T
2.	P	6.	E/M	10.	F	14.	T
3.	P	7.	P	11.	T	15.	T
4.	E/M	8.	P	12.	T		

CHAPTER 5

Test Your Knowledge

1.	T	14.	Data tracking
2.	T	15.	Retention of records
3.	T	16.	Compliance officer
4.	T	17.	Compliance plan elements
5.	F	18.	Hotline
6.	T	19.	Formal insurance course
7.	F	20.	Medical necessity
8.	T	21.	d
9.	T	22.	d
10.	T	23.	a
11.	Compliance	24.	a
12.	Fraud alert	25.	d
13.	OIG/HHS		

CHAPTER 6

Test Your Knowledge

1. 10-15
2. Frequency, errors
3. Analyzing
4. Results
5. CPT, HCPCS, ICD-9-CM
6. Countersigned
7. Medically
8. Coding, correct
9. Documentation
10. Without

CHAPTER 7

Test Your Knowledge

Case 1   Foghorn Leghorn (established patient/office)

History: Problem focused (99212)
  CC: recheck extremity swelling
  HPI: location: right leg
      timing: at all times
  ROS: none
  PMH: medications

Exam: Problem focused (99212) = 4 bullet documented
  Constitutional: 3 vitals documented
  Lungs: Clear
  Cardiovascular (2):   Sinus rhythm
      Exam of extremities

Medical Decision Making: Straightforward (99212)
  Diagnosis or Management Options: 1 established diagnosis—improving (minimal)
  Diagnostic Procedures: none (minimal)
  Risk: moderate
      presenting problems—1 stable illness (low)
      diagnostic procedures—none ordered (minimal)
      management options—prescription drug
        (moderate)

Level of E/M service documented: 99212
Other billable service(s) documented: J3420 (Vitamin B$_{12}$ injection—Medicare)
Diagnosis documented: Mild chronic edema (legs) 782.3
      Pernicious anemia 281.0

Case 2   Joan Deere (new patient/office)

History: Expanded problem focused (99202)
  CC: burning on urination and wants pregnancy test
  HPI: location: GU system
      quality: burning on urination
      duration: 3 days; stopped BC pills 3 months ago

modifying factors: stopped taking birth control pills

ROS: constitutional; gastrointestinal; genitourinary

Exam:

Expanded problem focused (99202) = 11 bullets documented

Constitutional (2):   vital signs; general appearance

Chest: palpation of breasts

Gastrointestinal (2): exam of abdomen; exam of rectum

Genitourinary (6):   pelvic exam including external genitalia and vagina; urethra; bladder; cervix; uterus; adnexa

Medical Decision Making: Moderate (99204)

Diagnosis or Management Options: 2 new problems (extensive)

Diagnostic Procedures: labs (minimal)

Risk: moderate

presenting problems—undiagnosed problem (moderate)

diagnostic procedures—labs (minimal)

management options—prescription drugs (moderate)

Level of E/M service documented: 99202

Other billable service(s) documented: 81002 (urine dip only)

Diagnoses documented: Dysuria 788.1 (do not code urethritis until confirmed in documentation)

Amenorrhea 626.0

Case 3   Sophia Lorenzo (new patient/office)

History:

Comprehensive (99204/99205)

CC: referral for cardiac problems/chest pain

HPI: location: substernal chest pain

timing: one week ago

context: after car accident

modifying factors: NTG; oxygen

associated signs and symptoms: nausea and vomiting; diaphoresis

ROS: complete: cardiovascular, respiratory, all other systems reviewed

PMH: current meds; prior illnesses/injuries

FH: negative for heart disease

SH: does not smoke or drink and exercises regularly

Exam:

Expanded problem focused (99202) = 14 bullets documented

Constitutional (2):   vital signs; general appearance

HEENT(2):   inspection of neck

exam of mucosa

Eyes: exam of conjunctiva

Respiratory: clear

Musculoskeletal (2): palpation of spine (back) and ribs (chest) in same bullet; inspection of digits and nails (no cyanosis or clubbing)

Cardiovascular (4):   palpation of heart; auscultation of heart; exam of femoral arteries; exam of extremities

Gastrointestinal: exam of abdomen

Nervous system: unremarkable

Medical Decision Making: Moderate (99204)
        Diagnosis or Management Options: 2 new problems (extensive)
        Diagnostic Procedures: labs; radiology; Medicine section (multiple)
        Risk: moderate
         presenting problems—2 or more stable conditions
          (moderate)
         diagnostic procedures—labs; x-rays; echo (minimal)
         management options—prescription drugs
          (moderate)

Level of E/M service documented: 99202
Other billable service(s) documented: 93000 (EKG with interpretation and report)
            36415 Venipuncture
Diagnoses documented: Angina (stable) 413.9
            Coronary artery disease 414.00
            Type 2 diabetes (not documented as uncontrolled) 250.00

Case 4 Jack Marison (established patient/office)

History: Problem focused (99212)
       CC: follow-up chronic conditions
       HPI: review of four chronic conditions
       ROS: none
       PMH: cataract surgery (operations and hospitalizations)
       SH: never used tobacco

Exam: Problem focused (99212) = 4 bullets documented
       Constitutional: vital signs
       Eyes: ophthalmoscopic exam
       Cardiovascular: exam of extremities
       Respiratory: chest clear

Medical Decision Making: Moderate (99214)
        Diagnosis or Management Options: 4 established diagnosis, stable (extensive)
        Diagnostic Procedures: labs (minimal)
        Risk: moderate
         presenting problems—2 or more stable chronic
          conditions (moderate)
         diagnostic procedures—labs (minimal)
         management options—prescription drugs
          (moderate)

Level of E/M service documented: 99212
Other billable service(s) documented: 36415 (Venipuncture—non-Medicare)
Diagnoses documented: Coronary artery disease 414.00
            Congestive heart failure 428.0
            Peripheral vascular disease 443.9
            Benign prostatic hypertrophy 600

Case 5   Mary Tyler (established patient/office)

History: Detailed (99214)

CC: chest pain

HPI: location: anterior chest
      quality: sharp, stabbing
      duration: 4–5 weeks
      context: with movement

ROS: Eyes; ENT; Cardiovascular; Respiratory; Gastrointestinal; Musculoskeletal; remaining systems negative

PMH: history of COPD; allergies; medications

Exam: Expanded problem focused (99213) = 11 bullets documented

Constitutional: general appearance
Skin: inspection of skin
Eyes (2):   exam conjunctiva; exam of pupils
ENT (2):   inspection of ears; exam of pharynx
Musculoskeletal: inspection and palpation of ribs (chest)
Respiratory: auscultation of lungs
Cardiovascular (2):   auscultation of heart; exam of extremities
Gastrointestinal: exam of abdomen

Medical Decision Making: moderate (99214)

Diagnosis or Management Options: 1 new problem, no additional workup (multiple)
Diagnostic Procedures: Medicine section—EKG (minimal)
Risk: moderate
    presenting problems—acute uncomplicated illness or injury (low)
    diagnostic procedures—EKG (minimal)
    management options—prescription drugs (moderate)

Level of E/M service documented: 99214
Other billable service(s) documented: 93000 (EKG with interpretation and report)
Diagnosis documented: Chest wall pain 786.52

Case 6   Martin Sharp (established patient/office)

History: Expanded problem focused (99213)

CC: ulcer left foot; elevated blood sugars

HPI: location: left foot
      quality: open necrotic ulcer
      severity: high blood sugars

ROS: Constitutional; Respiratory

PMH: history of coronary artery disease, CABG, myocardial infarction, chronic renal failure; current medications

Exam: Expanded problem focused (99213) = 10 bullets documented

Constitutional: vital signs
Cardiovascular (2):   exam of carotid arteries; auscultation
Neck: exam of neck
Respiratory: clear
Gastrointestinal (2):   exam of abdomen; liver, spleen
Musculoskeletal (2):   inspection of right lower extremity; inspection of left lower extremity
Skin: inspection of skin

Medical Decision Making: moderate complexity (99214)

Diagnosis or Management Options:	2 established problems worsening (extensive)
Diagnostic Procedures:	labs; radiology; Medicine section (multiple)
Risk:	high
	presenting problems—at least one chronic condition with severe exacerbation (high)
	diagnostic procedures—labs, CT scan, EKG (minimal)
	management options—prescription drugs (moderate)

Level of E/M service documented: 99213

Diagnoses documented:
Uncontrolled diabetes with diabetic peripheral vascular disease 250.73
Foot ulcer 707.1
Atherosclerotic heart disease 414.00
Carotid stenosis 433.10
Status post below the knee amputation V49.75
End-stage renal disease 585

Case 7   Jimmy Dugan (new patient/office)

History:
Expanded Problem Focused (99202)
CC: Unexplainable weight loss
HPI: duration: past year
quality: clear to yellow mucous
modifying factor: lost 20 pounds; spit up blood on one occasion
associated signs and symptoms: chronic fatigue
ROS: Constitutional
SH: divorced, lives alone somewhat of recluse, two-pack-a-day smoker, does not exercise much at all

Exam:
Expanded problem focused (99202) = 12 bullets documented
Constitutional (2):   vital signs; general appearance
HEENT (4):   exam of head, eyes, ears, nose, and throat within normal limits
Respiratory: exam of lungs
Cardiovascular (2):   exam of heart, peripheral edema
Gastrointestinal (3):   exam of abdomen, liver, kidney and spleen, rectal exam

Medical Decision Making: Moderate (99204)

Diagnosis or Management Options:	1 new diagnosis—additional workup planned (extensive)
Diagnostic Procedures (minimal):	chest CT
Risk:	Moderate
	presenting problems—at least one chronic condition
	diagnostic procedures—CT scan chest
	Management options—prescription drugs (moderate)

Level of E/M service documented: 99202—new patient

Diagnoses documented:
496 Chronic airway obstruction, not elsewhere classified
V15.82 Personal history of tobacco use, presenting hazards to health

Case 8   Tom Smith (established patient/office)

History: Detailed (99214)
                            CC: concerns of a productive cough
                            HPI: location: respiratory
                                   duration: three days
                                   quality: dark yellow secretions
                                   associated signs and symptoms: clear nasal secretions
                            ROS: constitutional; respiratory; cardiovascular; gastrointestinal
                            PMH: history of arteriosclerotic heart disease status post CABG

Exam: Expanded Problem Focused (99213) = 12 bullets documented
                            Constitutional: vital signs
                            Ears (3):   canals clear, tympanic membranes; nasal mucosa and turbinates;
                                                 oropharynx, tonsils
                            Neck (2):   lymph nodes (neck supple); thyroid
                            Respiratory (2):   Respiratory effort; auscultation of lungs
                            Cardiovascular (2): auscultation of heart; peripheral edema

Medical Decision Making: Moderate
                            Diagnosis or Management Options: 1 new diagnosis—no additional workup
                                                                   planned (extensive)
                            Diagnostic Procedures: none
                            Risk: Moderate
                                                                presenting problems—two chronic conditions;
                                                                   1 acute condition
                                                                diagnostic procedures—none
                                                                Management options—prescription drugs
                                                                   (moderate)

Level of E/M service documented: 99214 Detailed
Diagnoses Documented: Acute bronchitis 466.0
                                   Hypertension 401.9
                                   Personal history of other cardiovascular diseases V12.59

Case 9   Mary Smith (new patient/office)

History: Problem focused (99201)
                            CC: feels tired and extremely stressed
                            HPI: location: right upper arm
                                   timing: just before coming out here
                                   quality: mole irregular, deeply pigmented
                                   modifying factors: saw physician who cut into lesion
                            PMH: medications (albuterol inhaler), prior illnesses
                            SH: divorced, children, recent move

Exam: Expanded problem focused (99202) = 11 bullets documented
                            ENT (3):   canals; nose benign; throat benign
                            Neck (2):   supple, trachea midline; thyroid
                            Chest (2):   inspection of breasts; palpation of breasts and axilla
                            Respiratory: auscultation of lungs

Cardiovascular: auscultation of heart and sounds
Gastrointestinal (2):   exam of abdomen; liver, spleen

Medical Decision Making: Moderate (99204)

Diagnosis or Management Options:	3 new diagnoses—additional workup planned (extensive)
Diagnostic Procedures:	none (minimal)
Risk:	Moderate
	presenting problems—1 chronic condition, 2 self-limiting minor problems
	diagnostic procedures—labs
	Management options—prescription drugs (moderate)

Level of E/M service documented: 99201
Diagnoses documented:

        780.71   Chronic fatigue syndrome
        216.6   Benign neoplasm of skin of upper limb
        300.4   Neurotic depression

Case 10   Troy Dimly (established patient/office)

History: Problem focused (99212)

CC: comes in today in follow-up of recently diagnosed type II diabetes

HPI:
	location:	erectile dysfunction
	modifying factor:	hemoglobin A_{1c} 7.4%
	context:	lost 26 pounds
	timing:	since July

ROS: none

PFSH: none

Exam: Expanded problem focused (99213) = 9 bullets documented

Constitutional (2):	vital signs; general appearance (color good)
Eyes:	within normal limits
ENT (3):	Ears, nose, throat within normal limits
Respiratory:	exam of lungs (clear and stable)
Cardiovascular (2):	exam of heart (clear and stable); peripheral edema

Medical Decision Making: Moderate (99214)

Diagnosis or Management Options:	1 established problem—stable; 1 new problem—self-limited
Diagnostic Procedures:	none (minimal)
Risk:	low
	presenting problems—1 established problem—stable; 1 new problem—self-limited
	management options—prescription drugs (moderate)

Level of E/M service documented: 99213
Other procedures documented: 81015
Diagnoses documented:

        250.00   Type II diabetes mellitus
        302.72   Psychosexual dysfunction with inhibited sexual excitement

CHAPTER 8

Test Your Knowledge

1. Detailed review analysis
2. Monitoring
3. Corrective action
4. Audit
5. Upcoding
6. Summary report
7. Unbundling
8. Aggregate analysis report
9. Evaluation and management services
10. Training

CHAPTER 9

Test Your Knowledge

1. CPT, ICD-9-CM, HCPCS, audit tool, charge ticket, detailed review analysis, summary report, NCCI or CCI edits
2. Known as fragmenting bill, billing more than 1 code for more comprehensive code
3. Components of a more complex process and not usually identified separately
4. Modifier -51 exempt
5. Bill for only the therapeutic scope procedure
6. Type of audit/scope of audit, review operative note, report findings, educate
7. What is included in the total surgical procedure
8. The physician must provide 60 days of follow-up care after surgery
9. Any five of these: patient name, date of procedure, preoperative diagnosis, postoperative diagnosis, surgeon, anesthesia, procedure, description of procedure, physician signature
10. Make a copy of the operative report, underline/highlight important information, use medical references for unfamiliar terms, cross out non–coding-related documentation, check bundling issues, verify code sequencing when multiple procedures are performed, apply necessary modifiers

CHAPTER 10

Test Your Knowledge

Case 1   Brook Brinkman (established patient/office)

History: Detailed (99214)
            CC: left wrist pain for 1 year
            HPI: context: receiving physical therapy for 6 months
                 modifying factor: does not seem to be helping
                 location: wearing bilateral wrist supports
                 quality: helps to some extent

ROS: respiratory; cardiovascular
PMH: medications, allergies, past surgeries and illnesses

Exam: Expanded Problem Focused (99213) = 11 bullets
                Constitutional: general appearance
                Neck: supple
                Head: normocephalic
                Cardiovascular (2): carotid pulses; no murmurs, gallops, or rubs
                Respiratory (2):   clear to auscultation and percussion
                Abdomen: negative
                Musculoskeletal: left wrist weakness
                Skin: prominent mass on the palmar aspect of the left wrist

Medical Decision Making: Moderate (99214)
                Diagnosis or Management Options: 1 established diagnosis—worsening
                Diagnostic Procedures: none (minimal)
                Risk: moderate
                                                   presenting problems—1 chronic problem worsening
                                                      (moderate)
                                                   diagnostic procedures—none ordered (minimal)
                                                   management options—major surgery without
                                                      identified risk factors (moderate)

Level of E/M service documented: 99214
Diagnosis documented: Carpal tunnel 354.0

Case 2   Martha Stoops (established patient/office)

History: Expanded problem focused (99213)
                CC: follow up abdominal pain
                HPI: quality: pain seems to have dissipated
                       context: mild soreness that persists
                ROS: constitutional; gastrointestinal
                PFSH: none

Exam: Expanded Problem Focused (99213) = 6 bullets documented
                Respiratory (2):   clear to auscultation and percussion
                Cardiovascular (2): regular rate and rhythm; extremities—negative for edema
                Abdomen (2):   soft nontender without distention, no rebound or guarding

Medical Decision Making: Straightforward (99212)
                Diagnosis or Management Options: 1 established diagnosis—improved
                Diagnostic Procedures: none (minimal)
                Risk: moderate
                                                   presenting problems—limited
                                                   diagnostic procedures—none ordered (minimal)
                                                   management options—prescription drug
                                                      management (moderate)

Level of E/M service documented: 99213
Other billable service(s) documented: none
Diagnosis documented: gastroenteritis resolved 558.9

Case 3   Thomas Parker (new patient—hospital consultation)

History: Expanded problem focused (99252)
     CC: asked to consult hospital patient due to multiple medical problems
     HPI: location: fractured pelvis, bilateral lower amputee, ruptured spleen, lacerated liver
          modifying factor: sustained from a motor vehicle accident
     ROS: respiratory; cardiovascular; hematologic; musculoskeletal; ROS otherwise normal (counts as complete ROS)
     SH: patient does not smoke or drink, avid runner prior to accident
     PMH: no history of diabetes, hypertension, cardiac or respiratory disease

Exam: Detailed (99253) = 2 from 6 systems or body areas (21 bullets)
     Constitutional (2):   4 vitals; general appearance
     Eyes (2):   pupils are reactive to light and accommodation; no vessel changes, exudates, or hemorrhages noted
     ENT: oral mucosa normal; no lesions noted
     Neck: supple, no masses
     Respiratory (2):   normal—no wheezes or rubs appreciated; clear to auscultation
     Cardiovascular   normal sinus rhythm, no murmurs
     Abdomen (2):   no evidence of masses; no evidence of hernias
     Skin: laparotomy scar healing well, no signs of infection
     Musculoskeletal (4):   lower leg muscles flaccid, unable or will not move stumps; upper body within normal limits
          moves all upper extremities on command without difficulty range of motion good
     Neurological (2):   cranial nerves intact; hand grips strong bilaterally
     Psychiatric (3):   patient depressed (mood and affect)
          oriented to person, place, and time
          judgment impaired due to depression

Medical Decision Making: Moderate (99254)
     Diagnosis or Management Options: 1 new diagnosis to examining physician
     Diagnostic Procedures: none (minimal)
     Risk: moderate
          presenting problems—1 chronic problem stable
          diagnostic procedures—none ordered (minimal)
          management options—medication management (moderate)

Level of E/M service documented: 99252   *requires 3 of 3 key components
Other billable service(s) documented: none
Diagnosis documented: V49.75 Lower limb amputation status; below knee
                           309.0   Brief depressive reaction as adjustment reaction

Case 4   John Thoroson (new patient/office)

History: Expanded problem focused (99202)
     CC: patient's first visit, elevated temperature
     HPI: duration—past 12 hours
          severity—the high was 102
     ROS: GI
     PMH: no allergies or medications

SH: lives with parents

Exam: Expanded problem focused (99202) = 11 bullets documented
             Constitutional (2):   general appearance; vitals
             Eyes: normal
             ENT(2):   tonsils; ears, nose, and mouth normal
             Neck: supple
             Skin: negative
             Cardiovascular: normal rhythm, no murmurs
             Respiratory: lung sounds are normal
             Abdomen (2):   diffuse tenderness; no masses or organomegaly noted

Medical Decision Making: Moderate (99204)
             Diagnosis or Management Options: 1 new problem to presenting physician
             Diagnostic Procedures: labs; renal x-ray
             Risk: moderate
                                                presenting problems—moderate
                                                diagnostic procedures—minimal
                                                management options—prescription drug
                                                   management (moderate)

Level of E/M service documented: 99202
Other billable service(s) documented: Urine dip with microscopy 81000
                                        Venipuncture—36415
Diagnosis documented: 787.01 Nausea with vomiting
                                        590.10 Acute pyelonephritis
                                        041.4   *Escherichia coli (E. coli)*

Case 5   Nicholas Gristmeyer (established nursing home)

History: Expanded problem focused interval history (99312)
              CC: evaluated for left-sided cerebrovascular accident, right-sided paralysis
              HPI: duration: demented since stroke
                     modifying factors: opens eyes to name only
              ROS: does not answer questions (given comprehensive for attempt to obtain ROS)
              PMH: current medications

Exam: Expanded Problem Focused (99312) = 7 bullets documented
              Constitutional (2):   general appearance; vitals
              Eyes: cataracts bilaterally
              Cardiovascular: normal rhythm
              Respiratory (2):   clear to auscultation and percussion
              Abdomen: no masses or tenderness
              Psychiatric: responds to name only

Medical Decision Making: Moderate (99313)
              Diagnosis or Management Options: 1 established problem, worsening
              Diagnostic Procedures: none
              Risk: moderate
                                                 presenting problems—moderate
                                                 diagnostic procedures—(minimal)
                                                 management options—prescription drug
                                                    management (moderate)

Level of E/M service documented: 99312
Other billable service(s) documented: None

Diagnosis documented: 438.20 Hemiplegia affecting unspecified side due to cerebrovascular disease
263.9 Unspecified protein-calorie malnutrition
298.9 Unspecified psychosis

Case 6   Myrtle Byers (established patient/nursing home)

History   Detailed (99313)

CC:	follow-up for cellulitis	
HPI:	location:	left foot
	quality:	infection is about gone
	context:	recovering well
	modifying factors:	IV therapy for cellulitis
ROS:	respiratory; cardiovascular; musculoskeletal	
PMH:	history of IDDM, current medications	

Exam   Problem Focused (99311) = 4 bullets

Constitutional:	general appearance; vitals—3
Musculoskeletal:	left foot reddening upper surface
Skin:	infection decreased significantly

Note: no credit for "all other areas are normal": no indication of what was examined

Medical Decision Making: low complexity (99312)

Diagnosis or Management Options:	1 established diagnosis—improving
Diagnostic Procedures:	none (minimal)
Risk:	moderate
	presenting problems—1 chronic problem stable
	diagnostic procedures—none ordered (minimal)
	management options—prescription drug management (moderate)

Level of E/M service documented:	99312
Other billable service(s) documented:	none
Diagnosis documented:	682.7 Cellulitis
	250.01 IDDM

Case 7   Carlotta Maple (established patient/office)

History   Expanded problem focused (99213)

CC:	renew blood pressure medication and blood work	
HPI:	location:	bilateral knee pain
	quality:	tender and swollen
	modifying factors:	doing yard work on knees too long
ROS:	respiratory; cardiovascular	

Exam   Problem Focused (99212) = 5 bullets documented

Constitutional:	vitals
Neck:	within normal limits
Cardiovascular:	normal
Respiratory:	clear
Musculoskeletal:	knee appears swollen

Medical Decision Making: Moderate (99214)

        Diagnosis or Management Options: 1 new problem, no additional workup planned

        Diagnostic Procedures: none (minimal)

        Risk: moderate

        presenting problems—1 acute uncomplicated illness

        diagnostic procedures—none ordered (minimal)

        management options—prescription drug
           management (moderate)

Level of E/M service documented: 99213

Other billable service(s) documented: none

Diagnosis documented: 401.9   Hypertension, unspecified

        719.48 Pain in joint, other specified sites

Case 8   Martin Steiner (established patient/office)

History

Detailed (99214)

CC: check up hypertension

HPI: severity: severe headache pain

        location: head and face

        modifying factors: feeling more steady on feet

        timing: symptoms change with weather, today particularly bad day

ROS: respiratory; cardiovascular

PMH: recent hospitalization and CT and MRI scans

Exam

Problem Focused (99212) = 5 bullets documented

Cardiovascular (3): carotids without bruits

        regular rate and rhythm

        no edema

Respiratory (2):   lungs clear to A&P

Medical Decision Making: Moderate (99214)

        Diagnosis or Management Options: 2 established problems, worsening

        Diagnostic Procedures: EEG (minimal)

        Risk: moderate

        presenting problems—2 chronic with mild
           exacerbation

        diagnostic procedures - EEG (minimal)

        management options – prescription drug
           management (moderate)

Level of E/M service documented: 99214

Other billable service(s) documented: none

Diagnosis documented: Hypertension 401.9

        Headaches 784.0

Case 9   Rebecca Paulern (established patient/office)

History: Detailed (99214)
CC: ear pain
HPI: location: ears
context: pulling constantly on ears
duration: unable to sleep for 3 days
associated signs and symptoms: fever 101
PFSH: reviewed on form in chart—checked on form
ROS: ENT—ears; Psychiatric—temperament

Exam: Expanded Problem Focused (99213) = 12 bullets documented
Constitutional(2):   vitals—3; general appearance
Eyes: pupils
ENT(2)   nose; oropharynx
Neck (2)   supple; lymph nodes
Respiratory: effort
Cardiovascular: sounds, rate, rhythm
Abdomen: soft, nontender
Skin: color
Neurological: alert

Medical Decision Making: Straightforward (99212)
Diagnosis or Management Options: 1 new self-limited problem
Diagnostic Procedures: none (minimal)
Risk: moderate
presenting problems—1 self-limiting problem
diagnostic procedures—none ordered (minimal)
management options—prescription drug
management (moderate)

Level of E/M service documented: 99213
Other billable service(s) documented: none
Diagnosis documented: 380.10 Otitis xterna

Case 10   Maureen Bradfield (new patient/office)

History: Problem focused (99201)
CC: new patient visit, chief complaint vague, assume for Zoloft management
HPI: quality: depression has improved
PMH: depression (prior illnesses); S/P hysterectomy; medications
FH: heart disease

Exam: Expanded Problem Focused (99202) = 6 bullets documented
Constitutional: general appearance
Eyes: PERRLA
Respiratory: lungs clear
Cardiovascular (2):   heart regular; extremities without clubbing, cyanosis, or edema
Abdomen: soft, no CVA tenderness

Medical Decision Making: Moderate (99204)
Diagnosis or Management Options: 1 new problem to examining physician, no
additional workup planned
Diagnostic Procedures: none (minimal)

Risk: moderate
                                           presenting problems—1 stable chronic condition
                                           diagnostic procedures—none ordered (minimal)
                                           management options—prescription drug
                                               management (moderate)

Level of E/M service documented: 99201
Other billable service(s) documented: none
Diagnosis documented: 311 depression
                                      V17.3 family history of heart disease

PHYSICIAN MEDICAL RECORD REVIEW
SUMMARY REPORT

Physician: Harrison Brinklemeyer, MD   **Date of Review: 03/20/02**

Reviewer: Mark Thomas, CPC, CCS-P

Number of Charts Reviewed: 10

One service date was reviewed for each chart reviewed for appropriate coding and supporting documentation. Each chart was reviewed in detail for completeness.

E/M documentation appears to support service billed.	**7**
E/M documentation in the record appears to support a lower level of service than billed.	**2**
E/M documentation in the record appears to support a higher level of service than billed.	**1**

Other documentation coding issues:

1. On one patient encounter (Carlotta Maple) the physician did not appear to list hypertension on the fee ticket/charge ticket, but it was documented in the medical record.
2. One consultation for Thomas Parker did not contain enough documentation for a 99255 consultation. All three components appeared deficient in the documentation for the higher level of service.
3. On one date of service for Maureen Bradfield the physician did not appear to document enough information in the history. All three key components must be met for a new patient visit.
4. On one date of service for Martha Stoops, the physician documented a 99213 but billed the patient encounter as a 99212. Medical necessity supports a level 3 office visit for this encounter.

RECOMMENDATIONS

1. Review problem areas with physician.
2. Review E/M documentation guidelines with physician.
3. Review CMS documentation key component requirements for new and established patients.
4. Review consultation coding documentation requirements.
5. Conduct a medical record review in 6 months.

MEDICAL RECORD REVIEW
Principle Family Practice Group
DETAILED REVIEW ANALYSIS

Physician: Harrison Brinklemeyer   **Date of Review:**

Exam #	Patient Name	Service Date	Practice CPT® Code	History	Exam	Medical Decision Making	Documented CPT® Code
1	Brook Brinkman	02/01/02	99214	D	EPF	MOD	99214
2	Martha Stoops	02/10/02	99212	EPF	EPF	SF	99213
3	Thomas Parker	02/10/02	99255	EPF	D	MOD	99252
4	John Thoroson	03/15/02	99202 81000 36415	EPF	EPF	MOD	99202 81000 36415
5	Nicholas Gristmeyer	02/20/02	99312	EPF	EPF	MOD	99312
6	Myrtle Byers	02/12/02	99312	D	PF	LOW	99312
7	Carlotta Maple	02/10/02	99213	EPF	PF	MOD	99213
8	Martin Steiner	02/10/02	99214	D	PF	MOD	99214
9	Rebecca Paulern	02/10/02	99213	D	EPF	SF	99213
10	Maureen Bradfield	02/12/02	99202	PF	EPF	MOD	99201

Legend

PF—Problem Focused   SF—Straightforward Complexity
EPF—Expanded Problem Focused   LOW—Low Complexity
D—Detailed   MOD—Moderate Complexity
C—Comprehensive   HIGH—High Complexity

CHAPTER 11

Surgery Exam Cases

Patient	Procedure	Modifier	Diagnosis	Quantity
1. Martha Matson	66984	OS	336.9	1
2. Paul Binyion	25111		727.41	1
3. Michael Brunson	93510		414.01, 414.02, 429.3	1
	93539		414.01, 414.02, 429.3	1
	93540		414.01, 414.02, 429.3	1
	93543		414.01, 414.02, 429.3	1
	93545		414.01, 414.02, 429.3	1
	93555		414.01, 414.02, 429.3	1
	93556		414.01, 414.02, 429.3	1
4. Stanley Cox	66984	OD	366.9	1
5. Sarah Trotter	63042		722.10	1
	63060	-51	722.10	1
	69990	-51	722.10	1
6. Susan Dow	43235		787.2	1
	43450	-51	787.2	1
7. Emily Stanton	11642		173.3, 140.1	1
	13132	-51	173.3, 140.1	1
8. John Strait	31529		478.74	1
9. Tray Smith	29881		836.0	1
10. Howard Burns	30140		478.0	1

SUMMARY REPORT

Physician: Angela O'Graphy, MD   Date of Review: 03/30/2002

Reviewer: Marsha Briggs, RN, CPC, CPC-H, CCS, CCS-P

Number of Operative Notes Reviewed: 10

Page 1

Operative notes were reviewed for completeness and appropriateness of care along with coding documentation and medical necessity.

Documentation in the operative note appears to provide preoperative information	8
Surgery date appears to be documented in the note	9
Preoperative anesthesia appears to be documented in the note	8
Indication for procedure appears to be documented in the operative report	8
Preoperative diagnosis appears to be documented in the operative report	10
Postoperative diagnosis appears to be documented in the note and supported by findings	9
Surgeon/assistant/cosurgeons are listed in the operative note	N/A
Findings appear to be indicated in the operative report	10
Procedure details appear to be documented appropriately in the operative report	9
Postoperative condition of patient appears to be indicated in the operative report	7
The operative report appears to support procedure (CPT®/HCPCS)	7
The operative report appears to support medical necessity (ICD-9-CM)	10

Other Documentation and Coding Issues:

1. One date of service (Sarah Trotter) did not appear to document two additional procedures performed (63030 and 69990).
2. One date of service for Stanley Cox (66985) was billed for a cataract extraction and the correct code documented is 66984.
3. On one date of service for Emily Stanton, the physician did not bill the second procedure with modifier -51 (multiple procedures).
4. Two incorrect diagnoses for Stanley Cox (250.51 and 362.2) did not appear supported in the operative report.
5. On the date of service for Paul Binyion, the provider billed 25112 and the correct code is 25111 based on documentation in the operative report.
6. One date of service for John Strait, the provider billed 31528 and the correct code is 31529 based on documentation in the operative report.

SUMMARY REPORT (continued)

Page 2

RECOMMENDATIONS

1. Review problem areas with physician.
2. Review incorrect usage of diagnosis code(s) when not supported in operative report.
3. Review the importance of including the date of the procedure in the operative note.
4. Review format and what needs to be included in the operative note including the documentation of anesthesia, indications for the procedure, postoperative diagnosis, procedure details, and postoperative condition of the patient.
5. Conduct a surgical documentation review in 6 months.

GENERAL SURGICAL GROUP
DETAILED ANALYSIS

Physician: Angela O'Graphy, MD   Date of Review: 03/30/2002

Reviewer: Marsha Briggs, RN, CPC, CPC-H, CCS, CCS-P

Number of Operative Notes Reviewed: 10

		Billed			Documented		
Patient	Date of Service	CPT® Code	ICD-9-CM Code	MOD	CPT® Code	ICD-9-CM Code	MOD
Martha Matson	02/14/02	66984	336.9	OS	66984	366.9	OS
Paul Binyion	02/06/02	25112	727.41	-----	25111	727.41	-----
Michael Brunson	02/08/02	93510 93539 93540 93543 93545 93555 93556	414.01 414.02 429.3	-----	93510 93539 93540 93543 93545 93555 93556	414.01 414.02 429.3	-----
Stanley Cox	01/10/02	66985	366.9 362.2 250.51	OD	66984	366.9	OD
Sarah Trotter	02/10/02	63042	722.10	-----	63042 63060 69990	722.10	-51 -51
Susan Dow	02/18/02	43235 43450	787.2	-51	43235 43450	787.2	-51
Emily Stanton	02/15/02	11642 13132	173.3 140.1	-----	11642 13132	173.3 140.1	-51
John Strait	02/10/02	31528	478.74	-----	31529	478.74	-----
Tray Smith	02/06/02	29881	836.0	-----	29881	836.0	-----
Howard Burns	02/06/02	30140	478.1	-51	30140	478.1	Not required

Legend

OS—Left Eye
OD—Right Eye
-51—Multiple Modifiers